Avian Cellular Immunology

Editor

Jagdev M. Sharma, B.V.Sc., Ph.D.

Benjamin S. Pomeroy Chair in Avian Health
Department of Veterinary Pathobiology
College of Veterinary Medicine
University of Minnesota
St. Paul, Minnesota

CRC Press
Boca Raton Boston Ann Arbor

Library of Congress Cataloging-in-Publication Data

Avian cellular immunology/editor, Jagdev M. Sharma
    p. cm.
    Includes bibliographical references.
    Includes index.
    ISBN 0-8493-6833-2
    1. Chickens—Immunology. 2. Birds—Immunology. 3. Cellular
immunity. I. Sharma, Jagdev, M., 1941-
    [DNLM: 1. Bird Disease—immunology. 2. Birds—immunology.
3. Immunity, Cellular.   SF 995 A9565]
SF995.A94 1990
636.5'0896'079—dc20
DNLM/DLC   90-2494
for Library of Congress   CIP

To Sylvia, Dave, Susan
My Cheering Squad

PREFACE

The knowledge on avian cellular immunity has expanded rapidly within the last few years. It is now well accepted that cell-mediated immunity plays an important role in defense against neoplastic and nonneoplastic diseases of avian species. New data continue to accumulate as reproducible *in vitro* systems to assay immunity are adopted by an increasing number of laboratories. The advent of hybridoma technology has generated useful monoclonal antibody reagents that react against surface markers of avian lymphocytes. The use of these reagents has contributed significantly to new knowledge on the ontogeny and functional diversity of chicken lymphocytes. It has become apparent that surface markers and effector functions of lymphocytes known in the mammalian species are well conserved in birds. Some of the genes coding for lymphocyte surface marker proteins share sequence homology between mammals and birds.

Much of the work in avian immunity has been done with the chicken. Other members of the avian species have not been examined in adequate detail, and it remains to be seen if interesting comparative differences exist in the immune mechanisms within the species.

The objective in this volume was to bring together the information on various aspects of avian cellular immunity that now exists scattered in diverse journals. I am very hopeful that this objective has been adequately met because I had the good fortune of having the leading authorities in avian cellular immunity contribute chapters in their respective areas of expertise. It has been a real pleasure to collaborate with these individuals, and this experience has renewed my appreciation for the sense of cooperation that exists among my professional colleagues. I wish to express my heartfelt thanks to the contributors, to my friends and colleagues who didn't write chapters for this volume but helped me in other ways, and to the secretarial staff of my department at the University of Minnesota. A special word of thanks to Pamela Farr, Rosemary Finnegan, and Sean Harrington, who helped in word processing and literature search for the chapters I have coauthored.

This book comes on the heels of several publications based on proceedings of symposia on avian immunity and a recent two-volume CRC book, *Avian Immunology: Basis and Practice,* edited by Auli and Paavo Toivanen. Each of these publications has unique qualities. The Toivanens' excellent book, in particular, is a pioneering effort in compiling extensive emerging knowledge on diverse aspects of avian immunology. The present volume, in comparison, has a narrow focus on cellular immunity.

I believe this book will be of value to the students of avian cellular immunity involved in all areas of endeavor, i.e., students, teachers, research scientists, and industry scientists. In addition, the book may also serve as a resource for comparative immunologists.

J. M. Sharma
St. Paul, Minnesota
May 1990

THE EDITOR

Jagdev M. Sharma, B. V. Sc., Ph.D., holds the Benjamin S. Pomeroy Endowed Chair in Avian Health in the College of Veterinary Medicine, University of Minnesota, St. Paul.

Dr. Sharma received undergraduate training in Punjab, India and obtained his B.V.Sc. degree in 1961 from the College of Veterinary Science, Haryana Agricultural University, Hissar, India. He obtained his M.S. and Ph.D. degrees in 1964 and 1967, respectively, from the Department of Epidemiology and Preventive Medicine, College of Veterinary Medicine, University of California, Davis. In 1971, after completing postdoctoral work at Washington State University, Pullman, he was appointed Veterinary Medical Officer at the Regional Poultry Research Laboratory of the U.S. Department of Agriculture in East Lansing, Michigan. He remained in Michigan until his move in 1988 to accept the Endowed Professorship at the University of Minnesota. In 1976, he was appointed Clinical Assistant Professor in the Department of Veterinary Pathology of the Michigan State University, and promoted to Clinical Professor in 1982.

Dr. Sharma is a member of a number of professional societies, including the International Association of Comparative Research on Leukemia and Related Diseases, the World Veterinary Poultry Association, the American Veterinary Medical Association, the American Association of Avian Pathologists, the Conference of Research Workers in Animal Diseases, Sigma Xi, and Phi Zeta. He has been the recipient of a number of awards and citations, including the Upjohn Achievement Award conferred by the American Association of Avian Pathologists for distinguished research contributions in avian medicine.

Dr. Sharma has presented over 50 invited lectures at national and international meetings. He has published over 130 research papers, the majority of which are in the area of avian immunology. His current major research interests include the avian cellular immune mechanisms and the role of cellular immunity in neoplastic and nonneoplastic viral diseases.

CONTRIBUTORS

Stephen E. Bloom, Ph.D.
Professor of Cytogenetics
Department of Poultry and Avian
  Sciences
Cornell University
Ithaca, New York

Chen-lo H. Chen, Ph.D.
Research Associate Professor
Department of Microbiology and
  Immunology
Division of Developmental and Clinical
  Immunology
University of Alabama at Birmingham
Birmingham, Alabama

David S. Chi, Ph.D.
Professor
Department of Internal Medicine
East Tennessee State University
Johnson City, Tennessee

Max D. Cooper, M.D.
Professor
Departments of Pediatrics, Medicine,
  Microbiology, and Pathology
Howard Hughes Medical Institute
University of Alabama at Birmingham
Birmingham, Alabama

Rodney R. Dietert, Ph.D.
Professor of Immunogenetics
Department of Poultry and Avian
  Sciences
Cornell University
Ithaca, New York

Karen A. Golemboski, Ph.D.
Research Associate
Department of Poultry and Avian
  Sciences
Cornell University
Ithaca, New York

Mark H. Kaplan, B.Sc.
Graduate Assistant
Department of Immunology and
  Microbiology
Wayne State University School of
  Medicine
Detroit, Michigan

Jill M. Lahti, Ph.D
Postdoctoral Fellow
Department of Biochemistry
University of Alabama at Birmingham
Birmingham, Alabama

Hyun S. Lillehoj, Ph.D.
Immunologist
Protozoan Diseases Laboratory
Livestock and Poultry Institute
Agricultural Research Service
U.S. Department of Agriculture
Beltsville, Maryland

Haruo Matsuda, D.V.M., Ph.D.
Associate Professor
Department of Microbiology and Hygiene
Faculty of Applied Biological Science
Hiroshima University
Higashi-Hiroshima, Japan

Takeshi Mikami, D.V.M., Ph.D.
Professor
Department of Veterinary Microbiology
Faculty of Agriculture
University of Tokyo
Tokyo, Japan

James M. Pickel, B.A.
Graduate Fellow
Department of Microbiology and
  Immunology
Division of Developmental and Clinical
  Immunology
University of Alabama at Birmingham
Birmingham, Alabama

Stephen J. Prowse, Ph.D.
Principal Research Scientist
Division of Animal Health
CSIRO
Parkville, Victoria
Australia

Pascale Quéré, D.V.M., Ph.D.
Chargé de Rechercher
Station de Pathologie Aviaire
Institut National de la Recherche
  Agronomique
Tours, France

Muquarrab A. Qureshi, Ph.D.
Assistant Professor
Department of Poultry Science
North Carolina State University
Raleigh, North Carolina

Noel R. Rose, M.D., Ph.D.
Professor and Chairman
Department of Immunology and
  Infectious Diseases
School of Hygiene and Public Health
The Johns Hopkins University
Baltimore, Maryland

Karel A. Schat, D.V.M., Ph.D.
Professor
Department of Avian and Aquatic Animal
  Medicine
New York State College of Veterinary
  Medicine
Cornell University
Ithaca, New York

Jagdev M. Sharma, B.V.Sc., Ph.D.
Professor
Benjamin S. Pomeroy Chair
Department of Veterinary Pathobiology
College of Veterinary Medicine
University of Minnesota
St. Paul, Minnesota

Roy S. Sundick, Ph.D.
Associate Professor
Department of Immunology and
  Microbiology
Wayne State University School of
  Medicine
Detroit, Michigan

Constantine H. Tempelis, Ph.D.
Professor of Immunology
Department of Biomedical and
  Environmental Health Sciences
University of California
Berkeley, California

G. Jeanette Thorbecke, M.D., Ph.D.
Professor
Department of Pathology
New York University Medical Center
New York, New York

Paavo Toivanen, M.D.
Professor
Department of Medical Microbiology
Turku University
Turku, Finland

Timo Veromaa, M.D., Ph.D.
Research Associate
Department of Medical Microbiology
Turku University
Turku, Finland

Jennifer J. York, Ph.D.
Experimental Scientist
Division of Animal Health
CSIRO
Parkville, Victoria
Australia

TABLE OF CONTENTS

Chapter 1

SURFACE MARKERS ON AVIAN IMMUNE CELLS

Chen-lo H. Chen, James M. Pickel, Jill M. Lahti, and Max D. Cooper

TABLE OF CONTENTS

I. INTRODUCTION

Characterization of cell-surface differentiation antigens has been fundamental to understanding lymphocyte development. While most of the available information has been derived from studies in mammals, studies in birds first revealed the separate developmental pathways of T and B cells,[1] their hemopoietic stem-cell origin[2], and the seeding of the epithelial thymus by waves of blood-borne precursor cells.[3] Recent comparative analysis of T- and B-cell development using antibodies reactive with avian lymphocyte surface markers has revealed that the basic antigen recognition molecules are highly conserved in birds and mammals. The avian major histocompatibility complex (MHC) class I and II antigens, T-cell receptors, accessory T-cell molecules, and the immunoglobulins have been characterized. Several of the genes encoding these proteins have been cloned and shown to have sequence homology to their mammalian counterparts.

The phylogenetic distance between birds and mice has made it relatively easy to produce mouse monoclonal antibodies (mAb) to highly conserved cell-surface proteins on chicken lymphocytes. Novel antigens have thus been identified, many of which may well be found in mammals. This chapter outlines the information on the tissue distribution, structure, function, and genes of the immunologically important surface molecules that have been identified to date on chicken leukocytes.

II. MAJOR HISTOCOMPATIBILITY COMPLEX ANTIGENS

Chicken MHC was originally described as a blood-group B locus.[4] The availability of the first recombinant B haplotype[5] made it possible to propose a three-locus MHC model. These loci control the synthesis of at least three classes of antigens called B-F, B-L, and B-G.[6] B-F and B-L antigens correspond to the mammalian MHC class I and II antigens, respectively.[6] The B-G antigen, found only on erythrocytes, erythroid progenitor cells,[7] and thrombocytes,[8] has no known mammalian counterpart and has been named a MHC class IV antigen.[9] Only B-F and B-L antigens which are involved in the immune response, histocompatibility reactions, and disease resistance[9,10] will be reviewed here.

A. B-F ANTIGENS

B-F antigens are the chicken MHC class I gene products found on erythrocytes and leukocytes. Alloantisera and mAb against B-F antigens are available for haplotype determination and biochemical characterization[11,12] and have been reviewed recently.[9,13,14] Most of the available mAb recognize monomorphic determinants of these highly polymorphic antigens, although mAb which react with B-F determinants shared by only a few B haplotypes have also been obtained.[12] Two mAb that recognized B-F determinants, F21-2 (anti-α chain)[9] and F21-21 (anti-β_2-microglobulin),[15] cross-react with turkey cells, but not with *Xenopus*, rainbow trout, or human cells. Similar to their mammalian homologues, B-F antigens are composed of a membrane-bound glycosylated polymorphic heavy chain (α) of relative molecular mass (M_r) 40,000 to 45,000 noncovalently associated with the invariant light chain (β_2-microglobulin) of M_r 14,500.[15,16] Partial amino-acid sequence analysis has revealed considerable homology between chicken B-F molecules and mammalian class I antigens.[17,18]

B-F antigens are expressed on almost all cells in the central lymphoid organs of chickens. In the thymus, cortical cells are stained less strongly than medullary cells,[11,12] suggesting that the expression of class I antigens may increase during lymphocyte maturation. The presence of B-F antigens has not been demonstrated in brain or muscle.[11]

Expression of the B-F antigens has been examined most thoroughly using the mAb INN-CH-428.[19] This antibody has been reported to recognize B-F antigens in a hemagglutination assay, although it has not been shown to immunoprecipitate class I proteins. Using this antibody, it has been demonstrated that expression of B-F antigens begins relatively late in ontogeny. INN-CH-428 reactive molecules are not detected on red blood cells (RBC), peripheral blood leukocytes (PBL), or the cells from bursa and thymus on either embryonic day 18 (E18) or day 1 after hatching. The frequency of B-F$^+$ cells increases rapidly after hatching with almost 100% of the RBC, PBL, bursa and spleen cells expressing these antigens at 2 weeks of age. Medullary cells of the thymus were positive, while those in the cortical area were negative in these studies. In contrast to these results, expression of B-F antigens has been observed much earlier during ontogeny using other B-F specific mAb.[139,140] Further studies are thus needed to resolve this interesting discrepancy.

The sequence and structure of the B-F genes have been partially resolved. Two B-F transcripts have been sequenced. One was isolated by hybridizing tissue-specific complementary deoxyribonucleic acid (cDNA) probes to cosmid clones containing the B-L β genes,[20] indicating that these two loci are linked. The other was isolated by screening an expression vector cDNA library with an antisera prepared against purified B-F molecules.[8] The deduced B-F protein sequences from the two transcripts exhibit 84% similarity in the α_1 domain, 84% in the α_2 domain, 96% in the α_3 domain, and 100% in the transmembrane domain.[21] The amino acid sequence of B-F molecules showed 35 to 45% homology to mammalian class I antigens: maximal in the α_2 domain (40 to 52%), intermediate in the α_1 (32 to 47%) and cytoplasmic (27 to 45%) domains, and lower in the α_3 (32 to 36%) and transmembrane (24 to 38%) domains.[20] Although the divergence of B-F from the mammalian MHC class I antigens is striking, many of the amino acids directly involved in the secondary and tertiary structure are conserved in the chicken protein. Among the residues involved in the binding of β_2 microglobulin (β_2-m), four out of nine are substituted in the α_1 domain, one out of nine in the α_2 domain, and seven out of ten in the α_3 domain. Recently, β_2-m has been purified from chicken plasma and the N-terminal amino acid sequence determined.[16] A mixture of the corresponding oligonucleotide probes was used to isolate chicken β_2-m cDNA clones. The amino acid sequence of the chicken β_2-m showed 45 to 55% homology to its mammalian counterparts,[8] suggesting that residues involved in the binding of both chains have diverged together. It is interesting to note, however, that human β_2-m can exchange with β_2-m of the MHC class I molecules from chickens.[22]

B. B-L ANTIGENS

B-L antigens have been defined by alloantisera and mAb as the avian homologues of the mammalian class II antigens.[15,23-25] The available mAb have been reviewed previously.[9,13,14] Most of the antibodies recognize monomorphic determinants, as mouse mAb against polymorphic determinants of avian class II molecules are difficult to obtain. Immunoprecipitation and gel electrophoresis studies have revealed that the B-L antigen is a glycoprotein consisting of a single nonpolymorphic α chain of M_r 32,000 and one of the two polymorphic β chains of M_r 27,000.[24,25] In addition, the B-L heterodimer has been found to be associated with several basic invariant molecules in the cytoplasm but not on the cell surface.[25]

TABLE 1
Chicken T-Cell Antigens

Antigen	mAb (isotype)	% Cells expressing surface antigen			Molecular mass (kDa)	Ref.
		Thymus	Blood	Spleen		
CT1	CT1 (γ_1); CT1a (γ_3)	>90	<1	<1	65	33
CD2	2—4; 2—102	<95	60	60	40	29
CD3	CT3 (γ_1)	65—75	75—85	65—75	20,19,17	43,48
CD4	CT4 (γ_1)	80—85	35—45	15—20	64	40
	CTLA1 (γ_2); CTLA6 (γ_1)	59	22	16	65	38
	2—6; 2—35	80	40	20	64	29
CD5	CTLA5; CTLA8 (γ_1)	73	52	45	65,45	38
	3—58	90	65	70	56	29
CD8	CT8 (γ_1)	80—85	10—20	45—55	63 (34 dimer)	40
	CTLA3,4, and 9 (γ_1)	43	18	36	66 (33—35 dimer)	38
TCR1	TCR1 (γ_1)	5—15	15—25	15—25	90 (50,40 dimer)	43,48
TCR2	mAb 6 (γ_1)	45—55	45—55	35—40	90 (50,40 dimer)	47—49
TCR3	TCR3 (γ_1)	5—15	10—15	10—15	88 (48,40 dimer)	48,58
CD25 (IL-2R)	INN-CH-16 (μ)	<1	<1	<1	48—50	67

B-L antigens are expressed on B cells, cells of the monocyte-macrophage lineage, mitogen-stimulated T cells, and Marek's disease virus-induced T-cell tumors.[23-27] They have also been demonstrated on endothelial cells in bursal capillary blood vessels.[25] B-L antigens appear early during ontogeny, first being detectable on E12 bursa cells and on E13 macrophages and thymic dendritic cells.[23-26]

Using a probe encoding a human HLA-DQβ cDNA, the chicken B-L β genes have been cloned.[20,28] Five class II β genes defining two related isotypic families have been mapped to the B complex which is located on the 16th microchromosome. Exons encoding the β_1, β_2, and transmembrane domains of a B-L chain have been shown to have 63, 66, and 62% homology with the HLA-DQβ sequence, respectively. There are highly conserved regions in each domain which may play an important role in MHC class II function. However, many unique amino acid substitutions in the chicken β chain have also been detected, especially in the β_1 domain which is involved in antigen and T-cell recognition. The presence of B-L α genes in B-L β cosmids was investigated by chromosome walking.[20] Although several genes were localized, none of the identified genes have the transcriptional characteristics of a MHC class II α-chain gene, indicating that the B-L α gene(s) may not be associated with the B-L β genes. In contrast, the class II α-chain genes are always found closely linked to the β-chain gene in the HLA and H-2 complexes in mammals.[21]

III. LYMPHOCYTE ANTIGENS

A. T-CELL ANTIGENS

The characterization of avian T-cell development and function has lagged behind that of mammals partly because of the absence of antibodies that identify T-cell surface antigens. However, research in the last 5 years has begun to elucidate the T-cell differentiation pathway in chickens. These studies have revealed striking similarities between chicken T-cell surface molecules and those of their mammalian counterparts. The chicken T-cell system has also revealed interesting distinctions. The data available on T-cell surface antigens in chickens will be summarized here (Table 1), with particular emphasis on the similarities and differences between chickens and mammals.

1. CD2

The first antigen to be recognized on the surface of avian thymocytes during development is the avian homologue of CD2. This antigen is identified by mAb 2-4 and 2-102.[29] The CD2 molecule is expressed by thymocytes beginning around day 11 of embryonic life. CD2 expression is retained throughout adult life on both thymocytes and mature peripheral T cells, with the exception of γδ T cells which express the CD2 antigen only in the thymus.[29,140]

The chicken CD2 antigen is a M_r 40,000 single-chain protein.[29] Its cytoplasmic domain appears to exhibit considerable homology with the mammalian CD2 antigen, as a rabbit antiserum to a synthetic peptide from the cytoplasmic region of the human CD2 molecule is capable of immunoprecipitating the chicken CD2 homologue. The rabbit antibody also removes all of the CD2 reactive protein from chick thymic lysates in preclearance experiments.[29]

The mammalian CD2 molecule is expressed very early in ontogeny, in humans at the pro-T stage.[30] Due to the early appearance of this molecule, the CD2 antigen has been suggested to participate in T-cell growth and differentiation intrathymically. Mammalian studies have shown that CD2 is a cell-adhesion molecule that binds to LFA-3 molecules which are expressed by thymic epithelial cells and other cell types.[31] CD2 has also been shown to be involved in an alternate pathway of T-cell activation.[32] This alternate pathway appears to exist in the chicken as suboptimal doses of anti-CD2, and PMA (phorbol myristate acetate) can activate both embryonic and adult thymocytes and peripheral αβ T cells without involvement of the T-cell receptor (TCR) complex.[29] The early appearance of the CD2 antigen in conjunction with studies demonstrating the presence of an alternate activation pathway in chickens suggests that the avian CD2 analogue is functionally equivalent to its mammalian counterpart.

2. CT1

One of the next antigens to appear during chick embryonic development is the CT1 antigen.[33] This M_r 65,000 molecule, recognized by the CT1 and CT1a mAb, is first detectable on thymocytes on E11 to 12. By E15, CT1 is expressed by 97% of cortical thymocytes. The same molecule may also be recognized by the X.14[34] and TD1[35] antibodies, although the reported molecular weights of these antigens differ slightly. Another mAb, $T_{10}A_6$, reacts with a M_r 65,000 protein that has a similar ontogenetic pattern of expression in the thymus.[36] In contrast to CT1, however, this antigen is expressed by a subset of peripheral blood lymphocytes and splenocytes.

The function of the CT1 antigen is unknown although its tissue expression and ontogeny are similar to the mammalian CD1 antigen.[37] The CT1 molecule may not be the avian homologue of CD1 as the protein immunoprecipitated by the CT1 antibody has a M_r 65,000 as opposed to a M_r 40,000 of the CD1 antigen. In addition, the human CD1 antigen appears to be associated with β$_2$-m, which has not yet been identified in CT1 immunoprecipitates from chicken thymocytes. However, the recent characterization of a M_r 65,000 form of the human CD1 antigen using the mAB PHM3[37] leaves open the possibility that the CT1 antigen could be a chicken CD1 homologue.

3. CD5

An avian homologue of the CD5 antigen also appears on approximately E11 to 12. The CD5 antigen is identified by three different monoclonal antibodies: 3-58, CTLA5, and CTLA8.[29,38] This antigen is expressed on the majority of chick thymocytes and peripheral T lymphocytes, but its expression by the various T-cell subsets has not yet been reported. Incubation of chick splenocytes with anti-CD5 antibodies eliminates concanavalin A-responsive lymphocytes.[38] As in mammals,[39] the CD5 antigen is also expressed by a subpopulation of bursal lymphocytes and B cells (see Section III.B). Monoclonal antibodies CTLA5 and CTLA8 immunoprecipitate glycoproteins of M_r 65,000 and 45,000, while 3-58 immunoprecipitates a M_r 56,000 protein. These values are similar to the mouse CD5 protein, which has a M_r 67,000 and is associated with other, smaller proteins.[39]

4. CD4 and CD8

Expression of the avian homologues of both CD4 and CD8 begins in the thymus on E12 to 13.[40] Initially, the CD8 antigen is expressed by a small subpopulation of chick thymocytes before the CD4 antigen is expressed in detectable levels. The expression of both CD4 and CD8 then increases rapidly, with approximately 95% of the thymocytes expressing both by E17. After hatching, expression of these molecules is seen on 85 to 95% of the thymocytes. As in mammals, most cortical thymocytes express both CD4 and CD8, whereas mature thymocytes expressing either the CD4 or CD8 antigens are present in the thymic medulla and in the peripheral blood and spleen.[40]

Monoclonal antibodies reactive with the CD8 molecule have identified a M_r 63,000 protein under nonreducing conditions from thymocytes and T-cell membranes.[40] Under reducing conditions, a single protein band of M_r 34,000 has been observed, suggesting that the CD8 antigen is a disulfide-linked dimer. Another CD8 mAb also immunoprecipitates a protein of M_r 65,000, in addition to the M_r 33,000 to 35,000 dimer, under reducing conditions.[38] Whether this represents a CD8-associated molecule or nonreduced material remains unclear. The chicken CD4 antigen has been identified by mAb as a single chain polypeptide of M_r 64,000 from thymocytes, splenocytes, and peripheral T cells.[40] Three mAb reactive with CD4 molecules have been reported.[29,38,40]

The CD8 molecule in mammals is involved in signal transduction and TCR recognition probably by facilitating the interaction of T cells with class I MHC on antigen-presenting cells. The CD8 molecule also marks a sublineage of T cells with cytotoxic capabilities.[41,42] CD8 appears to function similarly in chickens and serves to delineate cytotoxic T cells.[38,40]

As in mammals,[41,42] the CD4+ T cells in the chicken have helper capabilities, mediated at least in part by lymphokine activity.[29,38,40] Avian CD4 mAb inhibit T-cell proliferative responses,[29,38,40] and this effect is synergistic with that of anti-class II MHC antibodies.[29]

5. T-Cell Receptors

a. Ontogeny and Tissue Localization of CD3/TCR Proteins

The CD3/TCR complex appears on thymocytes soon after the CD4 and CD8 molecules.[43] Elements of the CD3 complex, the invariant portion of the TCR, are first observed in the cytoplasm on E9, 3 d prior to CD3 expression on the cell surface.[44] As in mammals, the avian CD3 complex is always expressed on the cell surface in conjunction with the polymorphic T-cell receptor molecules.[43,45] The CD3 complex can be recognized by the CT3 mAb.[43] Three mutually exclusive sublineages of CT3+ cells are recognized by the TCR1,[46] TCR2,[47] and TCR3 mAb.[48] The first TCR isotype to appear in development is the γδ TCR (TCR1).[46,49] This TCR isotype appears on the surface of E12 thymocytes in conjunction with the CD3 complex. Relatively high levels of γδ TCR molecules ($>1 \times 10^4$) are present on the TCR1+ cells from the onset of their expression.[50] The TCR1 population expands rapidly to reach a peak of approximately 30% of the thymocyte pool on E15. The proportion of TCR1+ thymocytes declines thereafter to approximately 10%. TCR1+ cells rapidly traverse the thymus and can be seen in the spleen on E15.[44] In adult birds, approximately 20 to 50% of the peripheral blood lymphocytes and splenocytes express the TCR1 isotype.[46,51] While TCR1+ thymocytes rarely express either CD4 or CD8, most of the TCR1+ cells in both the spleen and intestine express the CD8 molecule.[49,52]

The vast majority of chicken thymocytes eventually express the TCR2 (αβ) isotype.[47,49] Expression of the TCR2 isotype begins on E15, 2 d after γδ+ cells are first observed, thus resembling the pattern observed in mammals.[53-55] The frequency of TCR2+ cells increases gradually until hatching when the majority of the thymocytes express this receptor isotype. In contrast to the TCR1+ cells, the initial level of TCR2 receptors is very low (approximately 600 per cell).[50] The density of TCR2 molecules then increases as these cells mature within the thymus. TCR2+ cells in the thymic cortex express both CD4 and CD8, whereas mature

TCR2$^+$ cells in the thymic medulla, peripheral blood, spleen, and intestine express either CD4 or CD8.[44,49] A difference in thymic transit time is also seen for TCR1$^+$ and TCR2$^+$ cells, with the former passing through the cortex within approximately 1 d as compared with a 3 to 4 d transient time for the latter.[44] All of these findings suggest differences in the process of thymic education for the two cell lineages.

The tissue localization of the two TCR isotypes also differs. TCR1$^+$ splenocytes are preferentially located in the splenic sinusoidal regions and in the intestinal epithelium in both birds and mammals.[52,56,57] Whereas TCR1$^+$ cells appear in the spleen by E15, TCR2$^+$ cells begin to enter the spleen on E19, where they are localized to the periarteriolar sheath regions. They reach the lamina propria of the intestine beginning on E20.[52]

One of the more interesting differences between the gallinaceous birds and mammals is the existence of a third sublineage of T cells.[58] These express a CD3-associated heterodimer that is not recognized by either the TCR1 or TCR2 mAb but recognized by the TCR3 mAb.[48] The TCR3$^+$ cells first appear in the thymus on E17, and their frequency increases slowly until the time of hatching when approximately 9% of the thymocytes express the TCR3 receptor.[48] Like the TCR2 population of thymocytes, the numbers of TCR3 molecules per cell increase gradually as these cells mature.[141] TCR3$^+$ cells in the thymic cortex express both CD4 and CD8. In the medullary region, a small percentage of these cells express either the CD4 or the CD8 molecules.[141] The TCR3$^+$ cells begin to seed to the periphery after hatching. In young adults, approximately 12 to 15% of the peripheral T cells express this receptor, 80% of these cells express CD4, and 20% express CD8.[48,58] The TCR3$^+$ cells are preferentially localized in the periarteriolar sheaths in the spleen, as are the TCR2$^+$ cells. In contrast, TCR3$^+$ cells are rarely found in the chicken intestine.[141]

b. Biochemical Characterization of the Chicken T-Cell Receptor Proteins

The CT3 mAb immunoprecipitates a complex of at least three proteins from T cells with M_r of 20,000, 19,000, and 17,000.[43] At least two of these proteins contain N-linked oligosaccharides. When the T-cell surface molecules are solubilized with a mild detergent, the TCR1, TCR2, and TCR3 heterodimers can be coprecipitated with the CT3 antibody.[43] Each heterodimer can also be immunoprecipitated with the TCR1,[46] TCR2,[49] or TCR3[48] mAb. Both TCR1 and TCR2 molecules are M_r 90,000 heterodimers composed of M_r 50,000 and 40,000 disulfide-linked glycoproteins.[49] Removal of the N-linked oligosaccharides reveals core proteins of M_r 36,000 and 33,000 from TCR1 and of M_r 34,000 and 29,000 from TCR2.[49] The TCR3 mAb immunoprecipitates a slightly smaller (M_r 88,000) heterodimer composed of M_r 48,000 and 40,000 polypeptides from T-cell lysates.[48] Removal of the N-linked sugar from the TCR3 molecules yields core proteins of M_r 31,000 and 34,000, clearly differentiating this TCR from TCR1.[58] The relationship between the TCR2 and TCR3 T-cell sublineages is more difficult to discern. Both TCR2 and TCR3 contain a core protein of M_r 34,000, and in addition, the M_r 50,000/48,000 peptides have similar isoelectric points (pI 6.2 to 7.6) as do the 40,000 chains (pI 5.7 to 7.0).[142] Deglycosylation of the isolated M_r 40,000 chains from both TCR2 and TCR3 immunoprecipitates yields M_r 34,000 core proteins. Peptide mapping data suggest that these two proteins are highly similar, but not the same.[58]

c. Lineage Relationships of the Cells Expressing the Different T-Cell Receptor Isotypes

The lineage relationships between the TCR1, TCR2, and TCR3 subpopulations have been examined in embryonic antibody-suppression experiments.[58,59,141] The results support the conclusion that all three subpopulations represent different T-cell sublineages. Injection of the TCR1 mAb selectively inhibits development of TCR1$^+$ cells without affecting development of either the TCR2$^+$ or TCR3$^+$ cells.[59] Combining the TCR1 mAb injection with neonatal thymectomy results in a dramatic permanent depletion of TCR1$^+$ cells, suggesting that this lineage of cells has a limited expansion capacity and requires prolonged seeding to fill the peripheral compartment. Embryonic injections of TCR2 and TCR3 mAb do not affect the development of the TCR1[+] cells.[51,58,141] Injection of the TCR2 mAb appears to abort the maturational process, as cells expressing high levels of TCR2 are not observed in treated birds.[143] If combined with thymectomy, repeated TCR2 mAb injections dramatically diminish the number of TCR2[+] cells.[51,58] This reduction of TCR2[+] cells is compensated by a dramatic increase in the frequency of TCR3[+] cells. Reciprocal results are obtained using the TCR3 mAb, suggesting that the TCR2[+] and TCR3[+] cells represent distinct sublineages.[141]

The waves of precursor cells for these three populations of T cells have been examined using the chicken-quail chimera system.[60] Transplantation of chicken E9 thymus containing the first wave of chicken stem cells into E3 quail embryos[61] resulted in the development of all three sublineages of chicken T cells, indicating that the first wave of precursor cells gives rise to all three sublineages of chicken T cells. Similarly, the second wave of thymic precursors also gives rise to these cell lineages. The results of these studies indicate that the thymus is the only site in which cells expressing TCR/CD3 complexes are generated.[61]

d. Functional Capability of Different T-Cell Receptor Isotypes

Functional studies on the different T-cell lineages are still limited. Preliminary studies indicate that both the TCR2[+] and TCR3[+] cells can elicit a graft vs. host response, but the frequencies of alloreactive cells differ in the two populations of T cells.[141] This suggests that the repertoire of the TCR2 and TCR3 cell lineages differs. The TCR1[+] cells frequently coexpress the CD8 antigen in the spleen and intestine, suggesting that they recognize antigen in association with class I and/or class I-like molecules which have been postulated to be involved in the recognition process in mammals.[62] Consistent with this view, the TCR1[+] cells are impotent in the graft vs. host assay[63] that depends on class II alloreactivity, whereas TCR1[+] cells from class I alloantigen-stimulated chickens exhibit specific T-cell cytotoxicity.[143] This can be inhibited by either anti-CD3 or anti-CD8 antibodies. Cross-linkage of the TCR1/CD3 complex with antibody has also been shown to elicit the cytotoxic capabilities of TCR1[+] cells.[144] TCR1[+]/CD8[+] cells may also be capable of suppressor activity.[64] These functional clues, in association with the preferential tissue localization patterns of TCR1[+] cells, suggest that these cells may play an important role in host defense. The large number of γδ cells relative to the mammal, moreover, makes the chicken an excellent model system to examine the function of the TCR1 lineage.

The TCR2[+] cell population appears to contain cells with both helper and cytotoxic capabilities. TCR2[+] cells exhibit proliferative responses to both conconavalin A and allogeneic cells. These cells produce lymphokines and are capable of cytotoxic responses to allogeneic target cells.[47]

While the *in vitro* responses of TCR3[+] cells have not been examined, TCR2-suppressed chickens, in which the percentage of TCR3[+] cells is increased, are capable of mounting antibody responses to sheep red blood cells,[140] suggesting that the TCR3[+] cells are capable of helper functions as well as graft vs. host potential.

e. A Third Lineage of Lymphocytes in Chickens

In the course of studies of T-cell development, we identified another lymphocyte lineage. These cells are characterized by cytoplasmic expression of a CD3 epitope even though they lack cell surface CD3/TCR.[65,66] These cells often express CD8 on their surface. We have named these cells TCR0 because they express some of the characteristic markers of T cells, but lack the capacity to express the T-cell receptor complex on their surface. They appear initially in the E8 spleen, prior to the appearance of cells expressing the CD3/TCR complex in the thymus. In studies of chick-quail chimeras, we have shown that TCR0 cells do not have the capacity to acquire cytoplasmic or surface expression of either immunoglobulin or

TCR proteins. In adults, TCR0 cells are found in the spleen (1% of the CT3$^+$ cells), intestine (30 to 40% of the CT3$^+$ cells), thymic medulla, and bursa.[66]

The origin of TCR0 cells has been examined in the chicken-quail chimera system.[65] These studies indicate that TCR0 cells are derived from splenic precursors prior to the migration of the first wave on stem cells to the thymus. Transplantation of E6 chicken spleen into E3 quail embryos resulted in the normal development and localization of chick TCR0 cells in the spleen, thymic medulla, bursa, and intestine, indicating that TCR0 cells represent a separate lineage of lymphoid cells.

6. Interleukin 2 Receptor

The chicken homologue of the interleukin 2 (IL-2) receptor, recognized by the mAb INN-CH-16,[67,68] is expressed only on activated T cells with >1% of the unstimulated splenocytes being reactive. The antibody stains less than 1% of the thymocytes and PBL. In immunized chickens, cells expressing the IL-2 receptor are primarily localized in the periarteriolar lymphatic sheath regions.

The IL-2 receptor mAb immunoprecipitates a M_r 48,000 to 50,000 protein under reducing conditions. This antibody has the ability to block mitogen-induced T-cell proliferation and to reduce IL-2 absorption by T lymphoblasts from conditioned media. The kinetics of the expression of IL-2 receptors are similar in birds and mammals.[67,68]

7. Other T-Cell Antigens

Several other T-cell surface antigens have been identified by mAb, but these antigens have not been characterized extensively and their functions are unknown. Three such antigens have been reported by Mazella and co-workers.[69] One of these has a M_r of 40,000 and is expressed by 95% of the thymocytes, but not by peripheral T cells or other splenocytes. This antigen is recognized by the TA3, TB1, and TB6 mAb. While the ontogenetic pattern of expression of this molecule has not been reported, its biochemical characteristics and tissue distribution are reminiscent of the mammalian CD1 antigen. Two additional antibodies reported by this group react with both thymocytes and subsets of peripheral T cells. One of these, TC4, identifies a cell-surface protein of M_r 110,000 expressed by 90% of the medullary thymocytes, 70 to 80% of the peripheral blood lymphocytes, and 60 to 70% of the splenocytes. The other antibody, TA1, recognizes a M_r 16,000 protein expressed by 40% of the thymocytes (60 to 70% of the medullary subpopulation), 30 to 35% of the peripheral blood lymphocytes, and 70 to 80% of the splenocytes. Two other anti-thymocyte antibodies, INN-CH/T51 and INN-CH/T53, have been reported.[70] These antibodies identify antigens of M_r 186,000 and 135,000, respectively. No other information on function, ontogeny, and tissue distribution has been reported.

B. B-CELL ANTIGENS

With the exception of immunoglobulins and a CD5 equivalent, the chicken B-lymphocyte antigens identified by mAb have no known mammalian homologues. Mouse mAb have identified chicken molecules that are antigenically divergent though their functional roles may prove to be conserved in vertebrates. These novel antigens thus may provide an opportunity to describe aspects of B-cell maturation and function that have not yet been revealed in mammalian systems. The patterns of expression and structural features of these proteins offer clues to their functional roles in B-cell development.

1. Immunoglobulins

Immunoglobulin (Ig) is the most conspicuous and well-understood protein on the surface of B lymphocytes. As in mammals, these antibody molecules define avian B cells as a function of their state of differentiation. Functional analogues of mammalian IgM, IgG, and IgA have been described,[71] and the genes encoding chicken IgM and IgG have been cloned.[72-76] Mouse mAb which react with chicken Ig have been produced,[13,77] and the structural features of the Ig proteins have been reviewed elsewhere.[78]

Chicken IgM, a pentameric molecule with a total mass of M_r 880,000 to 890,000, is composed of subunits of heavy and light chains of M_r 63,000 to 70,000 and M_r 22,000 to 24,000, respectively.[78] Virtually all bursal lymphocytes and the majority of circulating B lymphocytes express IgM on their surfaces.[79]

Chicken IgG is structurally distinct from the mammalian analogue, and some have proposed that a unique appellation, IgY, be used to acknowledge these differences.[80] Because the chicken IgG molecule contains an additional constant domain[75] when compared to the M_r 150,000 mammalian molecule, its weight is correspondingly higher at M_r 165,000 to 180,000. In adult spleen, 6% of the lymphocytes are surface IgG$^+$, while fewer cells express IgG in blood (1.6%) and in bursa (0.2%).[77] In the bursa, some IgG$^+$ cells also express IgM, evincing the sequential expression of IgM and then IgG by maturing B lymphocytes.[13,79]

IgA is expressed by fewer cells than IgG in spleen (0.6%), blood (0.2%), and bursa (0.1%).[77] Soluble IgA concentrations are increased in bile and in secretions from mucosal membranes.[81] A secretory component, which binds to chicken IgA, can be detected as a free protein in agammaglobulinemic birds, further suggesting the conservation of IgA function in avian species.[82,83]

An avian IgD candidate with a heavy chain of higher molecular weight (M_r 81,000) than that of μ chain has been identified. An anti-light-chain mAb immunoprecipitates the putative IgD molecules from B-cell lysates cleared of IgM, IgG, and IgA by immunoprecipitation with isotype specific mAb.[77] In addition, light chains were detected on the surface of cells from which IgM had been removed by modulation.[77] However, IgD-specific antibodies have not been produced, and an avian δ-chain constant region gene has not been identified.

Monoclonal antibodies have also been produced against Ig idiotypic epitopes. The CId-1, CId-2, and CId-3 antibodies recognize 0.3%, 0.2%, and 1% of the B cells in the bursa and 1%, 0.2%, and 1% of circulating B lymphocytes, respectively.[84,85] These mAb were produced against chicken antibodies to *N*-acetylglucosamine or *p*-aminobenzoic acid. The specificity of these mAb for variable determinants was demonstrated by immunochemical analysis. Lymphocytes expressing Ig with CId-1 and CId-2 idiotypes were increased fourfold and sixfold in birds which were immunized with the original antigens.[84]

While these anti-idiotypic mAb react with small populations of B cells, another mAb against the variable region of heavy chains, CV_H-1, binds up to one third of adult B cells and plasma cells expressing IgM, IgG, and IgA.[85]

The cloning and sequencing of immunoglobulin genes encoding λ light chains (probably the only light chain isotype in chickens) and heavy chains have recently been accomplished. These studies have shown that the mechanism for the generation of a repertoire of antigen-binding immunoglobulins is quite different from the mammalian system.[73-76,86-88] The λ and heavy chain loci both have a single functional variable region gene segment which is rearranged to J_λ (joining) or J_H and D_H (diversity) gene segments.[86,88] Untranslatable pseudogenes (25 ψV_λ and at least 45 ψV_H[88,88] contribute nucleotide sequence diversity to the intact and translated variable regions by a mechanism of copy replacement (gene conversion). However, the resulting immunoglobulin proteins are structurally similar to mammalian immunoglobulins; variation in the coding V_H and V_λ genes is confined to the complementarity determining regions (CDR).[73,88]

Allotypic markers of chicken IgM and IgG, defined by antisera, have also been useful in studies of B-cell development. Allelic exclusion was originally described in studies that took advantage of IgM allotype-specific antisera.[89] The dynamics of the peripheral B-cell population have also been examined by using immunoglobulin allotypic markers.[90] In a

TABLE 2
Chicken B-Cell Antigens

Antigen	mAb (isotype)	% Cells expressing surface antigen			Molecular mass (kDa)	Ref.
		Bursa	**Blood**	**Spleen**		
Bu-1a	L-22 (γ_2)	90—95	10—20	15—25	70	34
	21-1A (γ_1)				94	
Bu-1b	5-11G2 (γ_1)	85—90	2—18	15—27	70	94
Bu-2	Hy30 (γ_1)	98	17	35	66	98
CB1	A-21 (γ_1)	97	17	18	110 (55 dimer)	13
CB2	M2C2 (μ)	86	2	3	80—125	13
CB3	3—16 (γ_1)	62—83	20	26	50	13,99
CB4	5—15 (γ_1)	98	20	28	39,53,107	13
CB5	7—19 (μ)	96	16	23	167	13
CB7	7—10a2 (μ)	51	1	2		148
CB8	32c4 (μ)	90	15	10		148
CB9	65a3 (γ_3)	98	5	7	120 (65 dimer)	148
CB10	65b5 (γ_1)	97	5	10	220	148
CB11	31a6 (μ)	26	15	21	37	148

recent review, Benedict and Berestecky[78] have defined 11 allotypic markers for chicken immunoglobulin.

2. Nonimmunoglobulin Markers

Unlike the avian immunoglobulins, TCR and other T-cell antigens, a majority of B-cell antigens in chickens are novel, and their functional roles have not been defined. These antigens have been identified by mouse mAb, and their structures and patterns of expression are described (Table 2). One group of such mAb is designated the CB series because they react with chicken B cells. These are numbered in the order of their identification.

a. Bursal Lymphocyte Antigens

During the period of proliferation and clonal diversification that occurs in the bursa, B cells may express adhesion molecules, receptors for growth or differentiation factors, or enzymes. Two antigens expressed by all bursal lymphocytes, but not by peripheral B cells, are identified by the CB2 and HNK-1 mAb.

i. CB2

CB2, a cell-surface molecule of M_r 80,000 to 125,000, is expressed by all bursal lymphocytes.[13] The level of expression varies widely on individual cells, with some being only dimly positive while others are more than 100 times brighter in immunofluorescence assays. The level of CB2 expression is not related to cell size or to the precise location of the lymphocytes within the bursal follicles.

ii. HNK-1

The HNK-1 mAb[91] binds a myelin-associated glycoprotein on human neural and natural killer (NK) cells.[92] It also binds chicken neurons, cortical thymocytes, and bursal lymphocytes. The HNK-1 antigen is not expressed by peripheral lymphocytes in the chicken.[13] The antigen on bursal cells has a M_r of 110,000, the same molecular mass as the myelin-associated protein on neural cells,[92] suggesting that HNK-1 reactive molecules may play a role in governing the developmental patterns of cells in both the nervous and immune systems.

b. B-Cell Antigens

Of the markers listed in Table 2, several are expressed by virtually all B cells. These include Bu-1, Bu-2, CB1, CB3, CB4, and CB5. Others (CB7, CB8, CB9, CB10, and CB11) are detected by mAb only on subpopulations of B cells.

i. Bu-1

One of the best-studied B-cell markers is Bu-1. This M_r 70,000 antigen was detected first by alloantisera created by Gilmour and co-workers.[93] Xenoantisera and mouse mAb[93,94] were subsequently made against this cell-surface alloantigen. In young chickens, Bu-1 is expressed by virtually all bursal lymphocytes, as well as the peripheral B cells (Table 2), but is not found on plasma cells.[95] In the liver, macrophage-like cells express Bu-1, but these cells are not phagocytic, and cultured macrophages are not stained with a Bu-1 specific mAb.[34]

Allelic differences between Bu-1 molecules are recognized by alloantisera, and two alleles have been defined by mAb. The L22[34] and 21-1A4[94] mAb recognize Bu-1a allelic forms, while 511G2[94] recognizes Bu-1b molecules. While not genetically linked to the MHC, Bu-1 alleles appear to influence the level of expression of MHC class II (B-L) genes.[96] When these allelic differences were used to study B-cell development in the bursa,[95] the origin of precursors that colonize each follicle could be distinguished in chimeras of different Bu-1 allotypes. By scoring the number of follicles containing Bu-1a alone, Bu-1b alone, or mixtures of the two allotypes, it was possible to estimate the average number of precursors in each follicle at three or fewer.[97]

ii. Bu-2

The Bu-2 antigen, a protein of M_r 66,000, is expressed by bursal and peripheral B cells. The level of expression on B cells is high, but low levels of Bu-2 are also detected on macrophages and dendritic cells in the thymic medulla and in splenic periellipsoidal cuffs.[98] Though of similar molecular weight and tissue distribution, Bu-2 was shown to be distinct from the Bu-1 antigen by sequential immunoprecipitation, modulation studies, and two-color immunofluorescence of bone marrow where Bu-2 expression exceeds that of Bu-1.[98]

iii. CB3

The CB3 antigen is a glycoprotein of M_r 50,000 that is associated with the β_2 micro-globulin (β_2-m, M_r 14,000) on the surface of bursal and peripheral B lymphocytes.[99] Both CB3 and β_2-m are immunoprecipitated by mAb against one or the other protein. The anti-β_2-m antibody precipitates class I (B-F) heavy chains of M_r 45,000 as well as the CB3 heavy chain from B-cell lysates. The β_2-m associated with either class I or CB3 has an identical pI and molecular mass. In addition to the difference in molecular weight, the pI of CB3 (6.5 to 8.5) and the class I heavy chain (<5 to 6) are quite distinct.[99] Partial trypsin digestion of these heavy chains releases peptides of different sizes, indicating that the distribution of the basic amino acids is different in the two molecules. Although the CB3 molecule differs from class I molecules in both physical characteristics and tissue distribution, the association of CB3 with β_2-m suggests structural similarity to other β_2-m-associated class I-like proteins.

β_2-microglobulin-associated proteins in mammals, CD1, Qa, and TL may resemble class I molecules in their ability to present antigen. TL and Qa proteins can be recognized by TCR1$^+$ T cells ($\gamma\delta^+$).[100,101] CD1 is recognized by a TCR2$^+$ ($\alpha\beta$) CTL line which is CD4$^-$CD8$^-$.[102] The hypothetical functions of class I molecules include the presentation of specific antigens (possibly carbohydrates) to TCR1$^+$ cells.[62,103] The presentation of these antigens may occur in specific locations, such as the skin in the case of CD1$^+$ Langerhans cells.[62,103] A similar situation may exist in the intestinal epithelium of chickens where TCR1$^+$ cells are preferentially localized.[52] If CB3 functions as a class I-like molecule, B lymphocytes could present antigens to TCR1$^+$ cells in association with CB3 proteins, in addition to class I- and II-mediated recognition.

iv. Other B-Cell Antigens

CB1, CB4, and CB5[13] are also expressed in peripheral B cells, as well as in the bursa. The tissue distribution and molecular masses of these antigens are summarized in Table 2.

The CB1 antigen, M_r 110,000, was originally detected only on bursal lymphocytes and B-cell tumors. Recent evidence indicates that the CB1 mAb also reacts with normal peripheral B cells. In the bursa, the CB1 antigen is a disulfide-linked dimer composed of M_r 55,000 subunits whose pI are slightly different.[145] The CB4 antigen is a three chain structure with noncovalently associated subunits of M_r 107,000, 53,000, and 39,000. The CB5 antigen, a protein of M_r 167,000, is expressed on plasma cells as well as B cells.

c. Antigens of B-Cell Subpopulations

Subsets of B cells have been described in mammals.[39,104,105] In the chicken, CB8, CB9, and CB10 antigens are expressed on the majority of bursal lymphocytes, but only on a subset of peripheral B cells. CB8 is detected on approximately 60% of B lymphocytes in the blood and about 90% of IgM$^+$ lymphoblasts and plasma cells. In contrast, both CB9 and CB10 are expressed only by a small population of peripheral B lymphocytes. While CB9 is a single polypeptide of M_r 220,000, CB10 is a M_r 120,000 dimer consisting of two disulfide-linked M_r 65,000 chains. The CB8 molecule has not been characterized.

The CB11 antigen, although detected on the majority of peripheral B lymphocytes, is expressed only by a subset of bursal cells. In young chicks, CB7 is expressed on 51% of bursal cells and CB11 on 26%.[146] The distribution of these antigens in the bursa is striking. CB7$^+$ cells are located in the medulla, while CB11$^+$ cells are limited to the cortex and the surrounding interfollicular tissue. The mutually exclusive expression of these antigens by two physically and maturationally distinct populations of cells suggests different roles for these antigens in precise stages of differentiation. They also provide a convenient marker with which to distinguish these differentiation stages in single cell suspensions. CB11 is an antigen of M_r 37,000 while the molecular weight of CB7 has not been determined.

The CD5 mAb (Section III. A) recognizes a subpopulation of B lymphocytes. In the bursas of 8-week-old chickens, less than 10% of the lymphocytes bind these antibodies, but by 3 months betwenn 30 and 50% of bursal cells are stained.[38] Between 55 and 65% of peripheral B cells express CD5.[29,38] Whether these CD5$^+$ B cells represent an independent lineage with a specific tissue distribution, as has been proposed in mammals,[39] has not been explored.

d. Antigens of Nonlymphoid Bursal Elements

Interactions of developing bursal lymphocytes with nonlymphoid cells in the bursa are likely to be important, but these are not yet understood. One approach toward gaining the relevant information is to make monoclonal antibodies against cell-surface molecules on nonlymphoid bursal cells that may be involved in their interaction with developing B cells. Two mAb, BEP-1 and BEP-2, mark antigens on bursal epithelial cells.[106] BEP-1 appears on all epithelial cells in the bursa: plical epithelium, basement membrane-associated epithelium, cortico-medullary epithelium, and, sparsely, on the follical-associated epithelium (FAE). BEP-2 is a cytoplasmic antigen that is secreted by plical and medullary epithelium in bursa, thymus, and goblet cells in the intestine.

The B.2 mAb recognizes another nonlymphoid antigen that is expressed by Ig$^-$ cells in the bursa.[107] B.2 also binds the basement membrane, the cortico-medullary epithelium, FAE (but not the rest of the plical membrane), and a mesh work of reticular cells in the medulla.[107] Most phagocytic cells in the bursa express B.2 as do scattered cells in the spleen and thymus. High endothelial venules and skeletal and smooth muscle are also reactive with this antibody.

The B.3 mAb reacts with cells in the medulla region of bursal follicles, as well as thymic and intestinal epithelium.[108] Other antigens have been identified with antisera raised against bursal cells: bursa reticular fiber antigen (CBRFA) and gut-associated mucin antigen (CGAMA).[109] These markers may provide the ligands which mediate the communication of B lymphocytes with the extracellular environment during the critical bursal phase of development.

3. Developmental Expression of B-Cell Antigens

The bursa is colonized by lymphocyte precursors only between E7 and E14.[110] IgM is first evident both in the cytoplasm and on the surface of the bursal lymphocytes around E12.[76,111] Immunoglobulin gene rearrangements can be detected between E10 and E12,[112] but the accumulation of somatic changes in the transcribed V_λ and V_H gene segments continues beyond the third week after hatching.[76,86,88,112] Immunoglobulin gene rearrangement, modification, and translation can thus be used as hallmarks for the different stages in B-cell maturation, and the expression of other B-cell antigens can be placed within this framework. As the percentage of IgM^+ cells increases in the embryonic bursa, there is a concordant increase in the percentages of cells that express most of the other B-cell antigens. The level of their expression appears to be higher than IgM. An exception is the CB2 antigen which is expressed by only a subpopulation of IgM^+ cells until late in ontogeny when all of the IgM^+ cells become $CB2^+$.[145]

An intriguing recent finding suggests that Ig gene rearrangement may also occur in extra-bursal cells present in the E10 to 12 spleen, liver, and bone marrow.[112] Because these rearrangements are very rare, it is not yet clear whether these are precursors of B cells or if they are emigrants that have already traversed the bursal microenvironment.[113] Several of the mAb that mark B cells in adults also react with Ig^- cells in embryonic spleen. Bu-1,[114] 319-D3,[115,116] CB3, CB4, CB8, CB9, CB10, and CB11[145,146] are expressed by embryonic spleen cells that do not express immunoglobulin. The frequency of cells expressing these antigens decreases just before hatching when the frequency of Ig^+ cells in the periphery begins to increase.

IV. LEUKOCYTE COMMON ANTIGENS AND MYELOID ANTIGENS

Leukocyte common antigens (LCA; CD45; and T200) are expressed by virtually all chicken leukocytes, but not by nonhemopoietic tissues. The LCA glycoproteins expressed on different lymphocyte populations in mammals vary in apparent molecular weight from 180,000 to 220,000 as a function of their differentiation status and lineage.[117] The size heterogeneity is due to differential mRNA splicing and glycosylation status.[118] Certain LCA epitopes are lineage-restricted, and mAb against these can be used to separate functionally important subsets of lymphoid cells.[119] The large cytoplasmic domain of this highly conserved molecule (~700 amino acids) contains multiple serine phosphorylation sites. Amino acid sequence analysis has recently revealed striking homology between a major protein tyrosine phosphatase (PTPase 1B) and the tandem C-terminal homologous domains of LCA.[120] LCA is now thought to function in specific signal transduction pathways via protein tyrosine dephosphorylation.[121]

LCA molecules have also been identified on the cells of avian species by mAb, most of which are chicken specific. The L-17 mAb reacts with all myeloid and lymphoid cells in blood and lymphoid organs, but not with erythrocytes or thrombocytes.[34] The L-17 antigens have molecular weights of approximately 180,000 on thymocytes and 190,000 and 210,000 on bursal lymphocytes. Other antibodies reactive with similar molecules include the CL-1[122] and CLA3 mAb.[146] A lineage-restricted mAb, CLA-1, which reacts with T cells, early B cells, and myeloid cells,[13] precipitates a glycoprotein composed of noncovalently linked chains of M_r 180,000 and 195,000. The specificity of this LCA mAb appears to be similar to the BC10 mAb which recognizes human leukocytes.[123] Few studies have addressed the structure and function of the avian LCA.

Other nonlineage restricted mAb which may identify LCA or other leukocyte molecules have also been reported, but the antigens have not been well characterized. The 56-3-C mAb reacts with cell lines of myeloid and lymphoid origin, normal thymus and bursa cells, and erythroblasts.[124] HIS-C7 reacts with a membrane-bound determinant present on T and B lymphocytes, granulocytes, monocytes, and macrophages.[125] The 17-B-2 mAb, which identifies a M_r 30,000 protein,[124] and L-43, which detects a molecule of M_r 23,000,[14] are clearly different from the LCA mAb, but are similar to CAMPATH-1 which identifies a M_r 23,000 to 30,000 glycoprotein expressed on most lymphoid cells and monocytes in humans.[123] Another mAb, MB-1, reacts with quail, but not chicken, hemopoietic and endothelial cells.[126,127] The differential species-specific reactivity of these mAb is useful to study stem cell differentiation in quail-chick chimeras.

Another family of structurally related leukocyte glycoproteins in mammals includes molecules that mediate cellular adhesion in virtually all phases of the immune response. These adhesion molecules share a common β unit (M_r 95,000) that associates noncovalently with a series of different α chains of molecular weights ranging from 150,000 to 180,000.[128,129] None of the avian antigens have been clearly characterized as homologues of these adhesion proteins. We have produced a mAb, CLA-2, that reacts with most of the leukocytes and precipitates a heterodimer consisting of M_r 180,000 and 100,000 chains.[140] CLA-2 may thus be a candidate for a chicken adhesion molecule. Several mAb reactive with monocytes/macrophages have been generated. Four such antibodies react predominantly with immature myeloid cells and detect glycoproteins of M_r 100,000 to 190,000.[124] CVI-ChNL-68.1 reacts with monocytes, macrophages, and interdigitating cells.[130] K-1 reacts with adherent monocytes from spleen and peripheral blood and a virus-transformed monocytic cell line.[131]

Several mAb against human myeloid cells react with NK cells. NK cells represent a small fraction of peripheral blood mononuclear cells that are phenotypically and functionally heterogenous.[132] Both CD3− and CD3+ lymphocytic clones with NK activity have been defined.[133] NK cells in birds have been defined only by their spontaneously killing of tumor cells *in vitro*.[134,135] Recently, the K-14 and K-24 mAb were reported to stain 7 to 10% of the splenocytes, 8 to 10% of blood leukocytes, and <2% of the thymus and bursal lymphocytes. Pretreatment of spleen cells with either the K-14 or K-24 mAb abrogated NK-cell activity, suggesting that these mAb react with molecules expressed on NK cells.[131] The biochemical nature of these molecules is presently unknown.

V. CONCLUSION

The avian model has contributed to our understanding of the embryonic development of lymphocyte populations in the primary lymphoid organs and their peripheral migration. Cooperation between T and B cells and the functions of these cells follow many of the same rules in birds and mammals. However, study of the relevant cell interactions and structure-function relationships has been limited by the absence of suitable markers of the avian lymphocytes. Availability of the mAb and lymphocyte gene probes outlined in this review may enable the avian model to contribute new insight into the immune system.

The MHC class I and class II antigens, immunoglobulins, T-cell receptors, and their accessory molecules on chicken lymphocytes are the best characterized surface markers of avian cells. The biochemical characteristics of the identified molecules are highly conserved in birds and mammals. The most unusual feature of the chicken MHC is the very small size of the introns flanking the MHC genes.[20,21,25] The B-L βII gene is only 1.7 kb long compared to 8 kb for HLA-DQ β and up to 20 kb for HLA-DP β genes. The B-F and B-L β genes are also two orders of magnitude closer than are the class I and class II genes in the mammalian MHC complex. This may account for the absence of B-F/B-L recombinants.

Like the MHC antigens, the basic antigen recognition molecules and the differentiation pathways defined for mammalian T cells also appear to be conserved in birds. The sequential development of avian TCR1$^+$ and TCR2$^+$ cells during ontogeny parallels that noted for the $\gamma\delta$ and $\alpha\beta$ T cells in mammals. However, the subsequent generation of a third TCR3-bearing lineage of T cells in birds is an unprecedented finding. Our data suggest that the M_r 40,000 chain of TCR2 and TCR3 represent a shared α chain, while the M_r 50,000 chain of TCR2 and M_r 48,000 chain of TCR3 represent distinctive β chains. Molecular cloning of chicken TCR is in progress to determine the genetic basis for the sequential generation of these two sublineages of $\alpha\beta$ T cells.

The avian CD3 antigen has been used to identify a novel population of cytoplasmic CD3$^+$ lymphocytes that lack the TCR/CD3 receptor complex on their surface. These so-called TCR0 cells are abundant in the intestine and may represent a primitive lymphoid cell that plays an important local role in body defense. In support of this idea, gut-associated lymphoid tissue is found in all vertebrates and in some invertebrates.[136] A subpopulation of human lymphocytes capable of specific lysis of allogeneic target cells expresses the CD3 ϵ protein in the absence of other elements of the TCR/CD3 complex.[137] The expression of CD3 ζ chain has also been noted in human CD3$^-$ NK cells.[138] It remains to be determined whether the avian TCR0 cells have NK activity or represent a novel lineage of cells.

Chicken immunoglobulins resemble their mammalian counterparts in both structure and function. However, mechanisms for generating these molecules, as well as the site of origin of the cells that produce them, differ from the mammalian model in many respects. The bursa of Fabricius, which is required for normal avian B-cell development, has no anatomical equivalent in mammals. Cells with the pre-B phenotype (cytoplasmic μ heavy chain but no light chain expression), which are the hallmark of B-lymphopoietic sites in mammals, are not detected in the bursa. The primary role of the bursa is to expand the B-cell repertoire. Diversity is generated by a somatic mechanism of gene conversion in which a pool of V_H and V_L pseudogenes are used as donors of sequence to the productively rearranged variable gene segment.[86,87] At both the light chain and heavy chain gene loci, only a single variable gene segment is rearranged, and usually this occurs on only one allele. This strict constraint on rearrangement appears to limit aberrant rearrangements. This is an important safeguard since any non-functional rearrangements could be corrected by gene conversion events which occur continuously in the bursa, violating the principle of allelic exclusion.

Unlike immunoglobulins, most of the other B-cell markers identified so far have no known mammalian homologues. Studies of the structure, function, and genes encoding these novel antigens may be valuable in our understanding of the evolution of the immune system. The information obtained may also yield insight into the roles that analogous molecules play in mammals.

ACKNOWLEDGMENTS

We thank Mrs. E. A. Brookshire for her excellent secretarial assistance. This work has been supported by grants CA 16673 and CA 13148, awarded by the National Institutes of Health. MDC is an HHMI investigator.

REFERENCES

1. **Cooper, M. D., Peterson, D. A., and Good, R. A.,** Delineation of the thymic and bursal lymphoid systems in the chicken, *Nature (London),* 205, 143, 1965.
2. **Moore, M. A. S. and Owen, J. J.,** Stem cell migration in developing myeloid and lymphoid systems, *Lancet,* 2, 658, 1965.
3. **Le Douarin, N.,** Ontogeny of hematopoietic organs studied in avian embryo interspecific chimeras, in *Differentiation of Normal and Neoplastic Hematopoietic Cells,* Cold Spring Harbor Laboratory, Cold Spring Harbor, NY, 1978, 5.
4. **Briles, W. E., McGibbon, W. H., and Irwin, M. R.,** On multiple alleles affecting cellular antigens in the chicken, *Genetics,* 35, 633, 1950.
5. **Hala, K., Vilheimova, M., and Hartmanova, J.,** Probable crossing-over in the B blood group system of chickens, *Immunogenetics,* 3, 97, 1976.
6. **Pink, J. R. L., Droege, W., Hala, K., Miggiano, V. C., and Ziegler, A.,** A three-locus model for the chicken major histocompatibility complex, *Immunogenetics,* 5, 203, 1977.
7. **Longenecker, B. M. and Mosmann, T. R.,** Restricted expression of a MHC alloantigen in cells of the erythroid series, *J. Supramol. Struct.,* 13, 395, 1981.
8. **Kaufman, J., Thorpe, D., Skjodt, K., and Salomonsen, J.,** MHC proteins and genes in birds and reptiles, *Dev. Comp. Immunol.,* 13, 374, 1989.
9. **Crone, M. and Simonsen, M.,** Avian major histocompatibility complex, in *Avian Immunology: Basis and Practice,* Vol. 2, Toivanen, A. and Toivanen, P., Eds., CRC Press, Boca Raton, FL, 1987, 25.
10. **Vainio, O. and Toivanen, A.,** Cellular cooperation in immunity, in *Avian Immunology: Basis and Practice,* Vol. 2, Toivanen, A. and Toivanen, P., Eds., CRC Press, Boca Raton, FL, 1987, 1.
11. **Pink, J. R. L., Kieran, M. W., Rijnbeek, A.-M., and Longenecker, B. M.,** A monoclonal antibody against chicken MHC class I (B-F) antigens, *Immunogenetics,* 21, 293, 1985.
12. **Crone, M., Simonsen, M., Skjodt, K., Linnet, K., and Olsson, R.,** Mouse monoclonal antibodies to class I and class II antigens of chicken MHC. Evidence for at least two class I products of the B complex, *Immunogenetics,* 21, 181, 1985.
13. **Chen, C. H. and Cooper, M. D.,** Identification of cell surface molecules on chicken lymphocytes with monoclonal antibodies, in *Avian Immunology, Basis and Practice,* Toivanen, A. and Toivanen, P., Eds., CRC Press, Boca Raton, FL, 1987, 137.
14. **Pink, J. R. L. and Gilmour, D. G.,** Surface antigens of avian blood, in *Differentiation Antigens in Lymphohemopoietic Tissues,* Miyasaka, M. and Trnka, Z., Eds., Marcel Dekker, New York, 1988, 361.
15. **Ziegler, A. and Pink, J. R. L.,** Chemical properties of two antigens controlled by the major histocompatibility complex of the chicken, *J. Biol. Chem.,* 251, 5391, 1976.
16. **Skjodt, K., Welinder, K. G., Crone, M., Verland, S., Salomonsen, J., and Simonsen, M.,** Isolation and characterization of chicken and turkey beta 2-microglobulin, *Mol. Immunol.,* 23, 1301, 1986.
17. **Vitetta, E. S., Uhr, J. W., Klein, J., Pazderka, F., Moticka, E. J., Ruth, R. F., and Capra, J. D.,** Homology of (murine) H-2 and (human) HLA with a chicken histocompatibility antigen, *Nature (London),* 270, 535, 1977.
18. **Huser, H., Ziegler, A., Knecht, R., and Pink, J. R. L.,** Partial aminoterminal amino acid sequences of chicken major histocompatibility antigens, *Immunogenetics,* 6, 301, 1978.
19. **Sgonc, R., Hala, K., and Wick, G.,** Relationship between the expression of class I antigen and reactivity of chicken thymocytes, *Immunogenetics,* 26, 150, 1987.
20. **Guillemot, F., Billault, A., Pourquié, O., Béhar, G., Chaussé, A.-M., Zoorob, R., Kreibich, G., and Auffray, C.,** A molecular map of the chicken major histocompatibility complex: the class II β genes are closely linked to the class I genes and the nucleolar organizer, *EMBO J.,* 7, 2715, 1988.
21. **Guillemot, F. and Auffray, C.,** Molecular biology of the chicken major histocompatibility complex, *Crit. Rev. Poult. Biol.,* 2, 255, 1989.
22. **Schmidt, W., Festenstein, H., Ward, P. J., and Sanderson, A. R.,** Interspecies exchange of beta 2-microglobulin and associated MHC and differentiation antigens, *Immunogenetics,* 13, 483, 1981.
23. **Ewert, D. L. and Cooper, M. D.,** Ia-like alloantigens in the chicken: serologic characterization and ontogeny of cellular expression, *Immunogenetics,* 7, 521, 1978.
24. **Ewert, D. L., Munchus, M. S., Chen, C. H., and Cooper, M. D.,** Analysis of structural properties and cellular distribution of avian Ia antigen by using monoclonal antibody to monomorphic determinants, *J. Immunol.,* 132, 2524, 1984.
25. **Guillemot, F. P., Oliver, P. D., Peault, B. M., and Le Douarin, N. M.,** Cells expressing Ia antigens in the avian thymus, *J. Exp. Med.,* 160, 1803, 1984.
26. **Oliver, P. D. and Le Douarin, N. M.,** Avian thymic accessory cells, *J. Immunol.,* 132, 1748, 1984.
27. **Schat, K. A., Chen, C. H., Shek, W. R., and Calnek, B. W.,** Surface antigens on Marek's disease lymphoblastoid tumor cell lines, *J. Natl. Cancer Inst.,* 69, 715, 1982.

28. **Bourlet, Y., Béhar, G., Guillemot, F., Fréchin, N., Billault, A., Chausse, A. M., Zoorob, R., and Auffray, C.,** Isolation of chicken major histocompatibility complex class II (B-L) β chain sequences: comparison with mammalian β chains and expression in lymphoid organs, *EMBO J.,* 7, 1031, 1988.

29. **Vainio, O., and Lassila, O.,** Chicken T cells: differentiation antigens and cell-cell interactions, *Crit. Rev. Poult. Biol.,* 2, 97, 1989.

30. **Haynes, B. F., Denning, S. M., Singer, K. H., and Kurtzberg, J.,** Ontogeny of T-cell precursors: a model for the initial stages of human T-cell development, *Immunol. Today,* 10, 87, 1989.

31. **Springer, T. A., Dustin, M. L., Kishimoto, T. K., and Marlin, S. D.,** The lymphocyte function-associated LFA-1, CD2 and LFA-3 molecules: cell adhesion receptors of the immune system, *Annu. Rev. Immunol.,* 5, 223, 1987.

32. **Meuer, S. C., Hussex, R. E., Fabbi, M., Fox, D., Acuto, A., Fitzgerald, K. A., Hodgson, J. C., Protentis, J. P., Schlossman, S. F., and Reinherz, E. L.,** An alternative pathway of T-cell activation: a functional role of the 50 KD T11 sheep erythrocyte receptor protein, *Cell,* 36, 897, 1984.

33. **Chen, C. H., Chanh, T. C., and Cooper, M. D.,** Chicken thymocyte-specific antigen identified by monoclonal antibodies: ontogeny, tissue distribution, and biochemical characterization, *Eur. J. Immunol.,* 14, 385, 1984.

34. **Pink, J. R. L. and Rijnbeek, A. M.,** Monoclonal antibodies against chicken lymphocyte surface antigens, *Hybridoma,* 2, 287, 1983.

35. **Peault, B., Coltey, M., and Le Douarin, N. M.,** Tissue distribution and ontogentic emergence of differentiation antigens on avian T cells, *Eur. J. Immunol.,* 12, 1042, 1982.

36. **Houssaint, E., Diez, E., and Jotereau, F. V.,** Tissue distribution and ontogenic appearance of a chicken T lymphocyte differentiation antigen, *Eur. J. Immunol.,* 15, 385, 1985.

37. **McMichael, A. J. and Gotch, F. M.,** T-cell antigens: new and previously defined clusters, in *Leukocyte Typing III: White Cell Differentiation Antigens,* McMichael, A. J., Ed., Oxford University Press, Oxford, 1987, 31.

38. **Lillehoj, H. S., Lillehoj, E. P., Weinstock, D., and Schat, K. A.,** Functional and biochemical characterization of avian T lymphocyte antigens identified by monoclonal antibodies, *Eur. J. Immunol.,* 18, 2059, 1988.

39. **Herzenberg, L. A., Stall, A. M., Lalor, P. A., Sidman, C., Moore, W. A., Park, D. R., and Herzenberg, L. A.,** The Lyl B cell lineage, *Immunol. Res.,* 93, 81, 1986.

40. **Chan, M. M., Chen, C. H., Ager, L. L., and Cooper, M. D.,** Identification of the avian homologues of mammalian CD4 and CD8 antigens, *J. Immunol.,* 140, 2133, 1988.

41. **Littman, D. R.,** The structure of the CD4 and CD8 genes, *Annu. Rev. Immunol.,* 5, 561, 1987.

42. **Bierer, B. E., Sleckman, B. P., Ratnofsky, S. E., and Burakoff, S. J.,** The biological roles of CD2, CD4 and CD8 in T-cell activation, *Annu. Rev. Immunol.,* 7, 579, 1989.

43. **Chen, C. H., Ager, L. L., Gartland, G. L., and Cooper, M. D.,** Identification of a T3/T cell receptor complex in chickens, *J. Exp. Med.,* 164, 375, 1986.

44. **Bucy, R. P., Chen, C. H., and Cooper, M. D.,** Ontogeny of T cell receptors in the chicken thymus, *J. Immunol.,* 144, 1161, 1990.

45. **Clevers, H., Alacorn, B., Wileman, T., and Terhorst, C.,** The T cell receptor/CD3 complex: a dynamic protein ensemble, *Annu. Rev. Immunol.,* 6, 629, 1988.

46. **Sowder, J. T., Chen, C. H., Ager, L. L., Chan, M. M., and Cooper, M. D.,** A large subpopulation of avian T cells express a homologue of the mammalian Tγδ receptor, *J. Exp. Med.,* 167, 315, 1988.

47. **Cihak, J., Ziegler-Heitbrock, H. W. L., Trainer, H., Schranner, I., Merkenschlager, M., and Lösch, U.,** Characterization and functional properties of a novel monoclonal antibody which identifies a T cell receptor in chicken, *Eur. J. Immunol.,* 18, 533, 1988.

48. **Char, D., Chen, C. H., Bucy, R. P., and Cooper, M. D.,** Identification of a third T cell receptor (TCR3) in the chicken with a monoclonal antibody, *Fed. Proc.,* 3 (3), 1507, 1989.

49. **Chen, C. H., Cihak, J., Lösch, U., and Cooper, M. D.,** Differential expression of two T cell receptors TCR1 and TCR2 on chicken lymphocytes, *Eur. J. Immunol.,* 18, 538, 1988.

50. **George, J. F. and Cooper, M. D.,** Quantitative analysis of the cell surface expression of γδ TCR and αβ TCR in the chicken, *Fed. Proc.,* 3(3), 1506, 1989.

51. **Cihak, J., Ziegler-Heitbrock, L., Chen, C. H., Cooper, M. D., and Lósch, U.,** Expression of T cell antigen receptor molecules in the chicken, *7th Int. Congr. Immunol.,* 256, 1989.

52. **Bucy, R. P., Chen, C. H., Cihak, J., Lösch, U., and Cooper, M. D.,** Avian T cells expressing γδ receptors (TCR1) home to the splenic sinusoids and intestinal epithelium, *J. Immunol.,* 141, 2200, 1988.

53. **Pardoll, D. M., Fowlkes, B. J., Bluestone, J. A., Kruisbeek, A., Malby, W. L., Colligan, J. E., and Schwartz, R. H.,** Differential expression of two distinct T cell receptors during thymic development, *Nature (London),* 326, 79, 1987.

54. **Havran, W. L. and Allison, J. P.,** Developmentally ordered appearance of lymphocytes expressing different T cell antigen receptors, *Nature (London),* 335, 443, 1988.

55. **Haynes B. F., Singer, K. H., Denning, S. M., and Martin, M. E.,** Analysis of expression of CD2, CD3, and T cell receptor molecules during human fetal thymic development, *J. Immunol.,* 141, 3776, 1988.
56. **Goodman, T. and Lefrancois, L.,** Expression of gamma-delta T cell receptor on intestinal CD8⁺ intraepithelial lymphocytes, *Nature (London),* 333, 855, 1988.
57. **Bucy, R. P., Chen, C. H., and Cooper, M. D.,** Tissue localization and CD8 accessory molecule expression of T gamma-delta cells in humans, *J. Immunol.,* 142, 3045, 1989.
58. **Chen, C. H., Sowder, J. T., Lahti, J. M., Cihak, J., Lösch, U., and Cooper, M. D.,** TCR3: a third T cell receptor in the chicken, *Proc. Natl. Acad. Sci. U.S.A.* 88, 2352, 1989.
59. **Sowder, J. T., Chen, C. H., Cihak, J., Lösch, U., and Cooper, M. D.,** T cell ontogeny: suppressive effects of embryonic treatment with monoclonal antibodies to T3, TCR1 or TCR2, *Fed. Proc.,* 2, 874, 1988.
60. **Coltey, M., Jotereau, F. V., and Le Douarin, N. M.,** Evidence for a cyclic renewal of lymphocyte precursor cells in the embryonic chicken thymus, *Cell Differ.,* 22, 71, 1987.
61. **Coltey, M., Bucy, R. P., Chen, C. H., Cihak, J., Lösch, U., Char, D., Le Douarin, N. M., and Cooper, M. D.,** Analysis of the first two waves of thymic homing stem cells and their T cell progeny in chick-quail chimeras, *J. Exp. Med.,* 170, 543, 1989.
62. **Strominger, J.,** The gamma/delta T cell and class 1B MHC related proteins: enigmatic molecules of immune recognition, *Cell,* 57, 895, 1989.
63. **Simonsen, M.,** Graft versus host reactions. Their natural history, and applicability as tools of research, *Prog. Allergy,* 6, 349, 1962.
64. **Quere, P., Cooper, M. D., and Thorbecke, G. J.,** Suppressor cell properties in the chicken, *Fed. Proc.,* 3, 3374, 1989.
65. **Bucy, R. P., Coltey, M., Chen, C. H., Char, D., Le Douarin, N. M., and Cooper, M. D.,** Cytoplasmic CD3⁺ surface CD8⁺ lymphocytes develop as a thymus independent lineage in chick-quail chimeras, *Eur. J. Immunol.,* 19, 1449, 1989.
66. **Bucy, R. P., Chen, C. H., and Cooper, M. D.,** Development of cytoplasmic CD3⁺/TCR⁻ cells in the peripheral lymphoid tissues of chickens, *Eur. J. Immunol.,* 20, 1345, 1990.
67. **Hála, K., Schaunstein, K., Neu, N., Krömer, G., Wolf, H., Böck, G., and Wick, G.,** A monoclonal antibody reacting with a membrane determinant expressed on activated T lymphocytes, *Eur. J. Immunol.,* 16, 1331, 1986.
68. **Schauenstein, K., Krömer, G., Hála, K., Böck, G., and Wick, G.,** Chicken-activated T-lymphocyte-antigen (CATLA) recognized by monoclonal antibody INN-CH16 represents the IL-2 receptor, *Dev. Comp. Immunol.,* 12, 823, 1988.
69. **Mazella, O., Cauchy, L., Coudert, F., and Richard, J.,** Chicken thymocyte-specific antigens identified by monoclonal antibodies: characterization and distribution in normal tissues and in tumoral tissues from Marek's disease, *Hybridoma,* 5, 319, 1986.
70. **Wolf, H., Hála, K., Boyd, R. L., and Wick, G.,** MHC- and non-MHC-encoded surface antigens of chicken lymphoid and erythrocytes recognized by polyclonal xeno-, allo- and monoclonal antibodies, *Eur. J. Immunol.,* 14, 831, 1984.
71. **Yamaga, K. and Benedict, A. A.,** Class, amounts and affinities of anti-dinitrophenyl antibodies in chickens I. Production of 7S and 17S antibodies of equal affinity by intravenous injection of antigen, *J. Immunol.,* 115, 750, 1975.
72. **Dahan, A., Reynaud, C.-A., and Weill, J.-C.,** Nucleotide sequence of the constant region of a chicken mu heavy chain immunoglobulin mRNA, *Nucleic Acids Res.,* 11, 5381, 1983.
73. **Reynaud, C.-A., Anquez, V., Grimal, H., and Weill, J.-C.,** A hyperconversion mechanism generates the chicken light chain preimmune repertoire, *Cell,* 48, 379, 1987.
74. **Parvari, R., Ziv, E., Lantner, F., Tel-Or, S., Burstein, Y., and Schechter, I.,** A few germline genes encode the variable regions of chicken immunoglobulin light and gamma-heavy chains, *EMBO J.,* 6, 97, 1987.
75. **Parvari, R., Avivi, A., Lentner, F., Ziv, E., Tel-Or, S., Burstein, Y., and Schechter, I.,** Chicken immunoglobulin gamma-heavy chains: limited VH gene repertoire, combinatorial diversification by D gene segments and evolution of the heavy chain locus, *EMBO J.,* 7, 739, 1988.
76. **Reynaud, C.-A., Dahan, A., Anquez, V., and Weill, J.-C.,** Somatic hyperconversion diversifies the single V_H gene of the chicken with high incidence in the D region, *Cell,* 59, 171, 1989.
77. **Chen, C. H., Lehmeyer, J. E., and Cooper, M. D.,** Evidence for an IgD homologue on chicken lymphocytes, *J. Immunol.,* 129, 2580, 1982.
78. **Benedict, A. A. and Berestecky, J. M.,** Special features of avian immunoglobulins, in *Avian Immunology: Basis and Practice,* Toivanen, A. and Toivanen, P., Eds., CRC Press, Boca Raton, FL, 1987, 113.
79. **Kincade, P. W. and Cooper, M. D.,** Development and distribution of chicken immunoglobulin containing cells in chicken, *J. Immunol.,* 106, 371, 1971.

80. **Leslie, G. A. and Clem, L. W.,** Phylogeny of immunoglobulin structure and function. III. Immunoglobulins of the chicken, *J. Exp. Med.,* 130, 1337, 1969.
81. **Lebacq-Verheyden, A.-M., Vaerman, J.-P., and Heremans, J. F.,** Quantification and distribution of chicken immunoglobulins IgA, IgM and IgG in serum and secretions, *Immunology,* 27, 683, 1974.
82. **Porter, P. and Parry, S. H.,** Further characterization of IgA in chicken serum and secretions with evidence of a possible analogue of mammalian secretory component, *Immunology,* 31, 407, 1976.
83. **Parry, S. H. and Porter, P.,** Characterization and localization of secretory component in the chicken, *Immunology,* 34, 471, 1978.
84. **Chanh, T., Chen, C. H., and Cooper, M. D.,** Mouse monoclonal antibodies to chicken V_H idiotypic determinants reactivity with B and T cells, *J. Immunol.,* 129, 2541, 1982.
85. **Wright, J. T., Chen, C. H., Kubagawa, H., and Cooper, M. D.,** Avian B cell diversity examined with monoclonal anti-V_H antibodies, in *Avian Immunology,* Weber, W. T. and Ewert, D. L., Eds., Alan R. Liss, New York, 1987, 81.
86. **Weill, J.-C. and Reynaud, C.-A.,** The chicken B cell compartment, *Science,* 238, 1054, 1987.
87. **Maizels, N.,** Diversity achieved by diverse mechanisms in developing B cells of the chicken, *Cell,* 48, 359, 1987.
88. **Thompson, C. and Neiman, P.,** Somatic diversification of the chicken immunoglobulin light chain gene is limited to the rearranged variable gene segment, *Cell,* 48, 369, 1987.
89. **Ivanyi, J. and Hudson, L.,** Allelic exclusion of M1 (IgM) allotype on the surface of chicken B cells, *Immunology,* 35, 941, 1979.
90. **Ratcliffe, M. J. H. and Ivanyi, J.,** Allotype suppression in the chicken. III. Analysis of the recovery from suppression by neonatally injected or maternal antibodies, *Eur. J. Immunol.,* 11, 301, 1981.
91. **Abo, T. and Balch, C. M.,** A differentiation antigen of human NK and K cells identified by a monoclonal antibody (HNK-1), *J. Immunol.,* 127, 1024, 1981.
92. **Peault, B., Chen, C. H., Cooper, M. D., Barbu, M., Lipinski, M., and Le Douarin, N. M.,** Phylogenetically conserved antigen on nerve cells and lymphocytes resembles myelin-associated glycoprotein, *Proc. Natl. Acad. Sci. U.S.A.,* 84, 814, 1987.
93. **Gilmour, D. G., Brand, A., Donnelly, N., and Stone, H.,** Bu-1 and Th-1, two loci determining surface antigens of B and T lymphocytes in chickens, *Immunogenetics,* 3, 549, 1976.
94. **Veromaa, T., Vainio, O., Eerola, E., and Toivanen, P.,** Monoclonal antibodies against chicken Bu-1a and Bu-1b alloantigens, *Hybridoma,* 7, 41, 1989.
95. **Houssaint, E., Diez, E., and Pink, J. R. L.,** Ontogeny and tissue distribution of the chicken Bu-1a antigen, *Immunology,* 62, 463, 1987.
96. **Fredericksen, T. L. and Gilmour, D. G.,** Influence of genotypes at a non-MHC B lymphocyte alloantigen locus (Bu-1) on expression of Ia (B-L) antigen on chicken bursal lymphocytes, *J. Immunol.,* 134, 754, 1985.
97. **Pink, J. R. L., Vainio, O., and Rijnbeek, A.-M.,** Clones of B lymphocytes in individual follicles of the bursa of Fabricius, *Eur. J. Immunol.,* 15, 83, 1985.
98. **Huffnagel, G. B., Ratcliffe, M. J. H., and Humphries, E. H.,** Bu-2, a novel avian cell surface antigen on B cells and a population of non-lymphoid cells is expressed homogeneously in germinal centers, *Hybridoma.* 8. 589. 1989.
99. **Pickel, J. M., Chen, C. H., and Cooper, M. D.,** An avian B lymphocyte protein associated with β_2 microglobulin, *Immunogenetics,* in press.
100. **Vidovic, D., Roglic, M., McKune, K., Guerder, S., MacKay, C., and Dembic, Z.,** Qa-1 restricted recognition of foreign antigens by a (gamma delta) T-cell hybridoma, *Nature (London),* 340, 646, 1989.
101. **Bonneville, M., Ito, K., Krecko, E. G., Itohara, S., Kappes, D., Ishida, I., Kanagawa, O., Janeway, C. A., Murphy, D. B., and Tonegawa, S.,** Recognition of a self major histocompatibility complex TL region product by gamma delta T cell receptors, *Proc. Natl. Acad. Sci. U.S.A.* 86, 5928, 1989.
102. **Porcelli, S., Brenner, M. B., Greenstein, J. L., Balk, S. P., Terhorst, C., and Bleicher, P. A.,** Recognition of a cluster of differentiation 1 antigen by human CD4⁻ CD8⁻ cytolytic T lymphocytes, *Nature (London),* 341, 447, 1989.
103. **Raulet, D. H.,** Antigens for gamma/delta cells, *Nature (London),* 339, 342, 1989.
104. **Linton, P.-J., Decker, D. J., and Klinman, N. R.,** Primary antibody-forming cells and secondary B cells are generated from separate precursor stem cell subpopulations, *Cell,* 59, 1049, 1989.
105. **Herzenberg, L. A. and Herzenberg, L. A.,** Toward a layered immune system, *Cell,* 59, 953, 1989.
106. **Houssaint, E., Diez, E., and Hallet, M.-M.,** The bursal microenvironment: phenotypic characterization of the epithelial component of the bursa of Fabricius with the use of monoclonal antibodies, *Immunology,* 58, 43, 1986.
107. **Domingo, M., Reinacher, M., Burkhardt, E., and Weiss, E.,** Monoclonal antibodies directed towards the two major cell populations in the bursa of Fabricius of the chicken, *Vet. Immunol. Immunopathol.,* 11, 305, 1986.
108. **Spencer, J. S. and Benedict, A. A.,** Two chicken epithelial and bursal cell antigens detected by monoclonal antibodies, *Fed. Proc.,* 45, 1001, 1986.

109. **Boyd, R. L., Ward, H. A., and Muller, H. K.,** Antiserum specific for reticulin of the bursa of fabricius, *Int. Arch. Allergy Appl. Immunol.,* 50, 129, 1976.
110. **Le Douarin, N. M., Houssaint, E., Jotereau, F. V., and Belo, M.,** Origin of hemopoietic stem cells in the embryonic bursa of Fabricius and bone marrow studied through interspecific chimeras, *Proc. Natl. Acad. Sci. U.S.A.,* 72, 2701, 1975.
111. **Lydyard, P., Grossi, C., and Cooper, M. D.,** Ontogeny of B cells in the chicken, *J. Exp. Med.,* 144, 79, 1976.
112. **McCormack, W. T., Tjoelker, L. W., Barth, C. F., Carlson, L., Petryniak, B., Humphries, E. H., and Thompson, C. B.,** Selection of B cells with productive IgL gene rearrangement occurs in the bursa of Fabricius during chicken embryonic development, *Genes Dev.,* 3, 838, 1989.
113. **Ratcliffe, M. J. H., Lassila, O., Pink, J. R. L., and Vainio, O.,** Avian B cell precursors: surface immunoglobulin expression is an early, possibly bursa-independent event, *Eur. J. Immunol.,* 16, 129, 1986.
114. **Houssaint, E., Lassila, O., and Vainio, O.,** Bu-1 antigen expression as a marker for B cell precursors in chicken embryos, *Eur. J. Immunol.,* 19, 239, 1989.
115. **Kumbaniduwa, F.,** Application des anticorps monclonaux a l'ontogenese des lymphocytes B chez le poulet, Université Pierre et Marie Curie, Thesis, Paris, 1985.
116. **Yassine, F., Fedecka-Bruner, B., and Dieterlen-Lievre, F.,** Ontogeny of the chick embryo spleen-a cytological study, *Cell. Differ. Dev.,* 27, 29, 1989.
117. **Thomas, M. L.,** The leucocyte common antigens family, *Annu. Rev. Immunol.,* 7, 339, 1989.
118. **Thomas, M. L. and Lefrancois, L.,** Differential expression of the leucocyte-common antigen family, *Immunol. Today,* 9, 320, 1988.
119. **Jing, S., Ralph, S., Thomas, M., Head, A., Chain, A., and Trowbridge, I.,** Structural studies of the transferrin receptor and T200 glycoprotein (CD45), in *Leucocyte Typing III, White Cell Differentiation Antigens,* McMichael, A. J., Ed., Oxford University Press, Oxford, 1987, 899.
120. **Charbonneau, H., Tonks, N. K., Walsh, K. A., and Fischer, E. H.,** The leukocyte common antigen (CD45): a putative receptor-linked protein tyrosine phosphatase, *Proc. Natl. Acad. Sci. U.S.A.,* 85, 7182, 1988.
121. **Tonks, N. K., Charbonneau, H., Diltz, C. D., Fischer, E. H., and Walsh, K. K.,** Demonstration that the leukocyte common antigen CD45 is a protein tyrosine phosphatase, *Biochemistry,* 27, 8695, 1988.
122. **Houssaint, E., Tobin, S., Cihak, J., and Lösch, U.,** A chicken leukocyte common antigen: biochemical characterization and ontogenetic study, *Eur. J. Immunol.,* 17, 287, 1987.
123. **Cobbold, S., Hale, G., and Waldmann, H.,** Non-lineage, LFA-1 family, and leukocyte common antigens: new and previously defined clusters, in *Leukocyte Typing III, White Cell Differentiation Antigens,* McMichael, A. J., Ed., Oxford University Press, Oxford, 1987, 788.
124. **Kornfeld, S., Beug, H., Doederlin, G., and Graf, T.,** Detection of avain haematopoietic cell surface antigens with monoclonal antibodies to myeloid cells, *Exp. Cell Res.,* 143, 383, 1983.
125. **Jeurissen, S., Janse, E. M., Ekino, S., Nieuwenhuis, P., Koch, G., and de Boer, G. F.,** Monoclonal antibodies as probes for defining cellular subsets in the bone marrow, thymus, bursa of Fabricius and spleen of the chicken, *Vet. Immunol. Immunopathol.,* 19, 225, 1988.
126. **Peault, B. M., Thiery, J.-P., and Le Douarin, N. M.,** Surface marker for hemopoietic and endothelial cell lineages in quail that is defined by a monoclonal antibody, *Proc. Natl. Acad. Sci. U.S.A.,* 80, 2976, 1983.
127. **Labastie, M., Poole, T. J., Peault, B. M., and LeDouarin, N. M.,** MB1, a quail leukocyte endothelium antigen: partial characterization of the cell surface and secreted forms in cultured endothelial cells, *Proc. Natl. Acad. Sci. U.S.A.,* 83, 9016, 1986.
128. **Kishimoto, T. K., Miller, L. J., and Springer, T. A.,** Homology of LFA-1, Mac-1, and p150,95 with the extracellular matrix receptors defines a novel supergene family of adhesion proteins, in *Leukocyte Typing III, White Cell Differentiation Antigens,* McMichael, A. J., Ed., Oxford University Press, Oxford, 1987, 896.
129. **Hogg, N.,** The leukocyte integrins, *Immunol. Today,* 10, 111, 1989.
130. **Jeurissen, S. H. M., Jause, E. M., Koch, G., and de Boer, G. F.,** The monoclonal antibody CVI-CHNL-68.1 recognizes cells of the monocyte-macrophage lineage in chickens, *Dev. Comp. Immunol.,* 12, 855, 1988.
131. **Chung, K. S. and Lillehoj, H.,** Functional and biochemical characterization of monoclonal antibodies detecting avian T, macrophage and natural killer cell antigens, *Immunobiology,* 4 (Suppl.), 39, 1989.
132. **Trinchieri, G.,** Biology of natural killer cells, *Adv. Immunol.,* 47, 187, 1989.
133. **Lanier, L. L., Phillips, J. H., Hackett, J., Jr., Tutt, M., and Kumar, V.,** Opinion—natural killer cells: definition of a cell type rather than a function, *J. Immunol.,* 137, 2735, 1986.
134. **Fahey, K.-J. and York, J. J.,** Cytotoxic activity of avian lymphoid cells, in *Avian Immunology: Basis and Practice,* Toivanen, A. and Toivanen, P., Eds., CRC Press, Boca Raton, FL, 1987, 179.
135. **Sharma, J. M. and Schat, K. A.,** Natural immune functions, in *Avian Cellular Immunology,* Sharma, J. M., Ed., CRC Press, Boca Raton, FL, 1990.

136. **DuPasquier, L. and Schwager, J.,** Evolution of the immune system, in *Progress in Immunology,* Melchers, F., Ed., Springer-Verlag, Berlin, 1989, 1246.

137. **Ciccone, E., Viale, O., Pende, D., Malnati, M., Biassoni, R., Melioli, M., Moretta, A., Long, E. O., and Moretta, L.,** Specific lysis of allogeneic cells after activation of CD3⁻ lymphocyte culture, *J. Exp. Med.,* 168, 2403, 1988.

138. **Anderson, P., Caligiuri, M., Ritz, J., and Schlossman, S. F.,** CD3-negative natural killer cells express ζTCR as part of a novel molecular complex, *Nature (London),* 341, 159, 1989.

139. **Kaufman, J.,** personal communication.

140. **Chen, C. H. and Cooper, M. D.,** unpublished observations.

141. **Char, D. et al.,** manuscript in preparation.

142. **Sanchez, P. et al.,** manuscript in preparation.

143. **Cihak, J. et al.,** manuscript in preparation.

144. **Chan, M. M.,** unpublished data.

145. **Pickel, J. M. et al.,** manuscript in preparation.

146. **Olson, W. C. and Ewert, D. L.,** personal communication.

Chapter 2

CELLULAR COOPERATION IN IMMUNE RESPONSE AND ROLE OF MHC

Timo Veromaa and Paavo Toivanen

TABLE OF CONTENTS

I. INTRODUCTION

Glick and co-workers[1,2] serendipitiously discovered that surgical removal of the bursa of Fabricius in the chicken 2 weeks after hatching results in impaired antibody formation against bacterial antigens. Following this, several groups independently established the relationship between impaired immune functions and neonatal thymectomy.[3-5] The functions of both the bursa and the thymus in lymphocyte differentiation were later further characterized by bursectomy and thymectomy in combination with irradiation.[6-8] These findings eventually led to the understanding of the duality of the immune response with thymus-dependent cell-mediated immune functions and bursa or bursa equivalent-dependent antibody-mediated immune functions also in mammals.

Due to separate organs for B- and T-cell development, the chicken offers unparalleled experimental opportunities to study the ontogeny of cells responsible for antibody-mediated and cell-mediated immune functions.[9] However, complex regulatory mechanisms govern an individual's response to foreign antigens. The immune response is a result of interactions between B cells, T cells, and antigen-presenting cells. The purpose of this review is to summarize the existing data on cellular cooperation between these three types of cells in the chicken. We will also present a short overview on interactions between maturing lymphocytes and the epithelial structures of the bursa and the thymus because these interactions form the basis for collaboration of mature lymphocytes. Since some aspects are not dealt with in detail, the reader is kindly referred to recent reviews on avian T-cell differentiation[10] and on the avian major histocompatibility complex (MHC).[11,12]

II. CELLULAR COOPERATION DURING LYMPHOCYTE DEVELOPMENT

The bursa of Fabricius is a primary lymphoid organ having a central role in B-cell differentiation. Prebursal stem cells enter the bursa between days 8 and 15 of embryonation,[13-18] and only two to five *prebursal stem cells* colonize each bursal follicle.[19-21] These stem cells are committed to a distinct immunoglobulin (Ig) gene rearrangement at the very beginning of the embryonic bursal development.[22] Ig gene rearrangement occurs at the time of the entry of prebursal stem cells into the follicles or shortly thereafter.

Recently, Houssaint[23] has demonstrated that the colonization of the bursal epithelium by hemopoietic precursors is a two-step phenomenon. The first cells, representing macrophage/dendritic cell lineage, are responsible for the formation of the epithelial buds which, during the subsequent phase, are colonized by lymphoid precursors.[23]

Treating newly hatched chickens with cyclophosphamide, which destroys only the lymphoid cells in the bursa while leaving the bursal reticulum intact, Toivanen and Toivanen[24] have defined maturational stages of bursal lymphocytes. *Bursal stem cells* are immunologically immature cells, requiring the bursal microenvironment for further maturation.[24] They are defined by their ability to reconstitute lymphocyte numbers and bursal histology by homing into the empty follicles in bursae of recipients depleted of B cells by cyclophosphamide treatment.[24-26] These cells have been detected in chick embryos from day 13 of incubation up to 5 weeks of age.[24,27] In the bursa, spleen, and, to some extent, in the thymus and bone marrow, *early postbursal cells* are found at 3 to 6 weeks after hatching. Although quite capable of homing to the bursa, these cells can mature further independent of bursal influence.[24,28] After 6 weeks, the bursa and other lymphoid organs contain *postbursal cells,* which induce functional reconstitution in B-cell-depleted recipients without homing to the bursa. Seeded into periphery, these cells form the basis for a self-renewing B-cell population after the involution of the bursa.[26,29]

All the B lymphocytes in adult chickens have been thought to derive from bursal stem cells, as surgical bursectomy of 17 to 18-d embryo renders the hatched chickens virtually agammaglobulinemic.[30] Also, transfer of normal bursal cells from newly hatched chicks can totally reconstitute B-lymphocyte population and humoral immune responses in cyclophosphamide-treated, syngeneic recipients.[24] On the other hand, transfer of allogeneic cells does not reconstitute the humoral immune response to T-dependent antigens.[31] Functional reconstitution of the B-cell system requires at least one shared, common MHC haplotype.[28] However, following a secondary transfer back to the original host, allogeneically educated B-cells can also respond to both T-dependent and T-independent antigens.[32] The bursal microenvironment during maturation has no effect on the preference of B cells to cooperate successfully with only histocompatible T cells.[9,32,33]

The interactions between the thymic stem cells and stromal cells in the development of the thymus are dealt in more detail in Chapters 1 and 3 of this book. The reader is also referred to a recent review on the subject.[10]

It has been shown that chicken T-cell precursors can enter and proliferate in embryonic quail thymus rudiment providing that the quail thymic anlage has been grafted during a period of receptivity when it attracts T-cell precursors.[18] The functional capacity of these cells has not been analyzed in detail, but the results demonstrate that chicken T-cell progenitors are able to differentiate in a xenogeneic thymus.

Bursectomy has been reported to reduce cellularity of thymus.[34,35] However, we have demonstrated that in chickens bursectomized at 60 h of incubation—before the bursal colonization phase—the number of peripheral T cells is normal as analyzed with a T-cell-specific antiserum in immunofluorescence.[36] Furthermore, T cells from 14-week-old early bursectomized animals can induce normal graft vs. host (GVH) and mixed lymphocyte reactions (MLR). Their proliferative response to T-cell mitogens and specific antigens are normal as well as their ability to produce interleukin-2 (IL-2) in response to concanavalin A (ConA) stimulation. Taken together, these results demonstrate that the function of mature T-cells from bursaless birds is normal, although bursectomy may have an effect on the cellularity of the thymus.[36] Chicken thymus normally contains 5 to 15% surface immunoglobulin positive B cells,[37] and a possibility remains that the cells putatively depleted are B cells.

The effect of thymus on the development of the bursa was demonstrated by Hirota and Bito.[38] They observed that reconstitution of the bursal structure and B-cell function did not occur in cyclophosphamide-treated recipients which were surgically thymectomized. Confirmation for this observation came from experiments using cell recipients which had been treated with cyclophosphamide, surgically thymectomized, and irradiated. The transplanted bursa cells had to be supplemented with thymus cells in order to get a full morphological and functional reconstitution of the bursa-dependent immune system in these animals.[39] It is evident that T cells are required for the B-cell differentiation occurring in the bursa of Fabricius. As discussed in Section IV, this T-B collaboration is not MHC restricted, since the grafted bursa cells are capable of maturing even in an allogeneic bursa.

III. AVIAN MAJOR HISTOCOMPATIBILITY COMPLEX ANTIGENS

MHC is composed of several closely linked genes, the products of which are functionally involved in defense systems of the organism. In mammals the gene products of the MHC—all glycoproteins—are referred to as class I, class II, and class III antigens. Class I and II antigens are integrated membrane proteins, having a central role in the immune system, whereas class III antigens are components of the complement system.

The chicken MHC, originally described as a blood group system,[40,41] consists of three loci: B-F (class I), B-L (class II), and B-G (class IV).[42,43] In the chicken, genes encoding class III antigens or the complement components seem not to be linked to MHC (see Reference 44 for a review).

Similar to their mammalian counterparts, B-F or class I antigens consist of glycosylated polymorphic proteins of molecular weight from 40 to 45 kDa, noncovalently bound to avian β_2-microglobulin.[45] They are expressed on most nucleated cells, including the nucleated erythrocytes in contrast to mammals.[42] Monoclonal antibodies (mAbs) against B-F antigens have been produced, but none have proven to be haplotype-specific.[11,46,47] The B-F locus may encode more than one B-F antigen.[46] Recently, the B-F locus has been partially cloned and sequenced.[12,48]

The B-L or class II antigens in the chicken were first identified by Ziegler and Pink.[45] MAbs against the B-L antigens, all of which detect a monomorphic determinant on the B-L molecule, have been produced.[46,49-51] Using two-dimensional gel electrophoresis, Guillemot and co-workers[52] visualized a single acidic 34-kDa nonpolymorphic chain in all inbred chicken lines studied using mAb TaP1. Further, they detected two molecules differing in both isoelectric point (pI) and molecular weight, thus having classic characteristics of MHC class II β chains. The α-β heterodimer associates with several basic invariant molecules in the cytoplasm, but not on the cell surface, similar to man and mouse.[53,54] The existence of two β chains and one nonpolymorphic α chain suggests that each of the β chains can associate with the same α chain and generate two different α-β heterodimers.[52] Crone and co-workers[55] have presented evidence for two such populations of B-L molecules. Overall, the B-L antigens appear very similar to the HLA-DR antigens in man and I-E antigens in mouse.[52] Recently, one B-L β chain has been cloned and sequenced.[56]

As is the case in their mammalian counterparts, chicken B-L antigens are expressed on B cells as well as on some cells of the monocyte/macrophage series, but not on unstimulated T cells, thymocytes, or erythrocytes.[57] However, activated T cells are B-L$^+$.[49,58]

The first B-L$^+$ cells are found in 9-d embryos in the bursa, spleen, and mesonephrose.[49,57] In the bursa, B-L$^+$ cells increase from about 4% on day 9, to 30% on day 13, and 82% on day 18 of incubation; the 9 day embryonic spleen contains 34% of B-L$^+$ cells, decreasing slightly to 18% on day 13, and remaining unchanged on day 18 of incubation.[49] Two subpopulations of B-L$^+$ cells have been identified in the bursa; 40 to 60% of the large bursa cells exhibit brighter immunofluorescence reactivity than the relatively smaller bursal cells.[49] Interestingly, it has been reported that there are differences in the proportions of brightly staining B-L$^+$ bursa cells from different MHC homozygous chicken lines. The control of this difference has been proposed to associate with a non-MHC linked Bu-1 alloantigen locus.[59] However, in H.B14A chickens the difference at the Bu-1 locus does not have an influence on the level of expression of B-L antigen in bursal cells.[51]

The B-G (class IV) encoded polymorphic antigens have been described only in the avian species and are almost exclusively expressed on erythrocytes; however, evidence of their expression, at least on thrombocytes, exists. The B-G antigens consist of nonglycosylated proteins of apparent molecular weight of 46 to 48 kDa found on the cell surface as dimers or trimers. Interestingly, they seem not to be associated with histocompatibility reactions or other known immune functions,[60] although some controversy exists.[61,62] Recently, genes coding for B-G antigens have been cloned and sequenced,[63] allowing elucidation of the structure-function relationship within the chicken MHC in general and particularly within the B-G region.

IV. INTERACTIONS BETWEEN LYMPHOCYTES AND PROFESSIONAL ANTIGEN PRESENTING CELLS

The role of macrophages in the immune response is that of processing and presenting antigens and of secreting soluble factors. It is now well established that T cells bearing α/β T-cell receptors (TCR) recognize peptide fragments that are derived from intracellular processing of the antigens. TCRs see the peptide bound to MHC molecules, either class I (B-F in the chicken) or class II (B-L in the chicken).

Recently, a series of experiments has been carried out at our laboratory in order to characterize the role of MHC antigens in the control of antigen-specific T-cell proliferation.[64] Peripheral blood leukocytes from chickens primed with keyhole limpet hemocyanin (KLH) *in vivo* were induced to synthesize DNA in an *in vitro* response to KLH. The responding cells were shown to be T cells as judged by immunofluorescence staining with a T-cell-specific MAb 11A9. The *in vivo* antigen-primed peripheral blood leukocytes were stimulated *in vitro* with specific antigen and further propagated in the presence of IL-2. Subsequent antigen-specific T-cell proliferation required the presence of antigen-pulsed peripheral blood adherent cells (hereafter referred to as antigen presenting cells, APC). First it was demonstrated that B-G antigens do not serve as restriction elements for the T-cell-APC interaction because KLH-primed T cells from animals of the recombinant strain H.B21r3 (see Table 1) were not induced to proliferate when antigen was presented to them on H.B15-type (class I/class II incompatible, class IV compatible) APC.

As the recombination frequency between class I and class II loci in the chicken is extremely low, it has been difcult to study the genetic requirements of immune cell co-operation. Therefore, we used "spontaneous" recombinants, CHA and H.B19, described by Crone and Simonsen.[11] CHA (B[12]) and H.B19 (B[19]) chickens have indistinguishable B-L antigen as judged by serology. In addition, restriction fragment length polymorphism analysis has failed to detect differences between the particular B-L[12] and B-L[19] loci.[65] Both H.B19 and CHA antigen-specific T cell can recognize the nominal antigen on either H.B19 or CHA APC. As the MHC class I antigens of these lines are clearly different, antigen presentation to avian T cells appears to be MHC class II antigen restricted. This conclusion is substantiated by the inhibition of the antigen-specific T-cell response by a mAb against chicken MHC class II gene products,[51] but not by a mAb against chicken MHC class I gene products.[47] It should be noted that Maccubbin and Schierman[66] have demonstrated that T-cell cytotoxicity is MHC restricted in the chicken by using reticuloendotheliosis virus-transformed lymphoid cell lines as targets. They could not, however, distinguish between class I or class II-restricted killing.

V. INTERACTIONS BETWEEN T CELLS AND B CELLS

Full functional reconstitution of the humoral immune response to T-dependent antigens can be induced with bursal cells having identical MHC class II antigens with the recipient, even if class I and class IV antigens differ.[67] This indicates that T-B cooperation in the chickens is MHC class II restricted as in mammals.[67]

Presently, it is established that B cells, like other APCs, are able to take up and process an antigen and that they are able to express antigen-derived peptides on the cell surface in association with MHC class II molecules.[68] B lymphocytes have even been proposed to be the principal APCs *in vivo* based mainly on *in vitro* experiments.[68,69] Lassila and co-workers[70] have tried to dissect the cellular components involved in antigen presentation *in vivo* by asking whether resting B lymphocytes are of major physiological importance as APCs in the initiation of immune responses *in vivo*. In the chickens it is possible, by cyclophosphamide treatment shortly after hatching, to destroy B-cell precursors but leave intact the precursors of T cells, macrophages, and other cells. Introduction of bursa cells from another newly hatched chicken results in the establishment of a stable chimeric bird (A→B) having T cells and "professional" APCs expressing one set of MHC alleles (B) and B cells expressing another (A). The injection of committed bursal stem cells from normal syngeneic bursae restores permanently the recipients' ability to mount full spectrum of B-cell responses.[28]

TABLE 1
Chicken Lines at the Department of Medical Microbiology, Turku University

Line	B-complex			Ig-allotypes		Bu-1 allotypes	Origin
	B-F (Class I)	B-L (Class II)	B-G (Class IV)	IgM-1	IgG-1		
H.B2	2	2	2			a	Hy-line
CHA	12	12	12	a	g	b	Beckenham
H.B14Aa	14	14	14	a	g	a	Beckenham
H.B14Ab	14	14	14	a	g	b	Turku
H.B14C	14	14	14	b	i	a	Beckenham
H.B14D	14	14	14	b	g	a	Beckenham
H.B15a	15	15	15			a	Hy-line
H.B15b	15	15	15			b	Turku
H.B19	19	12	19			a	Scandinavian
H.B21r3	21	21	15			a/b	Basel
H.B15r1	15	15	21			a/b	Basel
H.Bw3	w4	w3	w4			b	Copenhagen
H.Bw4	w4	w4	w4			a	Copenhagen

Chimeric, MHC-disparate A→B chickens are tolerant of donor alloantigens.[31,71] The allogeneically reconstituted chickens respond normally to T-independent antigens such as *Brucella*, although their T-dependent antibody responses are totally deficient.[31,70] These results indicate that there is no T-B communication in these A→B chimeras. This is evidently due to the inability of resting B cells to present antigen to unprimed helper T cells. However, the T-dependent responses are restored if irradiated spleen cells of the same MHC type as B cells are added along with the antigen.[70] Based on these results it seems clear that non-B APCs initiate antigen-specific T-cell activation, which is also consistent with recent results obtained from MHC class II transgenic mice.[72] Furthermore, T-cell function as measured by alloreactivity, lymphokine production, or *in vitro* antigen-specific proliferation is normal in B-cell deficient chickens bursectomized early in ontogeny.[51] However, the significance of particular types of APC is probably variable, perhaps depending on particular responses against different antigens.

VI. CELLULAR MECHANISMS OF TOLERANCE TO MHC ANTIGENS IN THE CHICKEN

The avian species provides an excellent tool for the experimental manipulation and study of normal lymphoid ontogenesis. The chicken is an especially good model to study the function of class I and class II gene products in the induction of immune tolerance.

It is becoming evident that the major mechanism for immune tolerance is deletion of specific T-cell clones in the thymus. These T cells have α/β TCRs specific for "self" peptides bound to MHC molecules on the dendritic cells (see Reference 73 for a review). The clonal deletion does not, however, remove all autoreactive T cells, but these cells must be kept functionally inactive via largely unknown peripheral suppression mechanisms. The deletion process involves recognition of class I and class II molecules by CD4[+] and CD8[+] developing T cells. With the help of CD4 and CD8 molecules, T cells are also positively selected for recognition of the particular allelic forms of MHC molecules expressed on the thymic epithelial cells.[73] During this selection process, CD4[+] (mostly helper) and CD8[+] (mostly cytotoxic) T cells become restricted to class II and class I antigens, respectively. In alloreactivity, the primary targets for cytotoxic T cells are class I antigens, whereas class II antigens are the main stimulators of helper T cells.[74] Accordingly, the requirements for the induction of tolerance to class I and class II antigens may be different based on their different physiological roles in alloreactivity.[75]

The transfer of bursal cells to cyclophosphamide-treated recipients is a unique model for tolerance induction.[31] Bursal cells are committed to B-cell lineage and are unable to induce GVH disease. Recently, we have carried out a series of experiments aiming at clarifying the mechanisms of tolerance induction in B-cell-chimeric chickens reconstituted with class I or class II incompatible bursa cells. Firstly, Lehtonen and co-workers[71] demonstrated that both bursal stem cells and postbursal cells are able to induce specific transplantation tolerance to donor MHC antigens in cyclophosphamide-treated recipients, measured with skin-graft acceptance, MLR, and GVH splenomegaly assay. There is no difference in the tolerance-inducing capacity of class I, class II, or total MHC incompatible bursa cells.[76-78] On the contrary, tolerance was not induced in irradiated recipients; likewise, no chimerism was induced in these animals, suggesting that irradiation damages the bursal stroma and framework and thus prevents the homing of transplanted bursal cells into it.[79]

The cellular mechanisms of tolerance in B-cell-chimeric chickens have been studied by mixing lymphocytes from tolerant animals with normal, syngeneic cells in *in vitro* assays. Another approach included transfer of lymphoid cells from tolerant birds into irradiated, syngeneic secondary recipients. No evidence for suppression-mediated maintenance of tolerance to total MHC incompatibility could be found by combining normal and tolerant cells in GVH assays or in MLR cocultures.[80] When spleen cells from tolerant donors were transferred to syngeneic secondary recipients, tolerance to class I antigen disparity was transferable even after depletion of chimeric cells, suggesting a functional suppression mechanism.[77] Tolerance to class II antigens only was transferable primarily in skin grafting.[78] Transferability of tolerance to total MHC disparity was dependent on the presence of chimeric B cells in the inoculum indicating that host-derived suppression mechanism is not involved. Taken together, it seems that bursal cells can induce immune unresponsiveness to donor MHC antigens via several optional pathways, possibly depending on the mutual immunogenicity of the donor and recipient MHC antigens.[81]

VII. CONCLUDING REMARKS

Taken together, even though the MHC class I and class II antigen families are smaller in chickens than in mammals, as suggested by available biochemical and molecular genetics data,[12] this has no obvious qualitative or quantitative consequences at the functional level. It is apparent that the function of avian immune system follows the same basic rules as its mammalian counterpart. In the future, more detailed analysis of the structure of genes and products of the B complex will provide the basis for better understanding of the complex structure-function relationship of MHC and other molecules involved in the immune response. Further, as the number of available reagents detecting avian T- and B-cell differentiation antigens is rapidly increasing, it may be concluded that the chicken will maintain its position as a unique model to study cellular cooperation in immune responsiveness and unresponsiveness.

ACKNOWLEDGMENTS

We thank Olli Lassila, M. D. and Olli Vainio, M. D. for critical reading of the manuscript and Eija Nordlund for kind and efficient secretarial assistance. Our original studies were supported by the Sigrid Jusélius Foundation.

REFERENCES

1. **Chang, T. S., Glick, B., and Winter, A. R.,** The significance of the bursa of Fabricius of chickens in antibody production, *Poult. Sci.,* 34, 1187, 1955, 7.
2. **Glick, B., Chang, T. S., and Jaap, R. G.,** The bursa of Fabricius and antibody production of the domestic fowl, *Poult. Sci.,* 35, 224, 1956.
3. **Miller, J. F. A. P.,** Immunological function of the thymus, *Lancet,* 2, 748, 1961.
4. **Archer, O. and Pierce, J. C.,** Role of thymus in development of the immune response, *Fed. Proc.,* 20, 26, 1961.
5. **Fichtelius, K.-E., Laurell, G., and Philipsson, L.,** The influence of thymectomy on antibody formation, *Acta Pathol-Microbiol. Scand.,* 51, 81, 1961.
6. **Cooper, M. D., Peterson, R. D. A., and Good, R. A.,** Delineation of the thymic and bursal lymphoid systems in the chicken, *Nature (London),* 205, 143, 1965.
7. **Cooper, M. D., Peterson, R. D. A., South, M. A., and Good, R. A.,** The functions of the thymus system and the bursa system in the chicken, *J. Exp. Med.,* 123, 75, 1966.
8. **Good, R. A., Gabrielsen, A. E., Peterson, R. D. A., and Cooper, M. D.,** The central lymphoid tissue in developmental immunobiology, *Trans. Stud. Coll. Physicians Philadelphia,* 33, 180, 1966.
9. **Vainio, O. and Toivanen, A.,** Cellular cooperation in immunity, in *Avian Immunology,* Vol. 2, Toivanen, A. and Toivanen, P., Eds., CRC Press, Boca Raton, FL, 1987, 1.
10. **Peault, B., Dieterlen-Liévre, F., and Le Douarin, N.,** Cellular interactions during primary lymphoid organ ontogeny in birds, in *Avian Immunology,* Vol. 1, Toivanen, A. and Toivanen, P., Eds., CRC Press, Boca Raton, FL, 1987, 39.

11. **Crone, M. and Simonsen, M.,** Avian major histocompatibility complex, in *Avian Immunology,* Vol. 2, Toivanen, A. and Toivanen, P., Eds., CRC Press, Boca Raton, FL, 1987, 25.
12. **Guillemot, F. and Auffray, C.,** Molecular biology of the chicken major histocompatibility complex, *Crit. Rev. Poult. Biol.,* in press.
13. **Lassila, O., Eskola, J., Toivanen, P., Martin, C., and Dieterlen-Liévre, F.,** The origin of lymphoid stem cells studied in chick yolk sac-embryo chimeras, *Nature (London),* 272, 353, 1978.
14. **Lassila, O., Martin, C., Dieterlen-Liévre, F., Nurmi, T. E. I., Eskola, J., and Toivanen, P.,** Is the yolk sac the primary origin of lymphoid stem cells?, *Transplant. Proc.,* 11, 1085, 1979.
15. **Lassila, O., Eskola, J., and Toivanen, P.,** Prebursal stem cells in the intraembryonic mesenchyme of the chick embryo at 7 days of incubation, *J. Immunol.,* 123, 2091, 1979.
16. **Houssaint, E., Belo, M., and Le Douarin, N. M.,** Investigations on cell lineage and tissue interactions in the developing bursa of Fabricius through interspecific chimeras, *Dev. Biol.,* 53, 250, 1976.
17. **Le Douarin, N. M.,** Ontogeny of hematopoietic organs studied in avian embryo interspecific chimeras, in *Differentiation of Normal and Neoplastic Hematopoietic Cells,* Book A, Clarkson, B., Marks, P. A., and Till, J. E., Eds., Cold Spring Harbor Laboratory, Cold Spring Harbor, NY, 1978, 5.
18. **Le Douarin, N. M., Dieterlein-Liévre, F., and Oliver, P. D.,** Ontogeny of primary lymphoid organs and lymphoid stem cells, *Am. J. Anat.,* 170, 261, 1984.
19. **Sorvari, T., Toivanen, A., and Toivanen, P.,** Transplantation of bursal stem cells into cyclophosphamide-treated chicks. Redevelopment of bursal follicles, *Transplantation,* 17, 584, 1974.
20. **Pink, J. R. L., Vainio, O., and Rijnbeek, A. M.,** Clones of B lymphocytes in individual follicles of the bursa of Fabricius, *Eur. J. Immunol.,* 15, 83, 1985.
21. **Pink, J. R. L., Ratcliffe, M. J. H., and Vainio, O.,** Immunoglobulin-bearing stem cells for clones of B (bursa-derived) lymphocytes, *Eur. J. Immunol.,* 15, 617, 1985.
22. **Weill, J.-C., Reynaud, C.-A., Lassila, O., and Pink, J. R. L.,** Rearrangement of chicken immunoglobulin genes is not an ongoing process in the embryonic bursa of Fabricius, *Proc. Natl. Acad. Sci. U.S.A.,* 83, 3336, 1986.
23. **Houssaint, E.,** Cell lineage segregation during bursa of Fabricius ontogeny, *J. Immunol.,* 138, 3626, 1987.
24. **Toivanen, P. and Toivanen, A.,** Bursal and postbursal stem cells in chicken. Functional characteristics, *Eur. J. Immunol.,* 3, 585, 1973.
25. **Toivanen, P., Toivanen, A., and Good, R. A.,** Ontogeny of bursal function in chicken. I. Embryonic stem cell for humoral immunity, *J. Immunol.,* 109, 1058, 1972.
26. **Toivanen, P., Toivanen, A., Linna, T. J., and Good, R. A.,** Ontogeny of bursal function in chicken. II. Postembryonic stem cell for humoral immunity, *J. Immunol.,* 109, 1071, 1972.
27. **Weber, W. T.,** Avian B lymphocyte subpopulations: origins and functional capacities, *Transplant. Rev.,* 24, 8, 1975.
28. **Toivanen, P., Toivanen, A., and Vainio, O.,** Complete restoration of bursa-dependent immune system after transplantation of semiallogeneic stem cells into immunodeficient chicks, *J. Exp. Med.,* 139, 1344, 1974.
29. **Toivanen, P., Naukkarinen, A., and Vainio, O.,** What is the function of bursa of Fabricius? in *Avian Immunology,* Vol. 1, Toivanen, A. and Toivanen, P., Eds., CRC Press, Boca Raton, FL, 1987, 79.
30. **Cooper, M. D., Cain, W. A., Van Alten, P. J., and Good, R. A.,** Development and function of the immunoglobulin producing system, *Int. Arch Allergy,* 35, 242, 1969.
31. **Toivanen, P., Toivanen, A., and Sorvari, T.,** Incomplete restoration of the bursa-dependent immune system after transplantation of allogeneic stem cells into immunodeficient chicks, *Proc. Natl. Acad. Sci. U.S.A.,* 71, 957, 1974.
32. **Vainio, O. and Toivanen, A.,** Maturation of bursal stem cells within allogeneic or syngeneic bursal microenvironment: acquisition of postbursal maturity, *J. Immunol.,* 123, 1960, 1979.
33. **Vainio, O. and Toivanen, A.,** B cell genotype determines interaction preference with T cells: no effect of maturation environment, *J. Immunol.,* 131, 9, 1983.
34. **Fitzsimmons, R. C., Garrod, E. M. F., and Garnett, I.,** Immunological responses following early embryonic surgical bursectomy, *Cell Immunol.,* 9, 377, 1973.
35. **Fitzsimmons, R. C., Dixon, D. K., and Kocal, E. M. F.,** The bursal-thymic interrelationship and ontogeny of the immune response in the chick embryo, in *Developmental Immunobiology,* Solomon, J. B. and Horton, J. D., Eds., Elsevier/North-Holland, Amsterdam, 1977, 387.
36. **Veromaa, T., Vainio, O., Eerola, E., Lehtonen, L., Jalkanen, S., and Toivanen, P.,** T cell function in chickens bursectomized at 60 hr of incubation, *Transplantation,* 43, 533, 1987.
37. **Ivanyi, J.,** Function of the B-lymphoid system in chickens, in *Avian Immunology,* Rose, M. E., Payne, L. N., and Freeman, B. M., Eds., British Poultry Science Ltd., Edinburgh, Scotland, 1981, 63.
38. **Hirota, Y. and Bito, Y.,** The role of thymus for maturation of transferred bursa cells into immunocompetent B cells in chickens treated with cyclophosphamide, *Immunology,* 35, 889, 1978.
39. **Hirota, Y., Vainio, O., and Toivanen, P.,** T cell dependent B cell differentiation in the chicken, *Acta Pathol. Microbiol. Scand. Sect. C,* 89, 145, 1981.

40. **Briles, W. E., McGibbon, W. H., and Irwin, M. R.,** On multiple alleles affecting cellular antigens in the chicken, *Genetics,* 35, 633, 1950.
41. **Gilmour, D. G.,** Segregation of genes determining red cell antigens at high levels of inbreeding in chickens, *Genetics,* 44, 14, 1959.
42. **Pink, J. R. L., Droege, W., Hala, K., Miggiano, V. C., and Ziegler, A.,** A three-locus model for the chicken major histocompatibility complex, *Immunogenetics,* 5, 203, 1977.
43. **Briles, W. E., Bumstead, N., Ewert, D. L., Gilmour, D. G., Gogusev, J., Hala, K., Koch, C., Longenecker, B. M., Nordskog, A. W., Pink, J. R. L., Schierman, L. W., Simonsen, M., Toivanen, A., Toivanen, P., Vainio, O., and Wick, G.,** Nomenclature for the chicken major histocompatibility (B) complex, *Immunogenetics,* 15, 441, 1982.
44. **Koch, C.,** Complement system in avian species, in *Avian Immunology,* Vol. 2, Toivanen, A. and Toivanen, P., Eds., CRC Press, Boca Raton, FL, 1987, 43.
45. **Ziegler, A. and Pink, R.,** Chemical properties of two antigens controlled by the major histocompatibility complex of the chicken, *J. Biol. Chem.,* 251, 5391, 1976.
46. **Crone, M., Simonsen, M., Skjodt, K., Linnet, K., and Olsson, L.,** Mouse monoclonal antibodies to class I and class II antigens of the chicken MHC. Evidence for at least two class I products of the B complex, *Immunogenetics,* 21, 181, 1985.
47. **Pink, J. R. L., Kieran, M. W., Rijnbeek, A. M., and Longenecker, B. M.,** A monoclonal antibody against chicken MHC class I (B-F) antigens, *Immunogenetics,* 21, 293, 1985.
48. **Guillemot, F. P., Billaut, A., Pourquié, O., Béhar, G., Chaussé, A. M., Zoorob, R., Kreibich, G., and Auffray, C.,** A molecular map of the chicken major histocompatibility complex: the class II beta genes are closely linked to the class I genes and the nucleolar organizer, *EMBO J.,* 7, 2775, 1988.
49. **Ewert, D. L., Munchus, M. S., Chen, C. L. H., and Cooper, M. D.,** Analysis of structural properties and cellular distribution of avian Ia antigen by using monoclonal antibody to monomorphic determinants, *J. Immunol.,* 132, 2524, 1984.
50. **Guillemot, F. P., Oliver, P. D., Peault, B. M., and Le Douarin, N. M.,** Cells expressing Ia antigens in the avian thymus, *J. Exp. Med.,* 160, 1803, 1984.
51. **Veromaa, T., Vainio, O., Jalkanen, S., Eerola, E., Granfors, K., and Toivanen, P.,** Expression of B-L and Bu-1 antigens in chickens bursectomized at 60 hr of incubation, *Eur. J. Immunol.,* 18, 225, 1988.
52. **Guillemot, F., Turmel, P., Charron, D., Le Douarin, N., and Auffray, C.,** Structure biosynthesis, and polymorphism of chicken MHC class II (B-L) antigens and associated molecules, *J. Immunol.,* 137, 1251, 1986.
53. **Jones, P. P., Murphy, D. B., Hewgill, D., and McDevitt, H. O.,** Detection of a common polypeptide chain in I-A and I-E subregion immunoprecipitates, *Mol. Immunol.,* 16, 51, 1979.
54. **Charron, D. J., Aellen-Schulz, M. F., St. Geme, J., III, Erlich, H. A., and McDevitt, H. O.,** Biochemical characterization of an invariant polypeptide associated with Ia antigens in human and mouse, *Mol. Immunol.,* 20, 21, 1983.
55. **Crone, M., Jensenius, J., and Koch, C.,** Evidence for two populations of B-L (Ia-like) molecules encoded by the chicken MHC, *Immunogenetics,* 13 381, 1981.
56. **Bourlet, Y., Béhar, G., Guillemot, F., Fréchin, N., Billault, A., Chaussé, A.-M., Zoorob, R., and Auffray, C.,** Isolation of chicken major histocompatibility complex class II (B-L) B chain sequences: comparison with mammalian B chains and expression in lymphoid organs, *EMBO J.,* 7, 1031, 1988.
57. **Ewert, D. L. and Cooper, M. D.,** Ia-like alloantigens in the chicken: serologic characterization and ontogeny of cellular expression, *Immunogenetics,* 7, 521, 1978.
58. **Crone, M., Jensenius, J. C., and Koch, C.,** B-L antigens (Ia-like antigens) of the chicken major histocompatibility complex, *Scand. J. Immunol.,* 14, 591, 1981.
59. **Fredericksen, T. L, and Gilmour, D. G.,** Influence of genotypes at a non-MHC B lymphocyte alloantigen locus (Bu-1) on expression of Ia (B-L) antigen on chicken bursal lymphocytes, *J. Immunol.,* 134, 754, 1985.
60. **Salomonsen, J., Skjodt, K., Crone, M., and Simonsen, M.,** The chicken erythrocyte-specific MHC antigen. Characterization and purification of the B-G antigen by monoclonal antibodies, *Immunogenetics,* 25, 373, 1987.
61. **Vilhelmová, M.,** Test of prolongation of skin graft survival by blood injections provides evidence for presence of a new histocompatibility locus in the B-G region of chicken MHC, *Tissue Antigens,* 29, 83, 1987.
62. **Plachy, J.,** An analysis of the response of recombinant congenic lines of chickens to RSV challenge provides evidence for further complexity of the genetic structure of the chicken MHC (B), *Folia Biol. (Prague),* 34, 170, 1988.
63. **Goto, R., Miyada, C. G., Young, S., Wallace, R. B., Abplanalp, H., Bloom, S. E., Briles, W. E., and Miller, M. M.,** Isolation of a cDNA clone from the B-G subregion of the chicken histocompatibility (B) complex, *Immunogenetics,* 27, 102, 1988.
64. **Vainio, O., Veromaa, T., Eerola, E., Toivanen, P., and Ratcliffe, M. J. H.,** Antigen presenting cell-T cell interaction in the chicken is class II MHC restricted, *J. Immunol.,* 140, 2864, 1988.

65. **Andersson, L., Lundberg, C., Rask, L., Gissel-Nielsen, B., and Simonsen, M.,** Analysis of class II genes of the chicken MHC (B) by use of human DNA probes, *Immunogenetics,* 26, 79, 1987.

66. **Maccubbin, D. L. and Schierman, L. W.,** MHC-restricted cytotoxic response of chicken T cells: expression, augmentation and clonal characterization, *J. Immunol.,* 136, 12, 1986.

67. **Vainio, O., Koch, C., and Toivanen, A.,** B-L antigens (class II) of the chicken major histocompatibility complex control T-B cell interaction, *Immunogenetics,* 19, 131, 1984.

68. **Chesnut, R. and Grey, H.,** Antigen presentation by B cells and its significance in T-B interactions, *Adv. Immunol.,* 39, 51, 1986.

69. **Ashwell, J. D.,** Are B lymphocytes the principal antigen-presenting cells *in vivo?*, *J. Immunol.,* 140, 3697, 1988.

70. **Lassila, O., Vainio, O., and Matzinger, P.,** Can B cells turn on virgin T cells? *Nature (London),* 334, 253, 1988.

71. **Lehtonen, L., Vainio, O., Eerola, E., and Toivanen, P.,** Lymphoid cell chimerism and transplantation tolerance induced by bursal and postbursal cells, *Transplantation,* 40, 398, 1985.

72. **Van Ewijk, W., Ron, Y., Monaco, J., Kappler, J., Marrack, P., Le Meur, M., Gerlinger, P., Durand, B., Benoist, C., and Mathis, D.,** Compartmentalization of MHC class II gene expression in transgenic mice, *Cell,* 53, 357, 1988.

73. **Schwartz, R.,** Acquisition of immunologic self-tolerance, *Cell,* 57, 1073, 1989.

74. **Bach, F. H. and Sachs, D. H.,** Transplantation immunology, *N. Engl. J. Med.,* 317, 489, 1987.

75. **Streilein, J. W.,** Neonatal tolerance: towards an immunogenetic definition of self, *Immunol. Rev.,* 46, 125, 1979.

76. **Lehtonen, L., Vainio, O., Veromaa, T., and Toivanen, P.,** Transplantation tolerance to MHC antigens in chicken B cell chimeras. Effect of chimerism on the transferability of tolerance, *Transplant. Proc.,* 21, 252, 1989.

77. **Lehtonen, L., Vainio, O., Veromaa, T., and Toivanen, P.,** Tolerance to class I MHC antigens in chicken B cell chimeras. Effect of B cell depletion on transferability of tolerance, *Eur. J. Immunol.,* 19, 425, 1989.

78. **Lehtonen, L., Vanio, O., Veromaa, T., and Toivanen, P.,** B cell-induced tolerance to class II MHC antigens in the chicken, *Transplantation,* 48, 646, 1989.

79. **Lehtonen, L., Vainio, O., and Toivanen, P.,** Difference in allograft tolerance induction in X-irradiated and cyclophosphamide-treated chickens, *Transplantation,* 47, 910, 1989.

80. **Lehtonen, L., Vainio, O., and Toivanen, P.,** Mechanisms of transplantation tolerance in B-cell-chimeric chickens. Impairment of tolerance by T cell growth factor, *Transplantation,* 42, 184, 1986.

81. **Madsen, J. C., Superina, R. A., Wood, K. J., and Morris, P. J.,** Immunological unresponsiveness induced by recipient cells transfected with donor MHC genes, *Nature (London),* 332, 161, 1988.

82. **Salomonsen, J.,** personal communication.

Chapter 3

T-CELL IMMUNITY: MECHANISMS AND SOLUBLE MEDIATORS

K.A. Schat

TABLE OF CONTENTS

I. INTRODUCTION

Cell-mediated immune (CMI) functions form a major part of the defense systems in mammalian and avian species and probably also in the lower classes of vertebrates. Although many different effector systems can be involved in these CMI functions, only the acquired T cell-mediated responses will be reviewed in this chapter. It has to be realized, however, that these responses do develop as part of a complex, immunological system in which macrophages (see Chapter 5), suppressor T cells, natural killer (NK) cells, and lymphokine-activated killer (LAK) cells (see Chapter 4) have important functions. Fahey and York[1] have recently reviewed some general aspects of cell-mediated cytotoxicity in chickens, while Chi and Thorbecke[2] compared suppressor T cells and allogeneic cytotoxic T cells (CTL).

Over the last decade it has become clear that the actual regulation of these and other immune functions depends on a small number of lymphokines and/or cytokines (if factors produced by other cells than lymphocytes are included). In 1979 it was decided to name these components interleukins (IL).[3,4] The developments leading to this unified nomenclature have recently been reviewed.[5] Some of the early work on avian lymphokines has been summarized by Schauenstein and Kromer[6] and Schauenstein et al.[7] The aim of this chapter is to relate the recent research developments on avian CTL and IL to the knowledge of mammalian CTL and IL.

II. INTERLEUKINS

A. MAMMALIAN INTERLEUKINS

There are currently at least seven ILs (Il-1 through IL-7) and some other cytokines recognized in mammalian immunology. The information on mammalian lymphokines has recently been reviewed and is summarized in Table 1.[5,8] The interested reader is referred to these review papers for additional information and references. It has to be realized that the knowledge on mammalian ILs is rapidly expanding. Moreover, different functions are often ascribed to the same IL, while subsequent research may show that these ILs were incompletely purified or that functions were incorrectly assigned to a given IL. This is clearly illustrated by several recent publications in which it was demonstrated that IL-5 may be important as a differentiation factor for cytotoxic T cells[9] and for the production of immunoglobulin A (IgA)-producing B cells.[10] On the other hand, recent data suggest that IL-6 is also a (or perhaps the only) lymphokine needed for high-rate synthesis of secretory IgA.[11] The recently described lymphokine IL-7 is probably a T-cell growth factor[12] and may play a role in the differentiation of T cells with the γ/δ T-cell receptor (TCR1).[13]

B. AVIAN INTERLEUKINS

Unfortunately, much less is known about avian than mammalian ILs. It is assumed, however, that activation and differentiation of avian T cells follow a pattern similar to that in mammals.[7] This assumption was based partly on the discovery of IL-1- and IL-2-like substances in chickens and the knowledge that avian B and T cells react to stimulation with lipopolysaccharides (LPS) and mitogens in a fashion similar to mammalian lymphocytes.

1. Interleukin 1

The presence of mammalian IL-1 in culture fluids is generally demonstrated by stimulation of thymocytes using suboptimal doses of mitogen. The addition of IL-1-containing medium to the cultures stimulates the production of IL-2, which causes increased stimulation compared to the use of suboptimal doses of mitogen alone.[14] Hayari et al.[15] used this technique to demonstrate the production of IL-1 by adherent avian spleen cells. Splenic cell suspensions were plated, nonadherent cells were washed away after 24 h, and the adherent cells were

TABLE 1
Characterization of Mammalian Interleukins[a]

Name	Mol wt (kDa)	Gene cloned	Produced by	Biological effects on B and T cells
IL-1α IL-1β	13—17	Yes	Macrophages, B-cell lines, T-cell lines, NK cells, and others	Maturation of thymocytes and B-cell precursors; activation of adenylate cyclase; costimulatory effects for growth of activated T cells and IL-2 and IL-4-induced proliferation of Th2; lymphokine release from activated T cells; increased proliferation of stimulated B cells.
IL-2	15.5	Yes	Helper T-cell type 1 (Th1), cytotoxic T cell (Tc)	Growth of activated Th1,Th2, and thymocytes; generation of Tc; proliferation of B cells stimulated with LPS and anti-Ig; proliferation and differentiation of B cells after antigen stimulation; induction of IgM production; inhibits cAMP production in cells induced to proliferate.
IL-3	28	Yes	Activated Th1 and Th2	Promotes the development and differentiation of hematopoietic stem cells, pre-B and pre-T cells, but IL-3 is not essential for normal hematopoesis; may serve to recruit more hematopoietic cells during immune responses.
IL-4	20	Yes	Activated Th2, mast cells	Costimulant for B cell proliferation; enhances expression of class II MHC and CD23 on resting B cells; primes these cells for increased response to other B-cell stimulators; increases IgG_1 and decreases IgG_3 and IgG_{2a} and IgG_{2b} production; growth factor for activated T cells, stimulates IL-2 and IL-2R production; γ-INF inhibits IL-4.
IL-5	45	Yes	Activated Th2	Differentiation factor for Tc together with IL-2; differentiation factor for committed IgA B cells; increased IgM and IgG and (with IL4) IgG_1 and IgE secretion by activated B cells.
IL-6	23—30	Yes	Activated T and B cells, macrophages, others	Often needs cofactors (IL-1); induction of IL-2R and T-cell stimulation, generation of specific Tc, induction of high rate IgA secretion; cofactor for development of plasmacytomas and myelomas?
IL-7	25	Yes	Stroma cells	Proliferation of $CD4^-/CD8^-$ thymocytes; comitogen factor for Con A induced proliferation of $CD4^+$ and $CD8^+$ subpopulations.
γ-IFN	20.5	Yes	Activated Th1 Tc	Differentiation factor for B cells; antagonist of IL-4 effects on B and T cells.

[a] See References 5 and 8 for detailed information.

pulsed for 4 h with LPS. The presence of IL-1 was demonstrated 72 h afterward. Unfortunately, they did not characterize the factor(s) responsible for the stimulation of the thymocytes. Klasing[16] used monocytes harvested from the abdominal cavity 24 and 48 h after injection of Sephadex® G-50. These activated monocytes were incubated with *Escherichia coli* endotoxin for 30 min, washed extensively, and incubated for 18 h. The supernatant fluid was partially purified and contained proteins with molecular weight ranges from 10 to 30 kDa. It was later found that adherent splenocytes were better for production of IL-1 than monocytes harvested from the peritoneal cavity or peripheral blood monocytes. The avian macrophage cell line HD11, which was established by transformation of macrophages with a defective avian leukemia virus,[17] was superior for the production of IL-1.[18] Stimulation with either heat-killed *Staphylococcus aureus* or *E. coli*-derived endotoxin resulted in IL-1 production. Better results were obtained when the HD11 cell line was cultivated at 42° C instead of 39° C. Likewise, stimulation of thymocytes with IL-1 was temperature-dependent and higher at 42° than at 39° C. Chicken thymocytes could not be stimulated with either human or murine IL-1, and chicken IL-1 did not stimulate mouse thymocytes. Thus far, there is a paucity of information on the characteristics of avian IL-1. IL-1 in serum of LPS-stimulated birds had a molecular weight of 30 kDa.[19] It is not clear if this is the mature form or the precursor protein, which have molecular weights of 13 to 17 kDa and 33 kDa, respectively, in mammalian species.[5] Avian IL-1 has not yet been cloned, nor has the receptor been identified.

Crude preparations of IL-1 were used to determine some of its physiological effects. Chickens inoculated with IL-1-containing supernatant fluid from activated peritoneal macrophages had decreased levels of zinc and iron in serum plasma, but increased levels in the liver. In addition, the concentration of metallothionein was increased in the liver. These changes are similar to endotoxin-induced changes as part of inflammatory processes.[16] These responses are compatible with the well-established effects of mammalian IL-1 in inflammatory processes.[5]

It has been suggested that stress from (sub) clinical infections can result in lower weight gains. Klasing et al.[19] tested the hypothesis that IL-1 is at least partly responsible for the lower weight gains. Daily injections with crude IL-1 resulted in significantly lower weight gains than injections with either saline or heated IL-1 preparations. IL-1 serum levels were increased after inoculation of chickens with LPS. These results implicate IL-1 as one of the mediators of immunological stress. This finding is not surprising, because similar data have been reported for mammalian IL-1[5]

2. Interleukin 2

IL-2, originally described as T-cell growth factor or TCGF, is produced *in vitro* by stimulation of avian T lymphocytes with mitogens.[20,21] Supernatant fluids from mitogen-stimulated lymphocytes with IL-2 is referred to in this chapter as conditioned medium (CM). Improved yields of IL-2 are obtained by using concanavalin A (Con A) bound to chicken red blood cells (RBC).[22] This technique was based on the publication by Powell,[23] in which he described increased mitogen stimulation of lymphocytes in the presence of chicken RBC. Kromer et al.[22] compared the production of IL-2 by stimulation with free Con A, RBC-bound Con A, and Sepharose®-bound Con A. The RBC-bound Con A consistently induced the highest production of IL-2. This procedure has, however, a major disadvantage: purification of IL-2 is complicated by the extra proteins released from damaged RBC.[24] Dialysis of CM to remove suppressor factors with a molecular weight of <10 kDa is recommended to improve its activity.[22]

Thus far, chicken IL-2 has been poorly characterized, which is in part due to the difficulty in its purification. As a consequence, cloning of the gene for IL-2 has not yet been reported. Schnetzler et al.[21] examined some of the parameters for production of IL-2, and they partially characterized the product. Peak activity of IL-2 was present in supernatant fluids of peripheral blood lymphocytes (PBL) and spleen cells 24 h after mitogen stimulation. Like Schauenstein et al.[20] they found that stimulation with Con A resulted in slightly higher titers than stimulation with phytohemagglutinin (PHA). CM was adsorbed with Con A-activated T cells and all IL-2 activity was removed. Adsorption with normal, resting PBL did not remove IL-2. Vainio et al.[25] also reported that IL-2 activity could be removed by adsorption to Con A blast cells as well as with long-term cultured T cells. These results suggest the presence of IL-2-specific receptors on these cells. Recent work by Schauenstein et al.[26] suggests that a previously described monoclonal antibody (mAB) INN-CH 16, which detects a chicken activated T-lymphocyte antigen (CATLA),[27] actually recognizes the β chain of the IL-2 receptor. This hypothesis is based on the following observations:

1. CATLA is maximally expressed on Con A-stimulated blast cells at 48 h poststimulation. Afterward, it gradually disappears, but can be reexpressed by a second stimulation with Con A after 5 d.
2. The presence of a high level of INN-CH 16 competitively inhibits the proliferative response of T lymphoblasts.
3. Absorption of CM with T lymphoblasts treated with INN-CH 16 does not remove IL-2 activity. If this mAB indeed detects the IL-2 receptor, it must be possible to purify the protein and clone the gene for the receptor. It could also be used for the purification of IL-2 and subsequent cloning attempts.

Schnetzler et al.[21] reported the molecular weight of IL-2 by gel filtration and polyacrylamide gel electrophoresis (PAGE). They found activity with two protein peaks after gel filtration. Protein(s) in peak I had a molecular weight range of 9 to 11 kDa; the second one had a molecular weight of 19.5 to 21.5 kDa. Analysis by sodium dodecyl sulfate (SDS)-PAGE suggested a molecular weight of 13 kDa, which is in line with estimates for mammalian IL-2.[5] Vanio et al.[25] reported a value of 13 kDa after gel filtration. They reported that IL-2 has a (pI) of 5.9. Fredericksen and Sharma[28] purified IL-2 and γ-interferon (γ-IFN) by a multistep approach (Figure 1). IL-2 was separated from IFN using phenyl-sepharose.® Proteins with high hydrophobicity bind on this column, while proteins with low hydrophobicity will pass through. In contrast to mouse IL-2, chicken IL-2 seems to have low hydrophobicity. IL-2 was further purified by anion exchange chromatography and high-resolution gel filtration chromatography. The IL-2 activity was associated with two fractions with molecular weights of 30 and 14 kDa (Figure 1). However, the authors mentioned in the text of the same paper that the high-molecular-weight protein with activity was 30 kDa by SDS-PAGE and 26 kDa by high-resolution gel filtration chromatography. Obviously, more work is needed to purify chicken IL-2, and cloning of the gene would be of tremendous importance for further progress in avian immunology.

Chicken IL-2 has been partially characterized for its biological properties. Apparently, it is specific for chicken blast cells, but to this author's knowledge it has not been tested on other avian blast cells. Murine and human blast cells cannot be stimulated with chicken IL-2.[6,20] Likewise, human and mouse IL-2 do not stimulate chicken blast cells.[6,29] The half-life of avian IL-2 is considerably shorter than that of mammalian IL-2.[6] Lehtonen et al.[30] added IL-2 to mixed lymphocyte reaction (MLR) cultures of thymocytes to determine if this would enhance the allogeneic responses. There was no effect of IL-2 on alloreactivity using embryonal thymocytes, but the addition did enhance the response to major histocompatibility complex (MHC) class I antigens and even syngeneic responses when lymphocytes from 4 to 8-week-old birds were used. It was suggested that this enhanced response may be important for the development of autoimmune diseases (e.g., autoimmune thyroiditis in Obese-strain chickens). Previously, it had been reported that lymphocytes from Obese-strain birds are

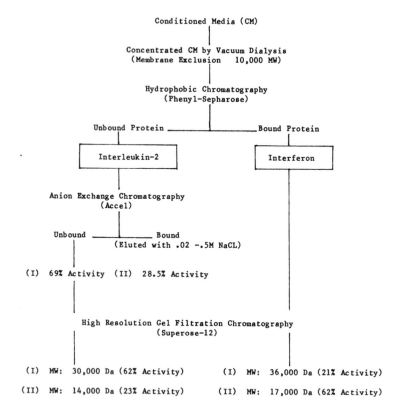

FIGURE 1.   The purification and separation protocol of IL-2 and γ-interferon from conditioned medium of Con A-activated spleen cells. (From Fredericksen, T. L. and Sharma, J. M., in *Progress in Clinical Biological Research,* Vol. 238, Alan R. Liss, New York, 1987, 145. With permission.)

more responsive to Con A than lymphocytes from their parent line (Cornell-C strain). As a consequence, the Obese birds have an increased production of IL-2.[31] The enhanced production of IL-2 is apparently the consequence of a diminished production of regulatory substances present in serum.[32]

3. γ-Interferon

In addition to ILs, activated T cells can produce some other substances which not only can activate other cells but also have the ability to induce resistance to viral infection. The best known group are the IFNs. Originally, these proteins were found after infection of cells with RNA viruses or treatment with interferon inducers such as polyinosinic-polycytidylic acid. Since then, it has become clear that similar proteins are produced after stimulation of lymphocytes. These proteins, named γ-IFN, or immune IFN, are important not only because they may induce resistance to virus infection in cells but also (and perhaps foremost) because they are important for the activation of macrophages and NK cells (see Chapter 4 for a more detailed description of the role of IFN in the activation of avian NK cells). The importance of γ-IFN for the regulation of cell-mediated immune responses in mammalian species has been reviewed.[33]

There is a paucity on information on avian γ-IFN. Von Bulow et al.[34] used crude supernatant fluids from Con A-stimulated thymocytes or spleen cells to examine the effects on macrophage activation. They used the induction of cytostasis in Marek's disease chicken cell line (MDCC)-RP1 and the effect on spreading of macrophages as criteria for the presence of γ-IFN. Supernatant fluids of Con A-stimulated spleen cells and thymocytes did contain factors causing spread of macrophages and induction of cytostatic activity. In addition, these CMs were able to induce antiviral resistance in chicken cell cultures but not in mouse L cells. The substance(s) was sensitive to treatment with heat, acid, and trypsin, thus resembling mammalian γ-IFN. Unfortunately, these studies do not rule out the presence of other substances causing similar effects. Pusztai et al.[35] examined the production of γ-IFN *in vitro* by stimulating PBL with Con A. Optimal levels of production were found after 96 h. Partially purified IFN with a molecular weight of 20.5 kDa had antiviral activity. In contrast, Fredericksen and Sharma[28] found two antiviral peaks with molecular weights at 17 and 36 kDa in CM prepared from spleen cells. Similar heterogeneity in molecular weight has been noted for mammalian γ-IFN.[29] The lower-molecular-weight fraction of avian IFN corresponds fairly well with the molecular weight of mammalian γ-IFN based on sequence analysis of IFN gene.[37] The heterogeneity of γ-IFN is probably the consequence of posttranslational changes. IFN, produced in chicken embryo fibroblasts (CEF) treated with inactivated Newcastle disease virus (NDV), had similar ranges in molecular weight.[38] However, sequence analysis of mammalian γ-IFN did not show any homology with α- or β-IFN.[37] There is some controversy over the species specificity of avian γ-IFN. Thacore et al.[39] found two types of IFN produced by lymphocytes in normal and genetically dystrophic chickens. One of these, which is heat labile, induced an antiviral state in human and simian cells but not in chicken cells, while the second, heat-stable IFN induced this effect only in chicken cells. On the other hand, Fredericksen and Sharma[28] reported that γ-IFN was not reactive in human cells.

4. Latency-Maintaining Factor

Recently, Buscaglia and Calneks[40] described a substance present in CM prepared from lymphocytes stimulated with Con A, which they named latency-maintaining factor (LMF). The addition of LMF to cultured spleen cells obtained from birds latently infected with Marek's disease virus (MDV) kept the virus infection latent. On the other hand, latency was not maintained when these cells were cultured in the absence of LMF. Thus far, LMF has not been characterized in great detail. The molecular weight is larger than 10 kDa, and it was susceptible to heating to 90°C for 5 min, but it has not yet been further defined. LMF was separated from γ-IFN using phenyl-Sepharose®. Although LMF and IL-2 came off this column in the same general peak, LMF was present only in the first part of the peak, while IL-2 was present in the second part. In addition, CM with high IL-2 titers did not always have high titers of LMF and vice versa. The finding of LMF may have important consequences for the understanding of the pathogenesis of Marek's disease (MD) and perhaps other herpesvirus-induced diseases. It has been well established that the early infection of MDV occurs in B lymphocytes. The cytolytic infection in these cells activates T cells as part of the immune response.[41,42] It is tempting to speculate that *in vivo* production of LMF, as a consequence of the T-cell activation, is a major factor for the maintenance of latency and perhaps the induction as well. It is of considerable interest that immunoincompetent chickens (e.g., those of young age or with induced immunosuppression) do not develop latent infections as readily, nor maintain latency as strongly, as do immunocompetent birds.[43] It will be of interest to determine if these birds produce lower titers of LMF than do immunocompetent birds.

5. Undefined Cytokines

Although there are several reports suggesting the presence of substances produced by leukocytes, there are two with possible relevance to the immune responses against virus infections.

Whitfill et al.[44] isolated a low-molecular-weight (<5 kDa) substance from blood sera from Rous sarcoma (RS)-regressor and RS-progressor chicken lines after challenge with RS virus (RSV). Inoculation of a mixture of LMW substance with RSV into wing webs of progressor-line chickens resulted in significantly lower levels of tumors than in birds inoculated with RSV alone. Subsequent studies demonstrated that incubation of RSV with LMW prior to inoculation enhanced the effect. It was suggested that the LMW substance is produced by either macrophages or T cells infiltrating the developing tumors. This substance was produced in regressor-line chickens as early as 4 d postchallenge.[45] The LMW substance seems to have a wider antiviral range than against RSV alone because it can also neutralize NDV.[46] It has to be emphasized that LMW has not been fully characterized and that it is not clear if it is produced by lymphocytes or monocytes.

A second undefined lymphokine is produced by the lymphoblastoid cell line MDCC-JMV-1 (JMV-1), which was developed from the MDV-induced transplantable tumor JMV. Both JMV and JMV-1 are unable to produce MDV (nonproducer cell line), but they contain the complete MDV genome.[47] Munch and Sevoian[48] and, later, Keller et al.[49] reported that JMV-1 produces a factor(s) which inhibited MDV replication and MD tumor-cell growth. Recently, it was reported that these factors were also able to reduce production of oocysts in chickens after challenge with *Eimeria tenella* or *E. acervulina*. Similar results were obtained with CM produced by Con A-stimulated T lymphocytes. These substances in JMV-1 supernatant fluids and CM were also able to inhibit intracellular replication of sporozoites in a bovine cell line and avian macrophages.[50] The nature of these lymphokines has not yet been elucidated. It is of interest that Con A-stimulated bovine peripheral blood lymphocytes also produce a lymphokine inhibiting the replication of *E. bovis* in a macrophage cell line.[51]

It is obvious that many lymphokines can be produced by avian lymphocytes, but there is a need for concerted effort to further characterize these ILs. Molecular cloning of these IL genes will be of great importance. Unfortunately, there seems to be a general lack in sequence homology between mammalian and avian IL genes. Efforts to cultivate avian lymphocytes and characterize the effects of the ILs on these cells will have to wait for the availability of purified or recombinant lymphokines.

III. DEVELOPMENT OF CYTOTOXIC T-CELL LINES

It is clear from the previous section that the lack of purified ILs has interfered with the development of IL-dependent cell lines. Yet, some cell lines have been developed using CM presumably containing IL-2. Schat et al.[52,53] developed lines with NK cell activity by culturing spleen cells obtained from specific pathogen-free chickens in the presence of CM. These cells did not require prior stimulation with Con A, were dependent on CM, and had the morphological appearance of large granular lymphocytes. The properties of the NK cell lines are reviewed in more detail in Chapter 4.

Two groups developed cell lines using splenocytes from antigen-primed chickens. Vainio et al.[25,54] used keyhole limpet hemocyanin (KLH) in complete Freund's adjuvant to prime chickens. Spleen cells were harvested after 13 d and stimulated *in vitro* with KLH. Blast cells were harvested after 5 d and cultivated up to 25 weeks in the presence of CM. The long-term cultured cells had the morphology of lymphoblasts, expressed T cell-specific antigen, and MHC class I and II antigens. The antigen presentation by antigen-presenting cells (APC) and subsequent proliferation of T cells were dependent on MHC class II compatibility, suggesting that these cells are CD4$^+$ helper T cells. The early antigen-driven proliferation was replaced by CM-driven replication after the initial 2 to 3 weeks. They proposed that the majority of the dividing cells in these cultures were expressing IL-2 receptors and responding to the IL-2 produced by the minority of antigen-driven cells. A similar mechanism was found earlier to be involved in the proliferation of antigen-specific stimulated mouse T cells.[55] A similar approach has been used by Bhogal et al.[56,57] Chickens were immunized by repeated oral inoculations of 5000 sporulated oocysts of *E. tenella*.

Nylon wool-nonadherent spleen cells from these chickens were stimulated *in vitro* for 4 d with *E. tenella* antigens prepared from oocysts or sporozoites. The blast cells were then propagated in CM-containing medium for an additional 4 to 5 d and restimulated with *E. tenella* in the presence of syngeneic, irradiated spleen cells as a source of APC. Several cloned cell lines were developed, some of which were kept in culture for at least 100 d. Some of these clones were able to provide helper T-cell functions for the *in vitro* production of *E. tenella*-specific antibody. Other clones produced factors able to activate macrophages. The activated macrophages had enhanced capacity to kill *E. tenella* sporozoites. The activation of macrophages by these clones suggests a delayed-type hypersensitivity (DTH) response. It was later shown that transfer of some of the clones into naive chickens induced DTH responses in the wattle after subsequent challenge with *E. tenella* antigens. The activation of macrophages by at least one of the clones was caused by the production of γ-IFN.[58]

Cell lines of cytotoxic/suppressor T cells have been developed in the course of studies on MD pathogenesis. The development of mAB specific for the avian homologues of CD4 and CD8 (see Chapter 1) was of importance to characterize lymphoblastoid cell lines derived from MDV-induced tumors. Schat et al.[59] demonstrated that the large majority of cell lines developed from tumors were CD4[+] and, thus, of the helper T-cell type. Recently, they found that at least some cell lines developed from local lesions were CD4[-]/CD8[+] (cytotoxic/suppressor T cells).[60] These cell lines were obtained by harvesting lymphocytes responding to inoculation of allogeneic, MDV-infected chick kidney cells between 4 and 19 d postinoculation.[61] The establishment of *in vitro* cultures did not require the use of CM. The initial proliferation was probably driven by ILs produced by the stimulation with MHC and/or MDV antigens. These cell lines were all positive for MDV genome when tested between 20 and 150 d in culture. It is not yet known if the CD4[-]/CD8[+] cell lines are able to lyse cells carrying the same MHC antigens as originally used for the inoculation of the birds. It is also possible that these cells are suppressor T cells, and it will be of interest to determine if some or all of the 19 CD4[-]/CD8[+] cell lines carry type II histamine receptors (H2R). Edelman et al.[62] described the presence of H2R on suppressor T cells in chickens with chemically induced fibrosarcomas. It had been previously shown in mice that suppressor cells carrying H2R regulated the response of cytotoxic T cells to histamine.[63]

Allogeneic cytotoxic T cells were also cultured from splenocytes obtained from chickens immunized with allogeneic RBC. The presence of CM was essential for the cultivation of these cells. At 20 d in culture the cells were still able to lyse allogeneic red blood cells.[64] Unfortunately, these cell lines have not been characterized for surface markers.

IV. CHARACTERIZATION OF EFFECTOR T CELLS

A. DELAYED-TYPE HYPERSENSITIVITY T CELLS

Several approaches can be used to study the development of T-cell-mediated immunity depending on the effector system to be examined. Many investigators have used the response of lymphocytes to mitogens to assess general immune responsiveness or have tested their response to specific antigens. In general, these assays measure nonspecific (mitogens) or specific (antigens) responses of helper T-cell populations, although mitogens can also stimulate other T-cell populations.[65]

DTH is a second type of immune reaction in which T cells are involved. DTH effector T cells produce lymphokines which activate other cells (e.g., macrophages).[65,66] The demonstration of DTH may be a good indication of relevant cell-mediated immune functions. Lee et al.[67] suggested that DTH reactions were important in the immune responses against *Salmonella typhimurium*. Bhogal et al.[58] studied CMI responses against *E. tenella* using DTH responses. Apparently, γ-IFN was produced by some of the cloned T-cell lines which were used for passive transfer of DTH against *Eimeria* antigens (see Section III). Interestingly, γ-IFN had been implicated in the control of coccidiosis in poultry.[68] Recent *in vivo* studies also suggest that γ-IFN may be important for protection against coccidiosis. Spleen cells cultured from chickens immunized with *E. tenella* produced γ-IFN within 24 h after stimulation with oocyst antigens. IFN production by stimulated spleen cells could be demonstrated shortly after antibodies were detected and lasted at least until 80 d after primary infection.[69] The role of γ-IFN in protective immunity has not been elucidated, but γ-IFN can activate NK cells, and a role for NK cells as part of the immune response against *Eimeria* species had been suggested.[70] Previously, Chi et al.[71] had shown that spleen cells obtained from birds immunized with human γ-globulin were able to transfer DTH reactions to naive birds. However, the experiments reported by Bhogal et al.[58] will allow a much better characterization of these effector cells and permit studies on their relevance in protective immunity.

B. CYTOTOXIC T CELLS

1. Introduction

It has been well documented that mammalian CTL lyse only antigen-positive cells carrying the same MHC antigens as the effector cells, while antigen-positive (but allogeneic) target cells are not lysed.[72] Binding of CTL to the target cells is a complicated process involving many molecules.[73] Adhesion molecules on the surface of CTL, such as CD2 and LFA-1, bind to proteins on the surface of the target cells. Most of the CTL are CD8+, and these molecules probably interact with the nonpolymorphic regions of class I MHC molecules. The foreign (viral, tumor, etc.,) antigens are recognized by the T-cell receptor (TCR) of the CD3/TCR complex. The CD3 part consists of at least five proteins which are responsible for signal transduction activating the lytic event. Originally, it was thought that all CTL were CD8 + and thus only able to lyse class I MHC-positive target cells. However, recently, antigen-specific CD4+ CTL, which are able to lyse class II MHC positive target cells, have been detected. The presence of CD4+ CTL has been described as part of the immune responses against herpes simplex virus type 1[74] and influenza virus.[75] It has been suggested that the generation of CD4+ vs. CD8+ CTL depends on the pathway of virus entry and antigen processing.[75,76]

2. Avian CTL

The role of CTL in antiviral or antitumor immunity in chickens has been poorly documented. MHC-restricted cytolysis has been reported for only a few virus infections. As a consequence, the effector cells have also been poorly characterized. The presence of cytotoxic T cells in chickens has been demonstrated by *in vivo* and *in vitro* assays.

a. In Vivo Assays

Three types of experiments for *in vivo* demonstration of effector cells have been used: passive transfer of immune cells followed by challenge, the Winn test,[77] and immunization with nonproducer MD lymphoblastoid tumor cell lines followed by challenge with virulent MDV. Passive transfer requires either the use of inactivated vaccines, especially if the immunizing agent can infect lymphocytes (e.g., MDV), or transfer followed by immediate challenge and a very short incubation period of the challenge virus. Powell et al.[78] used glutaraldehyde-inactivated, MDV-infected chick kidney cells to demonstrate the presence of immune lymphocytes. They eliminated the possibility of antibody-mediated cellular cytotoxicity by using bursectomized chickens. Fahey et al.[79] used immune and "hyperimmune" spleen cells from chickens immunized with live vaccine virus to transfer resistance to infectious laryngotracheitis (ILT) (caused by an α herpesvirus). Interestingly, they found better protection when birds were challenged at 7 d postimmunization than at 2 or 4 d. This suggests that mechanisms other than only the transfer of CTL may be involved in the induction of passive immunity. They were unable to demonstrate the transfer of the vaccine strain of ILT virus (ILTV), but a report by Bagust[80] suggested that ILTV can be latently present in tracheal tissue. In addition, von Bulow and Klasen[81] demonstrated that ILTV can replicate in macrophages. It is therefore possible that low numbers of infected cells were transferred. Neither of these two studies addressed the type of cells responsible for the transfer of resistance. These *in vivo* transfer studies are inherently complex and difficult to use for identification of specific cell types unless extremely pure populations of specific effector cells can be prepared. Perhaps *in vitro* stimulation of *in vivo*-primed CTL can be used in combination with mAB specific for CD8 and CD4 to obtain such populations for passive transfer studies. Cannon and Russell[82] demonstrated that *in vitro* restimulation of primed lymphocytes is feasible for avian lymphocytes. It would be of interest to test this approach.

Galton et al.[83,84] and others have used the Winn test to demonstrate immune responses against chemically induced fibrosarcomas. In this test, tumor cells are mixed with spleen cells from immune or control birds and injected into the wing web of 2- to 3-week-old recipients. Tumor growth is measured at regular intervals and differences between treatment groups are an indication of immune responses. This approach has the same disadvantages as the passive transfer followed by challenge described above: it requires noninfectious target cells and a mixture of effector cells can result in activation of host cells (e.g., DTH effector cells activating host macrophages) unless highly purified subpopulations of effector cells are used.

Schierman and co-workers[85-87] developed nonproducer MD lymphoblastoid cell lines from tumor transplants, which were developed in G-B1 ($B^{13}B^{13}$) and G-B2 (B^6B^6) birds. Inoculation with these cells resulted in a MHC-restricted protection against challenge with the original virulent tumor transplants. This finding is of interest because *in vitro* studies by Schat et al.[88] and Powell et al.[89] demonstrated significant lysis of allogeneic, but not syngeneic, MD cell lines after infection with SB-1 (a nononcogenic serotype 2 MDV strain used as a vaccine) and HPRS-16 (an oncogenic serotype 1 MDV strain), respectively. Similar *in vitro* findings were reported by Difronzo and Schierman.[86] Immunization with the non-producer cell lines also resulted in protection against virus infection, suggesting that MDV-specific antigens may be present in these nonproducer cell lines.[87] A potential candidate for this antigen is a virus-coded phosphorylated polypeptide that has been demonstrated in lytic MDV infections as well as in some producer and nonproducer MD cell lines.[90] Although these studies strongly suggest the presence of MHC-restricted effector cells, the CTL were not identified.

b. In Vitro *Assays*

CTL are most often demonstrated using *in vitro* isotope-release assays. The isotope of choice is ^{51}Cr, and the assay is commonly referred to as a chromium-release assay or CRA. Labeling procedures, preparation of effector cells, assay conditions, and the use of other isotopes are essentially similar to NK cell assays (see Chapter 4).

Thus far only a few studies have been published, in which avian MHC-restricted CTL have been described and/or characterized. Wainberg et al.[91] reported that syngeneic-restricted cytotoxicity could be detected using spleen cells from birds infected with the Schmidt-Ruppin strain, subgroup D, of avian sarcoma virus (ASV). The same birds, obtained from a closed flock, served often as donors for effector and target cells. With these experiments they confirmed their earlier work[92] that autochthonous immune lymphocytes were more effective in killing ASV-induced tumor cells than allogeneic immune lymphocytes. In addition, specific syngeneic cytolysis was detected using spleen cells from line 6 and line 7 chickens. Effector cells obtained from line 6 were able to lyse line 6-derived target cells but not line 7-derived target cells and vice versa.[91] It is of interest to note that line 6 and line 7 have both the B^2B^2 phenotype for the B-G antigens, but the MHC class I loci (B-F) are different for these lines based on skin-graft rejections.[93] The avian MHC and the linkage between B-G, B-L (MHC class II), and B-F has recently been reviewed.[94] Maccubbin and Schierman[95] provided further evidence for the presence of MHC-restricted CTL using reticuloendotheliosis virus (REV) in chickens. They developed three REV-transformed cell lines, RECC-UG5, UG6, and UG8 from G-B1 ($B^{13}B^{13}$), G-B2 (B^6B^6), and F$_1$ chickens, respectively. UG5 was lysed by effector cells from REV-infected G-B1 and F$_1$ chickens, but not by G-B2 spleen cells. On the other hand, UG6 was lysed by G-B2 and F$_1$, but not by G-B1, splenocytes. The effector cells were identified as T cells because treatment with polyclonal antithymocyte serum and complement significantly reduced the percent specific lysis. Neonatal treatment of chickens with cyclophosphamide caused an increase in specific lysis which they attributed to the absence of bursa-dependent suppressor T cells. This conclusion was not supported by Weinstock et al.[96] using spleen cells from REV-immunized, embryonally bursectomized chickens. They confirmed increased specific lysis in the absence of B cells, but they found that this was caused by the proportional increase of effector T cells in splenocytes from bursectomized vs. intact donors. In addition, they demonstrated that the effector cells were not only positive for class II MHC antigens,[96,97] but also that the effector T cells were CD4$^-$/CD8$^+$.[98] Thus, for the first time they demonstrated that CTL in chickens are CD8$^+$, and in analogy with mammalian systems, it can be concluded that these effector cells were restricted for viral antigen recognition in the context of MHC class I presentation. Weinstock et al.[96] also demonstrated that CTL were present at 6 d postinoculation and remained present in the spleens of infected birds for at least 3 weeks. They excluded the possibility of cytolysis of the target cells, RECC-CU60 ($B^{19}B^{19}$) and CU66 ($B^{17}B^{17}$), by virus-activated NK cells for two reasons: (1) REV infection did not induce increased lysis of LSCC-RP9, the target cells of choice for avian NK cell assays, and (2) the REV-induced cell lines were highly resistant to NK cell-induced lysis using NK cell lines.

Chubb et al.[99] developed an autochthonous assay system, in which they used short-term cultures of adherent macrophages for target cells. These cells were infected with either fowl pox virus or infectious bronchitis virus. After a 2-h incubation period, neutral red was added as an indicator for lysis and effector cells from immunized birds were added after an additional incubation of 30 min. They found specific lysis of virus-infected target cells only with the autochthonous combinations. Unfortunately, they did not have inbred lines of chickens available to further characterize the effector cells. It would be very interesting to determine if the CTL were CD4$^+$ or CD8$^+$. The former is certainly possible because the virus may not have replicated in the macrophages, but antigen processing may have occurred. The processing of antigen without virus replication tends to favor the presentation together with MHC class II rather than with class I antigens.[76]

Cannon and Russell[82] used *in vitro* stimulation of primed spleen cells to enhance the number of CTL against NDV. Spleen cells were cultured for 5 d in the presence of virus-infected peripheral blood lymphocytes. Blast cells were purified by centrifugation over Ficoll-hypaque and used as effector cells. Significant virus-antigen-specific lysis was detected, but syngeneic restriction was not demonstrated. Unfortunately, for target cells they used macrophages and PHA blasts only 1 h after infection with NDV. It may well be that they selected for CD4$^+$ effector cells, detecting a direct cytolytic effect by CD4$^+$ CTL or an indirect effect by DTH T cells or helper T cells. With the development of mAB specific for CD4, CD8, and TCR it will be possible to further characterize these cells.

V. CONCLUSIONS

It is obvious that the knowledge of avian lymphokines and CTL is still less than that of mammalian systems. It will be important to concentrate efforts on the cloning of IL genes so that purified soluble mediators become available. This will, in turn, provide the tools for developing CTL cell lines more efficiently. The development of the cell lines is needed for a better understanding of the mechanisms of CTL-induced cytolysis of virus-infected target cells and tumor cells. The fact that avian MHC-restricted cytotoxicity has been demonstrated in selected virus infections combined with the availability of relevant mAB is of great importance for the poultry industry. It may become possible to select genetic strains with increased cell-mediated immunity. In addition, the development of assay systems for CTL must be exploited to identify viral genes coding for antigens recognized by CD4$^+$ and/or CD8$^+$ CTL. It will be necessary to develop transfection systems to induce these genes in suitable target cells for CRA. Such an approach has been used successfully for the identification of antigens important for cell-mediated immune responses against murine cytomegalovirus.[100]

REFERENCES

1. **Fahey, K. J. and York, J. J.,** Cytotoxic activity of avian lymphoid cells, in *Avian Immunology: Basis and Practice,* Vol. 1, Toivanen, A. and Toivanen, P., Eds., CRC Press, Boca Raton, FL, 1986, 179.
2. **Chi, D. S. and Thorbecke, J.,** Suppressor cells and other T-lymphocytes, in *Avian Immunology: Basis and Practice,* Vol. 1, Toivanen, A. and Toivanen, P., Eds., CRC Press, Boca Raton, FL, 1986, 161.
3. **Aarden, L. A. et al.,** Revised nomenclature for antigen-nonspecific T cell proliferation and helper factors (letter), *J. Immunol.,* 123, 2928, 1979.
4. **Mizel, S. B. and Farrar, J. J.,** Revised nomenclature for antigen-nonspecific T-cell proliferation and helper factors (letter), *Cell. Immunol.,* 48, 433, 1979.
5. **Mizel, S. B.,** The interleukins, *FASEB J.,* 3, 2379, 1989.
6. **Schauenstein, K. and Kromer, G.,** Avian lymphokines, in *Avian Immunology: Basis and Practice,* Vol. 1, Toivanen, A. and Toivanen, P., Eds., CRC Press, Boca Raton, FL, 1986, 213.
7. **Schauenstein, K., Kromer, G., Fassler, R., and Wick, G.,** Implications of IL-2 in normal and disturbed immune functions in the chicken, in *Progress in Clinical Biological Research,* Vol. 238, Weber, W. T. and Ewert, D. L., Eds., Alan R. Liss, New York, 1987, 69.
8. **Vitetta, E. S., Fernandez-Botran, R., Myers, C. D., and Sanders, V. M.,** Cellular interactions in the humoral immune response, *Adv. Immunol.,* 45, 1, 1989.
9. **Ramos, T.,** Interleukin 5 is a differentiation factor for cytotoxic T lymphocytes, *Immunol. Lett.,* 21, 277, 1989.
10. **Schoenbeck, S., McKenzie, D. T., and Kagnoff, M. F.,** Interleukin 5 is a differentiation factor for IgA B cells, *Eur. J. Immunol.,* 19, 965, 1989.
11. **Beagley, K., Eldridge, J. H., Lee, F., Kiyono, H., Everson, M. P., Koopman, W. J., Hirano, T., Kishimoto, T., and McGhee, J. R.,** Interleukins and IgA synthesis. Human and murine interleukin 6 induce high rate IgA secretion in IgA-committed B cells, *J. Exp. Med.,* 169, 2133, 1989.
12. **Welch, P. A., Namen, A. E., Goodwin, R. G., Armitage, R., and Cooper, M. D.,** Human IL-7: a novel T cell growth factor, *J. Immunol.,* 143, 3562, 1989.
13. **Okazaki, H., Ito, M., Sudo, T., Hattori, M., Kano, S., Katsura, Y., and Minato, N.,** IL-7 promotes thymocyte proliferation and maintains immunocompetent thymocytes bearing $\alpha\beta$ or $\gamma\delta$ T cell receptors *in vitro*: synergism with IL-2, *J. Immunol.,* 143, 2917, 1989.
14. **Smith, K. A., Gilbride, K. J., and Favata, M. F.,** Interleukin 1-promoted interleukin 2 production, *Behring Inst. Mitt.,* 67, 4, 1980.
15. **Hayari, Y., Schauenstein, K., and Globerson, A.,** Avian lymphokines. II. Interleukin-1 activity in supernatants of stimulated adherent splenocytes of chickens, *Dev. Comp. Immunol.,* 6, 785, 1982.
16. **Klasing, K. C.,** Effect of inflammatory agents and interleukin 1 on iron and zinc metabolism, *Am. J. Physiol.,* 247, R901, 1984.
17. **Beug, H., von Kirchbach, A., Doederlein, G., Conscience, J.-F., and Graf, T.,** Chicken hematopoietic cells transformed by seven strains of defective avian leukemia viruses display three distinct phenotypes of differentiation, *Cell,* 18, 375, 1979.
18. **Klasing, K. C. and Peng, R. K.,** Influence of cell sources, stimulating agents, and incubation conditions on release of interleukin-1 from chicken macrophages, *Dev. Comp. Immunol.,* 11, 385, 1987.
19. **Klasing, K. C., Laurin, D. E., Peng, R. K., and Fry, D. M.,** Immunologically mediated growth depression in chicks: influence of feed intake, corticosterone and interleukin-1, *J. Nutr.,* 117, 1629, 1987.

20. **Schauenstein, K., Globerson, A., and Wick, G.,** Avian lymphokines. I. Thymic cell growth factor in supernatants of mitogen stimulated chicken spleen cells, *Dev. Comp. Immunol.,* 6, 533, 1982.

21. **Schnetzler, M., Oommen, A., Nowak, J. S., and Franklin, R. M.,** Characterization of chicken T cell growth factor, *Eur. J. Immunol.,* 13, 560, 1983.

22. **Kromer, G., Schauenstein, K., and Wick, G.,** Avian lymphokines: an improved method for chicken IL-2 production and assay. A con A-erythrocyte complex induces higher T cell proliferation and IL-2 production than does free mitogen, *J. Immunol. Methods,* 73, 273, 1984.

23. **Powell, P. C.,** The influence of erythrocytes on the stimulation of chicken lymphocytes by phytohaemagglutinin, *Avian Pathol.,* 9, 465, 1980.

24. **Buscaglia, C. and Schat, K. A.,** unpublished data, 1987.

25. **Vainio, O., Ratcliffe, M. J. H., and Leanderson, T.,** Chicken T-cell growth factor: use in the generation of a long-term cultured T-cell line and biochemical characterization, *Scand. J. Immunol.,* 23, 135, 1986.

26. **Schauenstein, K., Kromer, G., Hala, K., Bock, G., and Wick, G.,** Chicken-activated T-lymphocyte-antigen (CATLA) recognized by monoclonal antibody INN-CH 16 represents the IL-2 receptor, *Dev. Comp. Immunol.,* 12, 823, 1988.

27. **Hala, K., Schauenstein, K., Neu, N., Kromer, G., Wolf, H., Bock, G., and Wick, G.,** A monoclonal antibody reacting with a membrane determinant expressed on activated chicken T lymphocytes, *Eur. J. Immunol.,* 16, 1331, 1986.

28. **Fredericksen, T. L. and Sharma, J. M.,** Purification of avian T cell growth factor and immune interferon using gel filtration high resolution chromatography, in *Progress in Clinical Biological Research,* Vol. 238, Weber, W. T. and Ewert, D. L., Eds., Alan R. Liss, New York, 1987, 145.

29. **Schat, K. A. and Heller, E. D.,** unpublished data, 1985.

30. **Lehtonen, L., Vainio, O., and Toivanen, P.,** Ontogeny of alloreactivity in the chicken as measured by mixed lymphocyte reaction, *Dev. Comp. Immunol.,* 13, 187, 1989.

31. **Schauenstein, K., Kromer, G., Sundick, R. S., and Wick, G.,** Enhanced response to Con A and production of TCGF by lymphocytes of obese strain (OS) chickens with spontaneous autoimmune thyroiditis, *J. Immunol.,* 134, 872, 1985.

32. **Kromer, G., Schauenstein, K., Neu, N., Stricker, K., and Wick, G.,** *In vitro* T cell hyperreactivity in obese strain (OS) chickens is due to a defect in nonspecific suppressor mechanism(s), *J. Immunol.,* 135, 2458, 1985.

33. **Kirchner, H.,** The interferon system as an integral part of the defense system against infections, *Antiviral Res.,* 6, 1, 1986.

34. **von Bülow, V., Weiler, H., and Klasen, A.,** Activating effects of interferons, lymphokines and viruses on cultured chicken macrophages, *Avian Pathol.,* 13, 621, 1984.

35. **Pusztai, R., Tarodi, B., and Beladi, I.,** Production and characterization of interferon induced in chicken leukocytes by concanavalin A, *Acta Virol.,* 30, 131, 1986.

36. **Yip, Y. K., Barrowclough, B. S., Urban, C., and Vilcek, J.,** Purification of two subspecies of human gamma (immune) interferon, *Proc. Natl. Acad. Sci. U.S.A.,* 79, 1820, 1982.

37. **Gray, P. W. and Goeddel, D. V.,** Structure of the human immune interferon gene, *Nature,* 298, 859, 1982.

38. **Kohase, M., Moriya, H., Sato, T. A., Kohno, S., and Yamazaki, S.,** Purification and characterization of chick interferon induced by viruses, *J. Gen. Virol.,* 67, 215, 1986.

39. **Thacore, H. R., Kibler, P. K., Gregoria, C. C., Pollina, C. M., and Hudecki, M. S.,** Characterization of lymphocyte interferons with different species specificities from normal and genetically dystrophic chickens, *J. Interferon Res.,* 5, 279, 1985.

40. **Buscaglia, C. and Calnek, B. W.,** Maintenance of Marek's disease herpesvirus latency *in vitro* by a factor found in conditioned medium, *J. Gen. Virol.,* 69, 2809, 1988.

41. **Calnek, B. W.,** Marek's disease — a model for herpesvirus oncology, *Crit. Rev. Microbiol.,* 12, 293, 1986.

42. **Schat, K. A.,** Marek's disease: a model for protection against herpesvirus-induced tumours, *Cancer Surv.,* 6, 1, 1987.

43. **Buscaglia, C., Calnek, B. W., and Schat, K. A.,** Effect of immunocompetence on the establishment and maintenance of latency with Marek's disease herpesvirus, *J. Gen. Virol.,* 69, 1067, 1988.

44. **Whitfill, C. E., Allen, J., Gyles, N. R., Thoma, J., and Patterson, L. T.,** Isolation of high and low molecular weight components from chicken sera that have Rous sarcoma virus neutralizing activity, *Poult. Sci.,* 61, 1573, 1982.

45. **Whitfill, C., Weck, E., Blankenship, J., Gyles, N. R., and Thoma, J. A.,** Time course of production of low molecular weight viral-neutralizing substance(s) in chickens, *Immunogenetics,* 17, 387, 1983.

46. **Whitfill, C. E., Gyles, N. R., Horn, J., Skeeles, J. K., and Thoma, J. A.,** Antiviral substance in chicken sera, *J. Poult. Sci.,* 65, 143, 1986.

47. **Ross, L. J. N.,** personal communication, 1986.

48. **Munch, D. and Sevoian, M.,** Growth and characterization of, and immunological response of chickens to, a cell line established from JMV lymphoblastic leukemia, *Avian Dis.,* 24, 23, 1980.

49. **Keller, L. H., Belden, K. A., and Sevoian, M.,** Immunization of chickens against Marek's disease with cell-free supernatant from the JMV-1 lymphoblastoid cell line, in *Progress in Clinical Biological Research,* Vol. 238, Weber, W. T. and Ewert, D. L., Eds., Alan R. Liss, New York, 1987, 265.

50. **Lillehoj, H. S., Kang, S. Y., Keller, L., and Sevoian, M.,** *Eimeria tenella* and *E. acervulina*: lymphokines secreted by an avian T cell lymphoma or by sporozoite-stimulated immune T lymphocytes protect chickens against avian coccidiosis, *Exp. Parasitol.,* 69, 54, 1989.

51. **Hughes, H. P. A., Speer, C. A., Kyle, J. E., and Dubey, J. P.,** Activation of murine macrophages and a bovine monocyte cell line by bovine lymphokines to kill intracellular pathogens *(Eimeria. Toxoplasma),* *Infect. Immun.,* 55, 784, 1987.

52. **Schat, K. A., Calnek, B. W., and Weinstock, D.,** Cultivation and characterization of avian lymphocytes with natural killer cell activity, *Avian Pathol.,* 15, 539, 1986.

53. **Schat, K. A., Calnek, B. W., and Weinstock, D.,** Cultured avian lymphocytes with natural killer cell activity, in *Progress in Clinical Biological Research,* Vol. 238, Weber, W. T. and Ewert, D. L., Eds., Alan R. Liss, New York, 1987, 157.

54. **Vainio, O., Veromaa, T., Eerola, E., Toivanen, P., and Ratcliffe, M. J. H.,** Antigen presenting cell-T cell interaction in the chicken is MHC class II antigen restricted, *J. Immunol.,* 140, 2864, 1988.

55. **Augustin, A. A., Julius, M. H., and Cosenza, H.,** Antigen-specific stimulation and trans-stimulation of T cells in long term culture, *Eur. J. Immunol.,* 9, 665, 1979.

56. **Bhogal, B. S., Tse, H. Y., Jacobson, E. B., and Schmatz, D. M.,** Chicken T lymphocyte clones with specificity for *Eimeria tenella.* I. Generation and functional characterization, *J. Immunol.,* 137, 3318, 1986.

57. **Bhogal, B. S., Schmatz, D. M., Tse, H. Y., Ravino, O., and Jacobson, E. B.,** Generation and functional characterization of *Eimeria tenella* immune chicken T-cell clones, in *Progress in Clinical Biological Research,* Vol. 238, Weber, W. T. and Ewert, D. L., Eds., Alan R. Liss, New York, 1987, 127.

58. **Bhogal, B. S., Jacobson, E. B., Tse, H. Y., Schmatz, D. M., and Ravino, O. J.,** Parasite exposure elicits a preferential T-cell response involved in protective immunity against *Eimeria* species in chickens primed by an internal-image anti-idiotypic antibody, *Infect. Immun.,* 57, 2804, 1989.

59. **Schat, K. A., Chen, C.-L., Lillehoj, H., Calnek, B. W., and Weinstock, D.,** Characterization of Marek's disease cell lines with monoclonal antibodies specific for cytotoxic and helper T cells, in *Advances in Marek's Disease Research,* Kato, S., Horiuchi, T., Mikami, T., and Hirai, K., Eds., Japanese Association on Marek's Disease, Osaka, 1988, 220.

60. **Schat, K. A., Chen, C.-L., Char, D., and Calnek, B. W.,** Transformation of subsets of T lymphocytes by Marek's disease virus, manuscript in preparation, 1990.

61. **Calnek, B. W., Lucio, B., Schat, K. A., and Lillehoj, H. S.,** Pathogenesis of Marek's disease virus-induced local lesions. 1. Lesion characterization and cell line establishment, *Avian Dis.,* 33, 291, 1989.

62. **Edelman, A. S., Robinson, M. E., Sanchez, P., and Thorbecke, G. J.,** Suppressor T cells with histamine type II receptors in chickens bearing chemically induced fibrosarcomas, *Cell. Immunol.,* 110, 321, 1987.

63. **Khan, M. M., Sansoni, P., Engleman, E. G., and Melmon, K. L.,** Pharmacologic effects of autacoids on subsets of T cells, *J. Clin. Invest.,* 75, 1578, 1985.

64. **Chi, D. S.,** *In vitro* growth of chicken T cells using the supernatant from Con A-stimulated lymphoid cell cultures, *Int. J. Immunopharmacol.,* 4, 301, 1982.

65. **Sharma, J. M. and Tizard, I.,** Avian cellular immune effector mechanisms — a review, *Avian Pathol.,* 13, 357, 1984.

66. **Powell, P. C.,** Immune mechanisms in infections of poultry, *Vet. Immunol. Immunopathol.,* 15, 87, 1987.

67. **Lee, G. M., Jackson, G. D. F., and Cooper, G. N.,** The role of serum and biliary antibodies and cell-mediated immunity in the clearance of *S. typhimurium* from chickens, *Vet. Immunol. Immunopathol.,* 2, 233, 1981.

68. **Kogut, M. H. and Lange, C.,** Effect of lymphokine treatment on the invasion of cultured animal cells by *Eimeria tenella, Lymphokine Res.,* 7, 31, 1988.

69. **Prowse, S. J. and Pallister, J.,** Interferon release as a measure of the T-cell response to coccidial antigens in chickens, *Avian Pathol.,* 18, 619, 1989.

70. **Lillehoj, H. S.,** Intestinal intraepithelial and splenic natural killer cell responses to Eimerian infections in inbred chickens, *Infect. Immun.,* 57, 1879, 1989.

71. **Chi, D. S., Palladino, A., Romano, T., and Thorbecke, G. J.,** Transfer of delayed hypersensitivity in the chicken, *Dev. Comp. Immunol.,* 6, 541, 1982.

72. **Zinkernagel, R. M. and Doherty, P. C.,** MHC-restricted cytotoxic T cells: studies on the biological role of polymorphic major transplantation antigens determining T-cell restriction-specificity, function, and responsiveness, *Adv. Immunol.,* 27, 51, 1979.

73. **Clevers, H., Alarcon, B., Wileman, T., and Terhorst, C.,** The T cell receptor/CD3 complex: a dynamic protein ensemble, *Annu. Rev. Immunol.,* 6, 629, 1988.

74. **Schmid, D. S.,** The human MHC-restricted cellular response to herpes simplex virus type 1 is mediated by CD4$^+$, CD8$^-$ T cells and is restricted to the DR region of the MHC complex, *J. Immunol.,* 140, 3610, 1988.

75. **Morrison, L. A., Braciale, V. L., and Braciale, T. J.,** Antigen form influences induction and frequency of influenza-specific class I and class II MHC-restricted cytolytic T lymphocytes, *J. Immunol.,* 141, 363, 1988.

76. **Long, E. O. and Jacobson, S.,** Pathways of viral antigen processing and presentation to CTL: defined by the mode of virus entry?, *Immunol. Today,* 10, 45, 1989.

77. **Winn, H. J.,** Immune mechanisms in homotransplantation. II. Quantitative assay of the immunologic activity of lymphoid cells stimulated by tumor homografts, *J. Immunol.,* 86, 228, 1961.

78. **Powell, P. C., Rennie, M., Ross, L. J. N., and Mustill, B. M.,** The effect of bursectomy on the adoptive transfer of resistance to Marek's disease, *Int. J. Cancer,* 26, 681, 1980.

79. **Fahey, K. J., York, J. J., and Bagust, T. J.,** Laryngotracheitis herpesvirus infection in the chicken. II. The adoptive transfer of resistance with immune spleen cells, *Avian Pathol.,* 13, 265, 1984.

80. **Bagust, T. J.,** Laryngotracheitis (Gallid-1) herpesvirus infection in the chicken. IV. Latency establishment by wild and vaccine strains of ILT virus, *Avian Pathol.,* 15, 581, 1986.

81. **von Bulow, V. and Klasen, A.,** Effects of avian viruses on cultured chicken bone-marrow-derived macrophages, *Avian Pathol.,* 12, 179, 1983.

82. **Cannon, M. J. and Russell, P. H.,** Secondary *in vitro* stimulation of specific cytotoxic cells to Newcastle disease virus in chickens, *Avian Pathol.,* 15, 731, 1986.

83. **Galton, J. E., Palladino, M. A., Xue, B., Edelman, A. S., and Thorbecke, G. J.,** Immunity to carcinogen-induced transplantable fibrosarcoma in B2/B2 chickens. V. Relationship to tumor cell-specific delayed hypersensitivity and serum antibody, *Cell. Immunol.,* 73, 247, 1982.

84. **Edelman, A. S., Xue, B., Galton, J. E., Sanchez, P., and Thorbecke, G. J.,** Cross-reactive cellular and humoral immunity to carcinogen-induced chicken fibrosarcomas, *J. Immunol.,* 135, 2213, 1985.

85. **Schierman, L. W.,** Transplantable Marek's disease lymphomas. II. Variable tumor immunity induced by different lymphoblastoid cells, *J. Natl. Cancer Inst.,* 73, 423, 1984.

86. **DiFronzo, N. L. and Schierman, L. W.,** Transplantable Marek's disease lymphomas. III. Induction of MHC-restricted tumor immunity by lymphoblastoid cells in F1 hosts, *Int. J. Cancer,* 44, 474, 1989.

87. **Tseng, C. K., Fletcher, O. J., and Schierman, L. W.,** Preferential protection against Marek's disease pathogenesis by immunization with syngeneic virus-nonproducer lymphoblastoid cells, *Avian Pathol.,* 15, 557, 1986.

88. **Schat, K. A., Shek, W. R., Calnek, B. W., and Abplanalp, H.,** Syngeneic and allogeneic cell-mediated cytotoxicity against Marek's disease lymphoblastoid tumor cell lines, *Int. J. Cancer,* 29, 187, 1982.

89. **Powell, P. C., Mustill, B. M., and Rennie, M.,** The role of histocompatibility antigens in cell-mediated cytotoxicity against Marek's disease tumor-derived lymphoblastoid cell lines, *Avian Pathol.,* 12, 461, 1983.

90. **Ikuta, K., Nakajima, K., Naito, M., Ann, S. H., Ueda, S., Kato, S., and Hirai, K.,** Identification of Marek's disease virus-specific antigens in Marek's disease lymphoblastoid cell lines using monoclonal antibody against virus-specific phosphorylated polypeptides, *Int. J. Cancer,* 35, 257, 1985.

91. **Wainberg, M. A., Beiss, B., Beaupre, S., and Miron, L.,** Preferential lymphocyte-mediated cytotoxicity of syngeneic target cells in chickens bearing tumors induced by avian sarcoma virus, *Cancer Lett.,* 17, 23, 1985.

92. **Wainberg, M. A., Markson, Y., Weiss, D. W., and Doljanski, F.,** Cellular immunity against Rous sarcomas in chickens. Preferential reactivity against autochthonous target cells as determined by lymphocyte adherence and cytotoxicity tests *in vitro, Proc. Natl. Acad. Sci. U.S.A.,* 71, 3565, 1974.

93. **Stone, H. A.,** The Usefulness and Application of Highly Inbred Chickens to Research Programs, *Agric. Res. Serv. Tech. Bull. No. 1514.,* U.S. Department of Agriculture, Washington, D.C., 1975, 1.

94. **Crone, M. and Simonsen, M.,** Avian major histocompatibility complex, in *Avian Immunology: Basis and Practice,* Vol. 2, Toivanen, A. and Toivanen, P., Eds., CRC Press, Boca Raton, FL, 1987, 26.

95. **Maccubbin, D. L. and Schierman, L. W.,** MHC-restricted cytotoxic response of chicken T cells: expression, augmentation and clonal characterization, *J. Immunol.,* 136, 12, 1986.

96. **Weinstock, D., Schat, K. A., and Calnek, B. W.,** Cytotoxic T lymphocytes in reticuloendotheliosis virus-infected chickens, *Eur. J. Immunol.,* 19, 267, 1989.

97. **Weinstock, D. and Schat, K. A.,** Virus specific syngeneic killing of reticuloendotheliosis virus transformed cell line target cells by spleen cells, in *Progress in Clinical Biological Research,* Vol. 238, Weber, W. T. and Ewert, D. L., Eds., Alan R. Liss, New York, 1987, 253.

98. **Lillehoj, H. S., Lillehoj, E. P., Weinstock, D., and Schat, K. A.,** Functional and biochemical characterization of avian T lymphocyte antigens identified by monoclonal antibodies, *Eur. J. Immunol.,* 18, 2059, 1988.

99. **Chubb, R. C., Huynh, V., and Law, R.,** The detection of cytotoxic lymphocyte activity in chickens infected with infectious bronchitis virus or fowl pox virus, *Avian Pathol.,* 16, 395, 1987.

100. **Reddehase, M. J., Mutter, W., Munch, K., Buhring, H. J., and Koszinowski, U. H.,** CD8-positive T lymphocytes specific for murine cytomegalovirus immediate early antigens mediate protective immunity, *J. Virol.,* 61, 3102, 1987.

Chapter 4

NATURAL IMMUNE FUNCTIONS

J. M. Sharma and K. A. Schat

TABLE OF CONTENTS

I. INTRODUCTION

A number of cellular mechanisms provide natural defense against disease in normal, unimmunized individuals. Among these mechanisms, natural immunity mediated by natural killer (NK) cells, cells of antibody-dependent cell-mediated cytotoxicity (ADCC), and macrophages has been examined in some detail. The role of macrophages in cell-mediated immunity is being covered in detail in the next chapter, and therefore will not be discussed here. The purpose of this chapter is to review the available information on avian NK cells and discuss the role these cells may play in defense against neoplastic and nonneoplastic disease. ADCC will also be discussed briefly although this reactivity has not been studied in detail in birds.

Since their identification over 15 years ago, NK cells have been studied extensively in mammalian species in an effort to understand their role in natural defense and to explore their possible therapeutic potential in cancer and infectious disease. As their name implies, NK cells have the ability to lyse target cells. This cytotoxicity is not restricted by either class I or class II major histocompatibility complex (MHC) antigens. NK cells are reactive against a variety of target cells including virus-infected and undifferentiated cells, but the reactivity is particularly strong against neoplastically transformed target cells. Because of this, much effort has been expended in examining the role of NK cells in immune surveillance against certain types of cancer with encouraging experimental results.[1-3]

In mammalian species, NK activity is closely associated with a subpopulation of cells identified as large granular lymphocytes (LGL).[4] These cells are nonadherent and nonphagocytic and share surface antigens with T cells and cells of myelomonocytic series.[5,6] Mammalian NK cells may secrete cytokines and possess receptors for interleukin 2 (IL-2). IL-2-dependent lines of LGL have been developed.[7,8] The molecular biology of mammalian NK cells has recently been reviewed.[9]

In avian species, well-pronounced NK cell activity has been detected in chickens and quail. Chicken NK cell activity has been studied in some detail.

II. NATURAL KILLER CELL ACTIVITY IN CHICKENS

A. ASSAY SYSTEMS

NK-cell activity is most commonly measured by *in vitro* assays, although an *in vivo* assay has also been used. The latter technique was used by Lam and Linna;[10,11] chickens of line SC (B^2B^2) were used as donors and recipients. Lymphocytes from 8-week-old birds were transferred into 1-d-old recipients to demonstrate the presence of NK cells. These experiments are discussed further in Section IV.

In the *in vitro* assays, radioisotope-labeled target cells are incubated with effector cells. The following aspects of this assay will be briefly discussed: (1) selection of target cells, (2) selection of label and preparation of target cells, (3) preparation of effector cells, and (4) assay conditions.

1. Selection of Target Cells

The avian NK cell activity was first detected in specific-pathogen-free (SPF) chickens by using the Marek's disease (MD) lymphoblastoid cell line MDCC-MSB1 (MSB1).[12] It was later shown that LSCC-RP9 (RP9) cells were more susceptible to NK cell lysis than MSB1 cells.[13] The RP9 lymphoblastoid cell line was developed from a tumor in a B^2B^{15} chicken inoculated with the RAV-2 strain of avian leukosis virus (ALV).[14] At the present time, this cell line is used by most researchers studying avian NK cells. It is of interest to note that a virus-producing subline of RP9 is refractory to lysis by NK cells.[12]

Besides MSB1, most other MD-derived cell lines were refractory to NK cell lysis.[13,15]

The reason(s) for this resistance is unknown. All MD cell lines tested by Heller and Schat[15] were comprised of helper T cells positive for CD4.[16] It will be of interest to examine the susceptibility to NK cell lysis of the recently developed MD cell lines which are either cytotoxic/suppressor T cells (CD8[+]) or T cells lacking both the CD4 and CD8 surface markers.[17]

Mammalian cell targets susceptible to lysis by mammalian NK cells were generally refractory to avian NK cells. Leibold et al.[18] examined human (including K562, CEM, Jurkat, Daudi, Raji), monkey, mouse, and bovine cells as targets for avian NK cells. Specific cytotoxicity was noted sporadically. On the other hand, Fleischer[19] found that the human cell lines Raji and Ramos, as well as the mouse cell lines P3X63, 424 A11, and P815, were highly susceptible to lysis by chicken and Japanese quail NK cells. The human cell lines Molt-4 and BJAB, as well as the feline FES line, were less susceptible.

2. Selection of Label and Preparation of Target Cells

In most *in vitro* cytotoxicity assays for NK-cell activity, the target cells are labeled with $Na^{51}CrO_4$ although ^{75}Se[18], $^{111}Indium$,[20] or ^3H-proline[21] have also been employed. The level of NK-cell activity is often expressed as the percentage of the incorporated isotope label released into the supernatant fluid. In contrast, the ^3H-proline assay measures the survival of target cells by determining the amount of ^3H-proline left in the cells at the end of the assay period.

The method for labeling of avian lymphoblastoid target cells with ^{51}Cr has been published.[12,22,23] Optimal results (high uptake of isotope combined with low levels of spontaneous release) depend upon several factors. Target cells need to be actively replicating and are often subcultured 24 h prior to their use. Immediately before labeling, the cells are centrifuged over Ficoll Hypaque and counted; for optimal results the cell viability has to be >95%. The radioisotope is added, and the mixture is incubated for 45 to 60 min at 41°C. Extensive washing after the labeling period is needed to remove unincorporated isotope. We found it helpful to incubate the cells an additional 60 min prior to the last wash. To reduce cell damage, RPMI-1640 supplemented with 20% fetal bovine serum was used for all washes and incubations.

3. Preparation of Effector Cells

In general, spleen cell suspensions are used as the source of effector cells. Red blood cells are removed by centrifugation over Ficoll-Hypaque or by slow centrifugation. The disadvantage of the former technique is that there are many cell types present in these suspensions complicating the identification and characterization of effector cells. Differentiation of lymphocytes from thrombocytes is often difficult, and centrifugation over Ficoll-Hypaque may actually enrich for thrombocytes.[24] Peripheral blood lymphocytes (PBL) have been used as a source of NK cells but with limited success. Sharma and Coulson[12] and Wainberg et al.[25] reported the absence of NK cells in PBL while Fleischer[19] and Heller and Schat[15] found that PBL contain NK cells. Recently, cells with NK-like activity have been obtained from the intestinal epithelium.[26,27] These intestinal epithelial leukocytes (IELs) were able to lyse RP9, but not PR12, target cells in 4-h ^{51}Cr-release assays. The frequency of NK cells within the IEL population is unknown. Myers and Schat[28] confirmed the presence of NK cells in IEL preparations obtained from SPF chickens. They used RP9 cells as well as uninfected and rotavirus-infected, allogeneic and syngeneic chick kidney cells as targets. The NK cells lysed RP9 cells and rotavirus-infected cells, but not uninfected chick kidney cells or RECC-CU60 cells. The RECC-CU60 is an NK-resistant lymphoblastoid cell line transformed by reticuloendotheliosis virus.[29]

Thymocytes and bursa cells do not lyse NK-sensitive target cells in a 4-h ^{51}Cr-release assay although Lillehoj and Chai[27] reported that specific lysis was observed after 16 h of incubation. The possible role of macrophage-mediated lysis in the long-term assay needs to be established (see Section II.A.4).

4. Assay Conditions

Effector cells are mixed with target cells and incubated at 39 to 41°C for 4 h, which is long enough to detect acceptable levels of specific cytotoxicity (generally >5%). Prolonged assay periods may not only increase the level of specific release, but also result in increased nonspecific release of the radioisotope. In addition, other mechanisms of lysis can become important, especially macrophage-induced lysis.[30] It is therefore essential to remove all macrophages and monocytes from effector cell preparations if incubation periods longer than 4 to 6 h are required. The efficacy of macrophage removal should be examined by using macrophage-specific monoclonal antibody or by cultivating depleted cells and control cells and examining these cultures for adherent cells.

The ratio of effector to target cells (E:T) ratio is often 100:1 or 200:1. If possible, the effector and the target cells should be reacted at three different ratios so that regression line analysis can be used in facilitating statistical analysis of data. Ratios of 200:1 or 400:1 may enhance the possibility of interactions of target cells with cells other than NK cells. Two controls are important: (1) the use of "neutral" cells (e.g., thymocytes) at the same E:T ratio as used for the effector cells (these cells serve as a control for cell crowding in the cultures, and they help maintain suitable culture conditions); and (2) the use of NK-cell-resistant target cells. A high level of "specific" release in the latter indicates that factors (toxins?) other than NK cells may be the cause of cytotoxicity.

B. CHARACTERIZATION OF NATURAL KILLER CELLS

Several reports have indicated that treatment with either anti-B cell or anti-thymocyte serum and complement did not abrogate NK cell activity.[11,13] In addition, the NK cells used for *in vivo* protection studies were radioresistant.[11] In general, avian NK cells were found to be nonadherent to plastic or nylon wool.[10-13,30] Sharma[30] examined single-cell suspensions of local MD transplantable tumors for cytotoxic activity. Two types of cytotoxic cells were detected: (1) adherent cells that were cytotoxic in an 18-h assay and (2) nonadherent cells that were cytotoxic to RP9 cells in a 4-h assay. The adherent cytotoxic cells were characterized as macrophages and the nonadherent cells as NK cells. However, the possibility was not excluded that at least some of the nonadherent cells were macrophage precursors.[31,32] Recently, Mandi et al.[33] reported that relatively pure preparations of granulocytes obtained from spleen and PBL were able to lyse RP9 and LSCC-H32, an avian leukosis virus-transformed fibroblast cell line.[34] Infection of chickens with human adenovirus caused a marked increase in granulocyte-mediated cytotoxicity at 24 h postinoculation. The increase was followed by depressed NK cell responses for the next 14 d. During the first 24 h postinfection, there was also an increase in interferon (IFN) production. *In vitro* induction of IFN by adenovirus also increased the level of cytotoxicity of granulocytes. The addition of rabbit anti-chicken IFN serum reduced the adenovirus-induced increase, but did not change the level of cytotoxicity of nonstimulated granulocytes.[35] The addition of monoclonal antibodies specific for chicken granulocytes in combination with complement significantly reduced, but did not eliminate, lysis of target cells. In addition, this monoclonal antibody reduced ADCC.[36] It would be of interest to determine if this antibody detects the avian homologue of CD16 (FcR2) which consists of two proteins of 50 and 60 kDa, respectively. Ruiz-Cabello et al.[37] reported that CD16 is present on both human neutrophilic granulocytes and LGL with NK activity.

It appears that many cell types present in the spleen and PBL of chickens may lyse target cells in an NK fashion. The characterization of the effector cells depends, to a large degree, on the combination of preparation of effector cells, selection of target cells, and assay conditions.

C. *IN VITRO* PROPAGATION OF NATURAL KILLER CELLS

It has been well established that mammalian NK cells can be cultivated *in vitro* using purified or recombinant IL-2 or conditioned medium (CM).[7,8,38,39] The latter is often produced by stimulating lymphocytes with mitogens and may contain a number of growth factors in addition to IL-2. Most cell lines have only a limited life span and may lose their lytic activity during the later phase of their growth period.[40] It has been suggested that, in addition to IL-2, other factors may be needed to obtain truly continuous NK cell lines.[41] Recently, long-term NK cell cultures were established by initiating the culture of normal spleen cells in the presence of IL-2, followed by continuing culture in the presence of phytohemagglutinin (PHA) and IL-2. Stimulation of spleen cells with PHA prior to addition of IL-2 may selectively enhance the culture of T cells, which grow faster than NK cells. In contrast, NK cells may be preferentially stimulated by IL-2 in the absence of PHA. The addition of PHA to replicating NK cells provides the second stimulating factor.[42]

The establishment of cloned NK cell lines has both enhanced and complicated our understanding of NK cells. First, it was shown that cloned NK cell lines can have different target-cell specificities.[43] Second, it was discovered that IL-2 also activated another group of cells, the lymphokine-activated killer cells (LAK), lysed a wide range of target cells. Most of the LAK seem to have characteristics in common with NK cells, but some LAK may be derived from T cells.[43] The third complication is that cells with T-cell markers, as well as cells without T-cell markers, can be cultivated *in vitro* and behave as NK cells or LAK. Moretta et al.[44] demonstrated that human NK-cell clones also had allogeneic T-cell activity. Thurlow et al.[45] found that mature cytotoxic T cells (CTL) and NK-cell clones shared some antigens apparently unrelated to the CD8 antigen. Subsequently, Schmidt et al.[46] reported the presence in human peripheral blood of a small population of cells with phenotypic, morphologic, and functional characteristics typical of both NK and T cells. Minato et al.[47] established an LGL cell line directly from multipotential hematopoietic progenitor cells by using interleukin 3 (IL-3). Emerging colonies of cells required further cultivation in the presence of recombinant IL-2 and accessory macrophages. These cells became CD3$^+$ and expressed rearranged T-cell receptor (TCR) genes.

In contrast to the numerous reports on mammalian NK cell lines, there is a paucity of data on cultured avian NK cells. Schat et al.[48,49] reported the establishment of NK cell lines using nonstimulated spleen cells from SPF chickens. These cells were cultured in Leibovitz McCoy (LM) medium containing 2-mercaptoethanol, fetal bovine serum, chicken serum[50] and CM at 41°C for 50 to 60 d. The cells had the typical morphology of LGL with an eccentric nucleus, cytoplasmic vacuoles, and granules (Figures 1 and 3). In addition to LGL, a population of cells with a lymphoblastoid (LB) morphology was present (Figures 2 and 3). Cultures could be enriched for LB cells by using mitogen stimulation of spleen cells prior to the addition of CM and by storage in liquid nitrogen. LGL did not recover well from storage in liquid nitrogen.

Functionally, these LGL were highly effective in lysing RP9 and MSB1 at low E:T ratios of 10:1 and 5:1. In contrast, the NK-cell-resistant cell line MDCC-CU36 was resistant to lysis. Unfortunately, cloned cell lines were not established, which complicated a more definitive characterization of LGL and LB as cells with NK activity. Several of these cell lines were characterized for surface markers (Table 1). Most of the cells were positive for CLA-1. This antigen is present on B cells only prior to the development of surface immunoglobulin (Ig), and it remains present on T cells during their differentiation.[51] Expression of an antigen present on circulating T cells was only detected on LB cells derived from concanavalin A (Con A)-stimulated blast cells. Class II MHC (Ia) antigen was detected in variable percentages, but seemed to be correlated with the presence of LB. None of the cell lines stained with monoclonal antibodies against the μ chain of IgM and the thymocyte antigen CT-1. LGL were also positive for asialo-GM 1, an antigen commonly expressed on

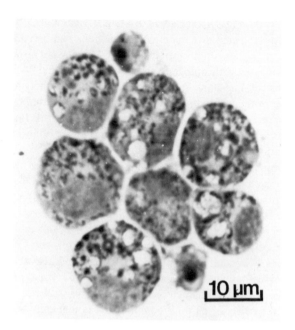

FIGURE 1.   Large granular lymphocyte line CU53 at 23
d in culture. The cells have a relatively uniform morphology
with an eccentric nucleus and cytoplasmic vacuoles and
granules. (Cytospin preparation, Wright-Giemsa stain.) (From
Schat, K. A., Calnek, B. W., and Weinstock, D., *Avian
Pathol.*, 15, 539, 1986. With permission.)

mammalian LGL. Interestingly, Lillehoj[52] reported an increase in asialo MG-1 expressing
intraepithelial lymphocytes after secondary infection with *Eimeria* species. The increased
expression correlated with increased NK-cell activity. Recently, two LGL preparations were
examined with monoclonal antibodies specific for CD4, CD5, CD8, and Ia. Both lines were
strongly positive for CD5 and negative for Ia. One line consisted of a mixed population
with 77% positive for CD4 and up to 19% positive for CD8; the other line was positive
only for CD4.[53] In another study, one LGL preparation was positive for CD8 and negative
for CD3 and CD4.[53a]

Since the development of LGL cell lines, Schat et al.[49] examined a small number of
SPF chickens for the presence of LGL and asialo-GM 1-positive cells in the spleen. We
detected a very low percentage of LGL (1% or less) and a slightly higher percentage of
cells positive for asialo GM 1. Low percentages of LGL in spleens of mammalian species
have also been reported.[54]

It is obvious from these limited data that the classification of cells with NK-cell activity
will be just as complicated in avian species as it has been in mammalian species. It will be
important to develop more efficient techniques for the cultivation and cloning of cells with
NK activity. One of the major impediments is the lack of purified or recombinant chicken
IL-2 and other lymphokines.

D. ENHANCEMENT OF NATURAL KILLER CELLS

There is extensive evidence that certain biological modifiers may modulate mammalian
NK cell expression *in vitro* and *in vivo*. For example, cultures of human and murine resting
NK-cell populations can be expanded by IL-2 or lectins.[55-57] IFN or IFN-inducers are perhaps
the predominant enhancers of NK-cell activity.[58-60]

Efforts have also been made to enhance NK-cell activity in the chicken although the

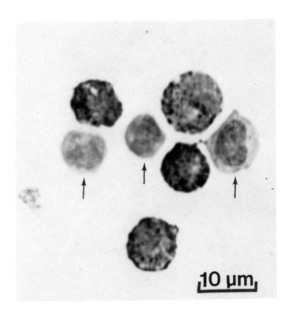

FIGURE 2. Four large granular lymphocytes (LGL) and three lymphoblastoid (LB, arrows) cells of 3830-3B at 29 d in culture. Note that the LBs are smaller than the LGLs and have a large nucleus to cytoplasm ratio. The LGLs appear smaller than those in Figure 1 because of the different preparative methods. (Air-dried preparation, Giemsa stain.) (From Schat, K. A., Calnek, B. W., and Weinstock, D., *Avian Pathol.*, 15, 539, 1986. With permission.)

data are not extensive. Recently, Ding and Lam[61] injected polyinosinic-polycytidylic acid (poly I:C) into chickens and examined the levels of NK cell activity in the spleen using an 18-h ^{51}Cr-release assay. Poly I:C is a potent inducer of IFN, and inoculation of this reagent into mice results in dramatic enhancement of NK activity.[59] In chickens, poly I:C elevated NK levels of spleen cells at a dosage level of 1.0 mg per animal. The augmentation of NK activity was quite rapid and was detected 3 h after administration of the drug. Successful induction of IFN in chickens by poly I:C is in conflict with the experience of several other laboratories that found this drug to be highly toxic for chickens or ineffective as an IFN booster of NK cells.[62-65] Portnoy and Merigan[62] showed that poly I:C induced IFN *in vitro* in cultures of chicken embryo fibroblast cells, but intravenous injection of this drug in as low a dose as 0.1 mg/kg rapidly killed 6-week-old noninbred chickens. Intratracheal deposition of poly I:C was also highly toxic at low doses. Intravenous inoculation of poly I:C at subtoxic doses did not induce detectable IFN in chickens.

A number of viruses induce IFN *in vivo* in chickens although the modulating effect of these viruses on NK activity has not been examined extensively. Inoculation of a strain of Newcastle disease virus that induced IFN *in vivo* also elevated NK levels in the spleen, whereas another non-IFN inducer strain of the virus did not have this effect.[61] On the other hand, infectious bursal disease virus (IBDV), a double-stranded RNA virus which is a potent IFN inducer,[66,67] did not alter NK levels in the spleen.[68] The failure to detect enhancement of NK activity in birds exposed to IBDV may be partly due to the assay procedure used. A 4-h ^{51}Cr-release assay was used in the trials with IBDV,[68] whereas elevated NK activity following Newcastle disease virus infection was detected in an 18-h assay.[61] In other studies, a 4-h ^{51}Cr-release assay detected significant elevation of NK activity in the spleen of SPF chickens exposed to turkey herpesvirus (HVT) or Marek's disease virus (MDV) serotypes

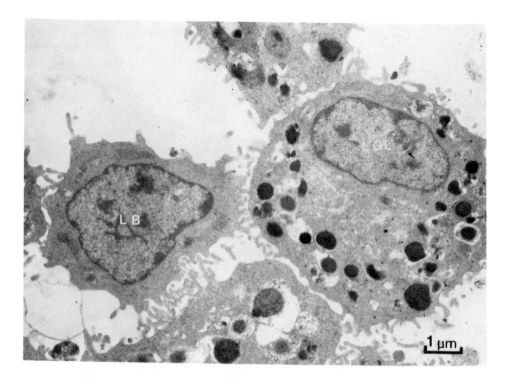

FIGURE 3.   Large granular lymphocyte (LGL) and lymphoblastoid cell (LB) in CU53 at 23 d in culture. Note the difference in size and ratio of nucleus to cytoplasm. LGLs contain many electron dense granules. (From Schat, K. A., Calnek, B. W., and Weinstock, D., *Avian Pathol.*, 15, 539, 1986. With permission.)

1 and 2[63,69,70] (Figure 4). Both of these herpesviruses induce IFN *in vivo* and *in vitro*.[71-76] The increase in NK levels in the spleen was detected within the first 3 weeks after virus exposure and appeared to be related to resistance of chickens against clinical MD.[69] Interestingly, this enhancement by SB-1, a serotype 2 strain of MDV, and HVT was found in young chickens only. Infection of older birds with these strains caused a decrease in NK-cell activity.[63] Heller and Schat[63] suggested that the enhanced level of NK activity in young birds could be the result of an enhanced maturation of the NK cells, while the decrease in older birds may be due to lymphokines causing a down-regulation. This hypothesis is supported by the finding that both HVT and SB-1 cause splenic enlargement,[77] which suggest that leukocytes become activated. Treatment of NK effector cells *in vitro* with extraneous IFN did not alter their cytotoxicity.[61]

E. INHIBITION OF NATURAL KILLER ACTIVITY

Several circumstances have been identified in which NK reactivity of chickens is inhibited. Inoculation of a pathogenic isolate of MDV in a highly susceptible genetic line of chickens resulted in progressive neoplastic disease and an accompanying decrease in NK levels in the spleen[69] (Figure 5). Hatchmates that were protected against clinical disease by vaccination did not experience NK cell inhibition. Thus, immunodepression accompanying progressive disease may also involve the NK system.

Studies in chickens and quail have revealed that NK activity is poorly expressed in young animals and that the activity becomes well-pronounced as the animals get older.[12,15,78] A similar age-dependent effect on NK cytotoxicity has been seen in rodents although, in contrast, NK cell activity has been detected in human fetuses during early stages of gestation[79] and high levels of activity are sustained through old age. There is preliminary evidence that

TABLE 1
Surface Markers on Cultured Lymphocytes with Natural Killer Cell Activity[48,49]

Cell line origin (genetic strain of chickens)	Treatment with Con A	Surface marker (no. lines positive/tested)[a]						
		CT-1	Circ. T cell	CLA-1	μ	Ia	Asialo GM1
P	−	0/4	0/6	6/6	0/5	2/6	—[b]
P2	+	—	1/1	1/1	—	1/1	—
N2	+	—	1/1	1/1	—	1/1	—
N2	−	—	—	—	—	—	3/3

[a] The percentages of positive cells/line varied, and not all lines were tested for all markers due to low cell numbers available. For explanation of surface markers, please see the text and References 48, 49, and 51.

[b] Not tested.

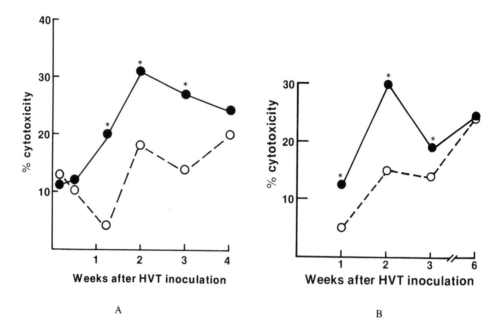

FIGURE 4. Natural cytotoxicity response in chickens inoculated with turkey herpesvirus (HVT) at 6 d of age. Five chickens were examined in each treatment group at each time, and cytotoxicity levels were averaged. Target cell-to-effector cell ratio was 1:400. ● Group inoculated with HVT; ○ uninoculated control group. Asterisks indicate statistically significant ($p < 0.05$) differences in cytotoxicity levels between inoculated and uninoculated groups. (A) Line-P chickens. (B) Line-N chickens. (From Sharma, J. M., *Avian Dis.*, 25, 882, 1981. With permission.)

the genetic background of chickens may also influence NK cell expression. In one study, genetic lines N, P, and 15 × 7 were compared for NK reactivity.[12] Of the three lines, chickens of line 15 × 7 had the lowest incidence of NK cytotoxicity, and the levels of cytotoxicity for positive chickens in this line were lower than those of lines N and P. Genetic background also seemed to influence the age-related expression of NK activity. In 15 × 7 chickens, NK activity was generally not detected before 9 weeks of age, whereas in line N, some chickens at 1 to 3 weeks of age had functional NK cells, and the mean cytotoxicity levels in chickens older than 7 to 9 weeks was higher in line N than in line 15 × 7.[12] In another study, no apparent differences in NK-cell reactivity were detected among lines N-2, P-2, and 003.[15] Likewise, Boyd and Wick[80] and Boyd et al.[81] did not detect differences in levels of spontaneous cytotoxicity using PBL from Obese and normal white leghorn chickens against tannic acid-treated chicken red blood cells.

The mechanism of reduced NK-cell activity at young age or in certain genetic lines of chickens is not known. It should be of interest to determine if suppressor cells play a part in natural inhibition of avian NK-cell expression as they do in the mouse.[82] Normal chicken embryos have well-developed suppressor cells that down-regulate the *in vitro* mitogenic response of functional T cells.[83,84] The effect of these suppressor cells on NK activity was not examined although it is unlikely that they inhibited NK expression in young chickens because the anti-T suppressor cells were not detected after hatching.[84] An alternate explanation may be that chicken fetal antigens (CFA) are responsible for the down-regulation of NK cells. Ohashi et al.[85] used an anti-CFA monoclonal antibody[86] to purify CFA from sodium deoxycholate-solubilized MSB1 cells using sodium deoxycholate. Both purified CFA and the solubilized MSB1 material were able to inhibit NK-cell activity by direct addition to the assay. Repeated inoculation of chickens with CFA at 2-d intervals also resulted in suppression of NK-cell activity. There is considerable evidence that CFA consists of a

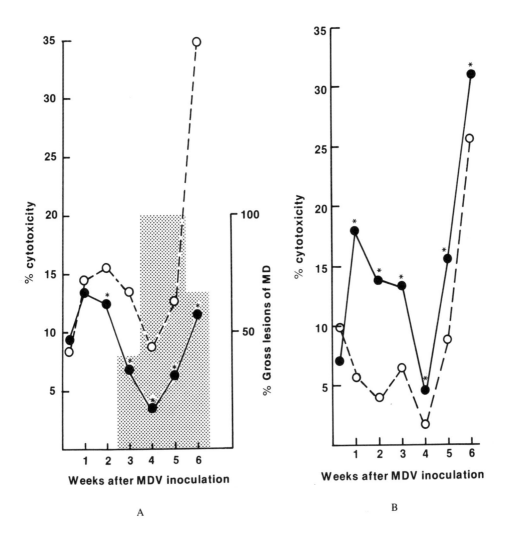

FIGURE 5. Natural cytotoxicity and gross lesion response in chickens inoculated with Marek's disease virus (MDV) at 6 d of age. Target cell-to-effector cell ratio was 1:400. ● Group inoculated with duck embryo fibroblasts (DEF) infected with MDV; ○ group inoculated with normal DEF. Asterisks indicate statistically significant ($p < 0.05$) differences in cytotoxicity levels between MDV and MDV-free groups. (A) Line-P chickens. Five chickens were examined in each treatment group at each time, except in MDV-infected group at 6 weeks, when only three survivors were left; responses were averaged. Histograms show percent chickens with gross lesions of Marek's Disease. (B) Line-N chickens. Five chickens were examined in each treatment group at each interval and responses were averaged. At both 3 and 5 weeks, 20% of chickens examined had microscopic lesions of Marek's Disease; gross lesions were not detected. (From Sharma, J. M., *Avian Dis.*, 25, 882, 1981. With permission.)

heterogeneous population of antigenic determinants that may occur in various combinations and are expressed in an age-dependent fashion.[87] Murthy et al.[88] noted the presence of CFA on a number of MD cell lines, and Powe.i et al.[89] and Trembicki et al.[90] reported that MD cell lines are heterogeneous for the expression of CFA determinants. It is not known if RP9 cells express CFA and how the CFA determinants on these cells are different from those on NK-cell-resistant cells.

The role of suppressor cells in inhibition of NK activity has been reported in Japanese quail.[91] Quail injected with chicken or quail amniotic fluid had reduced NK activity which was attributed to the inhibition of activity by suppressor cells stimulated by α-fetoprotein present in the amniotic fluid. The suppressor cells were nonadherent and were inactivated by treatment with antithymocyte serum and complement.[92] The mechanism of suppressor-cell action is not known, and possible effects of amniotic fluid on chicken NK reactivity has not been reported.

Quéré et al.[93] reported that thymulin, a nonapeptide involved in T-cell maturation and differentiation, suppressed NK-cell activity in MDV-infected birds. They inoculated female chickens of line GB1 ($B^{13}B^{13}$) with the oncogenic HPRS-16 strain of MDV and subsequently inoculated both infected and control birds with thymulin. This treatment reduced the level of NK activity against RP9 and the syngeneic MDCC-PA9 in MDV-infected, thymulin-treated birds compared to untreated MDV-infected birds or control birds. Injection with thymulin did not alter the development of tumors. These investigators[21,93,94] have consistently found cytotoxic activity against RP9 as well as allogeneic and syngeneic MD cell lines at the time of tumor development.

III. NATURAL KILLER CELL ACTIVITY IN AVIAN SPECIES OTHER THAN THE CHICKEN

Besides the chicken, the Japanese quail (*Coturnix coturnix japonica*) is the only other member of the avian species in which NK cells have been described.[18,78] Yamada et al.[78] used a microcytotoxicity assay in which target cells were adhered to the bottom of the wells of microtiter plates, and monolayers of target cells were incubated with effector cells for 16 h. After the end of the incubation period, the residual target cells in the wells were counted to quantitate the cytotoxic effect of the effector cells.

Spleen cells from normal, 4-week-old quail lysed a number of target-cell types which included normal quail embryo cells, quail embryo cells transformed with Schmidt-Ruppin strain of Rous sarcoma virus (RSV), established quail cell lines derived from cells transformed by defective Bryan high titer strain of RSV, and tumors induced by methylcholanthrene. The nature of the target antigen(s) against which NK cells reacted was not determined. The range of susceptible target cells indicated that the cytotoxicity may have been directed against embryonic antigens normally present in embryonic tissues or newly expressed on transformed cells.

The cytotoxic activity was higher in 4-week-old than in 1-week-old quail, and effector cells were nonadherent and were not inactivated by treatment with rabbit serum containing antibodies against quail T cells or quail immunoglobulins. As in chickens and mice,[12,95,96] quail NK cells were thermolabile, and treatment of the effector cells for 1 h at 56°C abrogated their cytotoxic activity. The level of activity of NK cells in the quail spleen significantly dropped if the quails were injected intravenously with amniotic fluid from quail embryos or from 8-d-old embryonating chicken eggs. The inhibition of NK activity was attributed to the appearance of suppressor cells in the spleen of amniotic fluid-treated quails. The suppressor-cell inducer was later identified to be α-fetoprotein present in the amniotic fluid.[91]

Fleischer[19] noted that PBL and spleen of normal quail were cytotoxic for a number of mammalian and avian target cells in a 4-h ^{51}Cr-release assay. The cytotoxicity was higher with PBL than with spleen cells. The relationship of this spontaneous cytotoxic activity to NK cells was not clear because the effector cells were adherent and phagocytic and thus resembled macrophages.

Although NK cells have been detected in quail, the role of these cells in defense against neoplastic or nonneoplastic diseases of quail needs to be examined further. Yamada and Hayami[91] noted that quail, treated with amniotic fluid of chicken or quail origin developed RSV-induced tumors with a shorter latent period than that observed in untreated quail. The rapid tumor development in the treated group was attributed to inhibition of NK activity by the amniotic fluid.

Presence of NK cells in chickens and quail indicates that this system may constitute an important line of natural defense in birds. Additional studies on the distribution of NK activity in other birds may be of value to ascertain the phylogenetic development of NK cells and the importance of this line of natural defense among members of the avian species.

IV. ROLE OF NATURAL KILLER CELLS IN DEFENSE AGAINST DISEASE

Much of the information on the possible role of NK-cell natural defense against disease has come from studies on viral or transplantable tumor systems in chickens. Possible involvement of NK cells in defense against nontumoral disease conditions has not been adequately examined in birds.

Lam and Linna[10,11] presented evidence that adoptive transfer of spleen cells containing NK cells protected chickens against metastatic progression of the JMV transplantable tumor. This tumor cell line was developed by rapidly passing cells of MDV-induced tumors in embryonated chicken eggs.[97] JMV cells lack detectable infectious MDV or viral antigens but contain MDV genome,[98] and a viral phosphorylated protein can be induced in these cells.[99] The inoculation of JMV cells results in rapidly metastasizing tumors that generally kill chickens within 5 to 10 d. Newly hatched chickens are most susceptible to the lethal effect of JMV; if inoculation with the tumor cell is delayed until the chickens are 4 weeks of age or older, the incidence of progressive tumors and mortality is much reduced.[100] Adoptive transfer of spleen cells from JMV-resistant 7- to 8-week-old chickens into newly hatched recipients resulted in resistance of the recipient chickens to a lethal dose of the JMV cells.[10,11] The protective spleen cells were nonadherent, radiosensitive, expressed surface Fc receptors, and resisted treatment with polyclonal anti-T-cell and anti-B-cell serums prepared in rabbits and complement. Based on the characteristics of the protective cells, the authors concluded that age-related resistance to the JMV transplant in chickens may be mediated by NK-like cells. Although these data suggest the presence of NK cells in spleens, the possibility cannot be excluded that some of the transferred cells (e.g., monocytes, dendritic cells) were able to enhance maturation of the recipient's immune system or produce antitumor products such as tumor necrosis factor.[101] It would be of interest to repeat the transfer experiments using antimacrophage monoclonal antibody[101] and fluorescence-activated cell-sorter to examine the possibility of macrophage involvement in protection against JMV. It is noteworthy that the JMV-derived RPL-1 cell line is poorly lysed by avian NK cells in *in vitro* assays.[12,15,19]

There is indirect evidence that NK cells may also regulate RSV-induced local tumor development in the wing-web of quail. As noted above, α-fetoprotein present in chicken amniotic fluid reduced NK cell activity of quail spleen cells below normal levels. When Yamada and Hayami[91] treated quail with α-fetoprotein before inoculating RSV into the wing-web, the tumors appeared at the site of virus inoculation faster than in quail that did not receive α-fetoprotein. Faster tumor development was attributed to inhibition of NK cell defense in treated quail. Additional evidence for a role of NK cells in RSV-induced local lesions was presented by Wainberg et al.[25] These authors cultured tumor cells from RSV-induced wing-web tumors and used the cultured cells as targets for NK cell lysis. The tumor target cells obtained from regressing tumors were sensitive to NK cell lysis, whereas target cells from progressing tumors were resistant. Progressing tumors contained appreciably higher numbers of virus-producing macrophage-like cells than did the regressing tumors.[102] The resistance of these tumors to NK lysis was not due to viral interference,[25] although others had suggested that production of ALV may make cells resistant to NK lysis (please see Section II.A.1). An alternate explanation may be that the macrophages present in the progressing tumors down-regulated NK cells. This result suggested that tumor regression may be regulated by intratumoral NK cell activity.

An interesting relationship between spleen NK activity and disease response was noted in resistant and susceptible chickens exposed to MDV. Marek's disease virus is a naturally occurring herpesvirus causing T-cell lymphomas in chickens.[103] Although most commercial chickens are susceptible to tumor induction by MDV, the susceptibility is influenced by several factors. Genetic background plays an important role in defense against the disease. Genetically resistant chickens become infected with MDV and develop persistent viremia but do not develop progressive tumors.[104] The susceptibility of chickens to MD tumors is also influenced by the age at which virus exposure occurs. Newly hatched chickens are most susceptible but become resistant as they become older.[105-107] Resistance against MD tumors may be induced by vaccinating chickens with HVT, a virus serologically related to MDV, or with serotype 2 MDV strains.[108] Sharma[69] compared NK levels in a 4-h ^{51}Cr-release assay in spleens of susceptible chickens undergoing progressive MD with those resistant to MD either due to genetic background or prior vaccination with HVT. Chickens of genetic line P (highly susceptible to MD) and line N (highly resistant to MD) were inoculated at 6 d of age with a pathogenic isolate of MDV and disease response, and NK levels of spleen cells were chronologically monitored. The virus caused progressive debilitating disease in line P chickens. Lesions characterized by extensive gross and microscopic lymphoid-cell proliferation in peripheral nerves and gonads were detected in most birds starting at 3 weeks after exposure. By 8 weeks after virus exposure, all line P chickens had died due to acute MD. Progressive disease in line P chickens was accompanied by a significant drop in NK-cell levels starting at 2 weeks after virus exposure and depressed NK reactivity of spleen cells persisted through the course of the disease. The inhibition of NK activity in diseased line P chickens was most prominent at 7 weeks of age, the age when NK expression in normal virus-free chickens had reached maximal levels.[12,15] In contrast with line P, MDV did not cause progressive disease in line N chickens, and these chickens developed elevated NK levels following virus exposure. On the other hand, Quéré and Dambrine,[94] using a ^{3}H-proline assay, noted that NK cell activity increased as MD tumors progressed. Differences in the experimental condition between the studies of Sharma[69] and Quéré and Dambrine[94] may be responsible for conflicting results.

A similar relationship of NK activity and resistance or susceptibility to MD was noted in chickens that were protected against MD by vaccination with HVT.[69] Line P chickens were vaccinated with HVT prior to inoculation with pathogenic MDV. Vaccination prevented progressive MD in line P chickens and caused persistently augmented NK levels. Inoculation of HVT alone in lines N and P chickens resulted in elevated NK-cell activity. Heller and Schat[63] noted that another MD vaccine virus, SB-1, also enhanced NK cell activity in chickens of lines N and P. In line N chickens, the NK cell enhancement was higher if HVT and SB-1 were given in combination than when either virus was given alone. Protection studies have shown that bivalent vaccines containing HVT and SB-1 act synergistically and are more protective than single vaccines against certain highly virulent field isolates of MDV.[108]

The above data suggest a relationship between NK cell expression in the spleen and resistance to MD. Elevated NK levels were associated with resistance and depressed NK levels with susceptibility to MD. It is not known if this is a cause or effect relationship. Several viral infections have been reported to alter NK cell activity in animals[61,109-111] and enhanced susceptibility to herpes simplex virus in humans may be associated with low NK cell reactivity.[112]

Functional NK cells were also detected in solid MD tumors.[30] Cells comprising solid metastatic tumors induced by MDV were compared with those comprising regressive tumors induced by local subcutaneous injections of MDCT-RP3, a transplantable cell line derived by serial *in vivo* passage of MDV-derived ovarian tumor.[113] Tumor masses from both types of tumors were dispersed by enzymatic treatment, and cells were tested for cytotoxic activity against RP9 target cells in a 4-h ^{51}Cr-release assay. NK cell reactivity was recovered from viral, as well as transplantable, tumors although the incidence and the levels of NK cell cytotoxicity were greater in the regressive tumors than in the progressive tumors. Furthermore, in the regressive tumors, the NK levels were higher in the tumor than in the spleen of tumor-bearing chickens. Lymphoid cells with diverse functions have been recovered from MD lymphomas,[30,114] and complex immune interactions may be involved in tumor regression. The presence of NK cells in regressing MD tumors indicates that these cells may be involved in tumor regression.

Infection with *Eimeria acervulina* and *E. maxima* may also influence the level of NK activity in the spleen and intestinal epithelium of chickens.[52] Splenic and IEL NK cell activity was generally suppressed during the first few days after infection, but increased above background levels between 7 and 14 d postinoculation. Secondary infection with *Eimeria* resulted in enhanced NK cell responses as early as 1 d postinoculation. It is of interest to note that FP strain chickens have a higher level of resistance to secondary *E. maxima* infection than do the SC strain of chickens.[115] The FP strain chickens also had a significantly higher level of NK cell activity after secondary challenge with *E. maxima* than did SC chickens.[52]

V. ANTIBODY-DEPENDENT CELL-MEDIATED CYTOTOXICITY

Cells mediating ADCC constitute another mechanism of natural defense against disease. This activity is quantitated by long-term ^{51}Cr-release assays. The effector cells, present in spleen or PBL of unstimulated animals, can kill target cells. Antibody plays a central role in mediating ADCC. The Fab end of the antibody attaches to the antigen on the surface of the target cell and the Fc end attaches to the Fc receptor present on the surface of the effector cell. Thus, the specificity of the ADCC reactivity is determined by the interaction of the antibody with the antigen(s) present on the target cells. The effector cells may have diverse characteristics and may resemble the LGL associated with NK activity.[116,117]

ADCC has been reported in chickens, quail, and duck.[19,118,119] The effector cells of chicken ADCC were adherent, Fc receptor-bearing, radiosensitive, and non-T, non-B cells.[119] The cells may be phagocytic or nonphagocytic.[19,118,120] ADCC reactivity was present in agammaglobulinemic chickens.[120,121]

The importance of ADCC in defense against disease in the avian species has not been examined in detail. ADCC activity has been reported in chickens infected with MDV, HVT, and human adenovirus.[122-124] Leukocyte-derived IFN may enhance ADCC.[125]

VI. SUMMARY

A well-developed NK cell system has been identified in normal, unimmunized chickens and quail. The effector cells of this natural immune reactivity are present in the spleen and PBL. There are conflicting data on the characteristics of avian NK effector cells. Several IL-2-dependent cell lines of chicken NK cells were maintained *in vitro* for several months. Studies on the characteristics of the *in vitro*-propagated NK cells have revealed that the cells are LGL and lack immunoglobulin receptors. Surface antigens expressed on these cells include CLA-1 and perhaps CD4, CD5, and CD8. A better definition of surface markers on avian NK cells must await development of cloned NK cell lines.

NK cell activity appears to be age dependent in chickens and quail. The rate of progressive increase in NK levels with increasing age may be genetically controlled. Infection with certain viruses elevates NK reactivity although the mechanism of elevation is not clear. Interferon, a potent booster of mammalian NK activity, does not seem to consistently affect avian NK cells. Progressive disease in chickens or suppressor cells induced by inoculation of α-fetoproteins in quail and CFA in chickens have been reported to depress NK cells. Data from studies with MD and RSV indicate that NK cells may play a protective role in natural defense against tumor progression in birds. In addition to NK cells, effector cells of ADCC have also been detected in chickens, quail, and ducks. The importance of ADCC in natural immune defense against disease in birds needs to be established.

ACKNOWLEDGMENTS

We are grateful to Ms. Pamela Farr and Mrs. Gwen Troise for assistance in preparation of this manuscript.

REFERENCES

1. **Kawase, I., Urdal, D.L., Brooks, C. G., and Henney, C. S.,** Selective depletion of NK cell activity *in vivo* and its effect on the growth of NK-sensitive and NK-resistant tumor cell variants, *Int. J. Cancer,* 29, 567, 1982.
2. **Riccardi, C., Pucceti, P., Santoni, A., and Herberman, R. B.,** Rapid *in vivo* assay of mouse natural killer cell activity, *J. Natl. Cancer Inst.,* 63, 1041, 1979.
3. **Warner, J. F. and Dennert, G.,** *In vivo* function of a cloned cell line with NK activity: effects on bone marrow transplants, tumor development and metastasis, *Nature (London),* 30, 31, 1982.
4. **Timonen, T., Ortaldo, J. R., and Herberman, R. B.,** Characteristics of human large granular lymphocytes and relationship to natural killer and K cells, *J. Exp. Med.,* 153, 569, 1982.
5. **Kaplan, J.,** NK cell lineage and target specificity: a unifying concept, *Immunol. Today,* 7, 10, 1986.
6. **London, L., Perussia, B., and Trinchiere, G.,** Surface phenotype of resting and activated human natural killer cells, in *Natural Immunity: Cancer and Biological Response Modification,* Lotzova, E. and Herberman, R. B., Eds., S. Karger, Basel, 1986, 1.
7. **Suzuki, R., Handa, K., Itoh, K., and Kumagai, K.,** Natural killer cells as a response to interleukin-2. I. Proliferative response and establishment of cloned cells, *J. Immunol.,* 130, 981, 1983.
8. **Timonen, T., Ortaldo, J., and Herberman, R. B.,** Cultures of purified human NK cells, in *NK Cells and Other Natural Effector Cells,* Herberman, R. B., Ed., Academic Press, New York, 1982, 821.
9. **Trinchieri, G.,** Biology of natural killer cells, *Adv. Immunol.,* 47, 187, 1989.
10. **Lam, K. M. and Linna, T. J.,** Transfer of natural resistance to Marek's disease (JMV) with non-immune spleen cells. I. Studies of cell population transferring resistance, *Int. J. Cancer,* 24, 662, 1979.
11. **Lam, K. M. and Linna, T. J.,** Transfer of natural resistance to Marek's disease (JMV) with non-immune spleen cells. II. Further characterization of protecting cell population, *J. Immunol.,* 125, 715, 1980.
12. **Sharma, J. M. and Coulson, B. D.,** Presence of natural killer cells in specific-pathogen-free chickens, *J. Natl. Cancer Inst.,* 63, 527, 1979.
13. **Sharma, J. M. and Okazaki, W.,** Natural killer cell activity in chickens: target cell analysis and effect of antithymocyte serum on effector cells, *Infect. Immun.,* 31, 1078, 1981.
14. **Okazaki, W., Witter, R. L., Romero, C., Nazerian, K., Sharma, J. M., Fadly, A., and Ewert, D.,** Induction of lymphoid leukosis transplantable tumours and the establishment of lymphoblastoid cell lines, *Avian Pathol.,* 9, 311, 1980.
15. **Heller, E. D. and Schat, K. A.,** Inhibition of natural killer activity in chickens by Marek's disease virus-transformed cell lines, in *Proc. 2nd Int. Symp. Marek's Disease,* Calnek, B. W. and Spencer, J. L., Eds., American Association of Avian Pathologists, Kennett Square, PA, 1985, 286.
16. **Schat, K. A., Chen, C.-L., Lillehoj, H., Calnek, B. W., and Weinstock, D.,** Characterization of Marek's disease cell lines with monoclonal antibodies specific for cytotoxic and helper T cells, in *Advances in Marek's Disease Research,* Kato, S., Horiuchi, T., Mikami, T., and Hirai, K., Eds., Proc. 3rd Int. Symp. Marek's Disease, Japanese Association on Marek's Disease, Osaka, Japan, 1988, 220.
17. **Schat, K. A., Chen, C. L. H., Char, D., and Calnek, B. W.,** manuscript in preparation.
18. **Leibold, W., Janotte, G., and Peter, H. H.,** Spontaneous cell-mediated cytotoxicity (SCMC) in various mammalian species and chickens: selective reaction pattern and different mechanisms, *Scand. J. Immunol.,* 11, 203, 1980.
19. **Fleischer, B.,** Effector cells in avian spontaneous and antibody-dependent cell-mediated cytotoxicity, *J. Immunol.,* 125, 1161, 1980.
20. **Waytes, T., Bacon, L., and Rose, N.,** Use of indium-111 in antibody-dependent complement-mediated cytotoxicity assay for the detection of B locus alloantigens on chicken lymphocytes, *Transplantation,* 29, 201, 1980.

21. **Dambrine, G., Coudert, F., and Cauchy, L.,** Cell-mediated cytotoxicity in chickens infected with Marek's disease virus and the herpes virus of turkeys, in *Resistance and Immunity to Marek's Disease*, Biggs, P. M., Ed., Commission of the European Communities, Luxembourg, 1980, 320.

22. **Schat, K. A. and Calnek, B. W.,** *In vitro* cytotoxicity of spleen lymphocytes against Marek's disease tumour cells: induction by SB-1, an apparently nononcogenic Marek's Disease virus, in *Resistance and Immunity to Marek's Disease*, Biggs, P. M., Ed., Commission of the European Communities, Luxembourg, 1980, 301.

23. **Schat, K. A. and Murthy, K. K.,** *In vitro* cytotoxicity against Marek's disease lymphoblastoid cell lines after enzymatic removal of Marek's disease tumor-associated surface antigen, *J. Virol.*, 34, 130, 1980.

24. **Traill, K. N., Bock, G., Boyd, R., and Wick, G.,** Chicken thrombocytes. Isolation, serological and functional characterization using the fluorescence activated cell sorter, *Dev. Comp. Immunol.*, 7, 11, 1983.

25. **Wainberg, M. A., Beaupre, S., Beiss, B., and Israel, E.,** Differential susceptibility of avian sarcoma cells from different periods of tumor growth to natural killer cell activity, *Cancer Res.*, 43, 4774, 1983.

26. **Chai, J. Y. and Lillehoj, H. S.,** Isolation and functional characterization of chicken intestinal intraepithelial lymphocytes showing natural killer cell activity against tumor target cells, *Immunology*, 63, 117, 1988.

27. **Lillehoj, H. S. and Chai, J. Y.,** Comparative natural killer cell activities of thymic, bursal, splenic and intestinal intraepithelial lymphocytes of chickens, *Dev. Comp. Immunol.*, 12, 629, 1988.

28. **Myers, T. J. and Schat, K. A.,** Natural killer cell activity of chicken intraepithelial leukocytes against rotavirus-infected target cells, *Vet. Immunol. Immunopathol.*, in press.

29. **Weinstock, D., Schat, K. A., and Calnek, B. W.,** Cytotoxic T lymphocytes in reticuloendotheliosis virus-infected chickens, *Eur. J. Immunol.*, 19, 267, 1989.

30. **Sharma, J. M.,** Presence of adherent cytotoxic cells and nonadherent natural killer cells in progressive and regressive Marek's disease tumors, *Vet. Immunol. Immunopathol.*, 5, 125, 1983.

31. **Baccarini, M., Hao, L., Decker, T., and Lohmann-Matthes, M. L.,** Macrophage precursors as natural killer cells against tumor cells and microorganisms, *Nat. Immun. Cell Growth Regul.*, 7, 316, 1988.

32. **Lohmann-Matthes, M. L., Domzig, W., Zahringer, M., and Lang, H.,** K cell and NK cell-like activity of macrophage precursor cells, *Behring Inst. Mitt.*, 65, 26, 1980.

33. **Mandi, Y., Seprenyi, G., Pusztai, R., and Beladi, I.,** Are granulocytes the main effector cells of natural cytotoxicity in chickens?, *Immunobiology*, 170, 284, 1985.

34. **Kaaden, O. R., Lange, S., and Stiburek, B.,** Establishment and characterization of chicken embryo fibroblast clone LSCC-H32, *In Vitro*, 18, 827, 1982.

35. **Mandi, Y., Pusztai, R., Baranji, K., Seprenyi, G., Tarodi, B., Bakay, M., and Beladi, I.,** The role of interferon in the adenovirus-induced augmentation of granulocyte-mediated cytotoxicity in chicken, *Immunobiology*, 174, 210, 1987.

36. **Mandi, Y., Veromaa, T., Baranji, K., Miczak, A., Beladi, I., and Toivanen, P.,** Granulocyte-specific monoclonal antibody inhibiting cytotoxicity reactions in the chicken, *Immunobiology*, 174, 292, 1987.

37. **Ruiz-Cabello, F., Nevot, M. A. L., Garrido, A., and Garrido, F.,** A study of GRM1 monoclonal antibody that reacts with natural killer cells and granulocytes, *Nat. Immun. Cell Growth Regul.*, 6, 99, 1987.

38. **Ting, C. C., Yang, S. S., and Hargrove, M. E.,** Effect of interleukin 2 on cytotoxic effectors, *Cell. Immunol.*, 73, 275, 1982.

39. **Kedar, E., Ikejiri, B. L., Sredni, B., Bonavida, B., and Herberman, R. B.,** Propagation of mouse cytotoxic clones with characteristics of natural killer (NK) cells, *Cell. Immunol.*, 69, 305, 1982.

40. **Sheehy, J. J., Quintieri, F. B., Leung, D. Y. M., Geha, R. S., Dubey, D. P., Limmer, C. E., and Yunis, E. J.,** A human large granular lymphocyte clone with natural killer-like activity and T cell-like surface markers, *J. Immunol.*, 130, 524, 1983.

41. **Olabuenaga, S. E., Brooks, C. G., Gillis, S., and Henney, C. S.,** Interleukin 2 is not sufficient for the continuous growth of cloned NK-like cytotoxic cell lines, *J. Immunol.*, 131, 2386, 1983.

42. **van de Griend, R. J., Goedegebuure, S. P., van Krimpen, B. A., and Bolhuis, R. L. H.,** Cloning of human CD3 + T cells and CD3 − natural killer cells and requirements for long-term expansion, *Transplantation*, 20, 149, 1988.

43. **Hercend, T. E. L., Reinherz, S., Meuer, S. F., Schlossman, S. F., and Ritz, J.,** Phenotypic and functional heterogeneity of human cloned natural killer cell lines, *Nature (London)*, 301, 158, 1983.

44. **Moretta, A., Pantaleo, G., Mingari, M. C., Melioli, G., Moretta, L., and Cerottini, J. C.,** Assignment of human natural killer (NK) like cells to the T cell lineage. Single allospecific T cell clones lyse specific or NK sensitive target cells via distinct recognition structure, *Eur. J. Immunol.*, 14, 121, 1984.

45. **Thurlow, P. J., McArthur, G., and McKenzie, I. F. C.,** Investigation of T and natural killer cell function with monoclonal antibodies, *Transplantation*, 41, 104, 1986.

46. **Schmidt, R. W., Murray, C., Daley, J. F., Schlossman, S. F., and Ritz, J.,** A subset of natural killer cells in peripheral blood displays a mature T cell phenotype, *J. Exp. Med.*, 164, 351, 1986.

47. **Minato, N., Hattori, M., Sudo, T., Kano, S., Miura, Y., Suda, J., and Suda, T.,** Differentiation *in vitro* of T3 + large granular lymphocytes with characteristic cytotoxic activity from an isolated hematopoietic progenitor colony, *J. Exp. Med.*, 167, 762, 1988.

48. **Schat, K. A., Calnek, B. W., and Weinstock, D.,** Cultivation and characterization of avian lymphocytes with natural killer cell activity, *Avian Pathol.*, 15, 539, 1986.

49. **Schat, K. A., Calnek, B. W., and Weinstock, D.,** Cultured avian lymphocytes with natural killer cell activity, in *Avian Immunology*, Vol. 238, Weber, W. T. and Ewert, D. L., Eds., Alan R. Liss, New York, 1987, 157.

50. **Calnek, B. W., Shek, W. R., and Schat, K. A.,** Latent infections with Marek's disease virus and turkey herpesvirus, *J. Natl. Cancer Inst.*, 66, 585, 1981.

51. **Chen, C. H. and Cooper, M. D.,** Identification of cell surface molecules on chicken lymphocytes with monoclonal antibodies, in *Avian Immunology: Basis and Practice*, Vol. 1, Toivanen, A. and Toivanen, P., Eds., CRC Press, Boca Raton, FL, 1987, 137.

52. **Lillehoj, H. S.,** Intestinal intraepithelial and splenic natural killer cell responses to Eimerian infections in inbred chickens, *Infect. Immun.*, 57, 1879, 1989.

53. **Lillehoj, H. S., Lillehoj, E. P., Weinstock, D., and Schat, K. A.,** Functional and biochemical characterization of avian T lymphocyte antigens identified by monoclonal antibodies, *Eur. J. Immunol.*, 18, 2059, 1988.

53a. **Nigro, R. P. and Schat, K. A.,** unpublished data.

54. **Hackett, J., Jr., Bennett, M., Koo, G. C., and Kumar, V.,** Origin and differentiation of natural killer cells. III. Relationship between the precursors and effectors of natural killer and natural cytotoxic activity, *Immunol. Res.*, 5, 16, 1986.

55. **Trinchieri, G., Matsumoto-Kobayashi, M., Clark, S. C., Seehra, J., London, L., and Perussia, B.,** Response of human peripheral blood natural killer cells to interleukin-2, *J. Exp. Med.*, 160, 1147, 1984.

56. **Phillips, H. J. and Lanier, L. L.,** A model for the differentiation of human natural killer cells, *J. Exp. Med.*, 161, 1464, 1985.

57. **Ortaldo, J. R., Mason, A. T., Jerard, J. P., Henderson, L. E., Farrar, W., Hopkins, R. F., III, Herberman, R. B., and Rabin, H.,** Effects of natural and recombinant IL-2 on regulation of interferon gamma production and natural killer activity: lack of involvement of the tac antigen for these immunoregulatory effects, *J. Immunol.*, 133, 779, 1984.

58. **Trinchieri, G., Santoli, G., and Koprowski, H.,** Spontaneous cell-mediated cytotoxicity in humans. Role of interferon and immunoglobulins, *J. Immunol.*, 120, 1849, 1978.

59. **Djeu, H. Y., Heinbaugh, J. A., Holden, H. T., and Herberman, R. B.,** Augmentation of mouse natural killer activity by interferon and interferon inducers, *J. Immunol.*, 122, 175, 1979.

60. **Gidlund, M., Oru, A., Wigzell, H., Senk, A., and Gresser, I.,** Enhanced NK cell activity in mice injected with interferon and interferon inducers, *Nature (London)*, 273, 759, 1978.

61. **Ding, A. H. J. and Lam, K. M.,** Enhancement by interferon of chicken splenocyte natural killer cell activity against Marek's disease tumor cells, *Vet. Immunol. Immunopathol.*, 11, 65, 1986.

62. **Portnoy, J. and Merigan, T. C.,** The effect of interferon and interferon inducers on avian influenza, *J. Infect. Dis.*, 124, 545, 1971.

63. **Heller, E. D. and Schat, K. A.,** Enhancement of natural killer cell activity by Marek's disease vaccines, *Avian Pathol.*, 16, 51, 1987.

64. **Sharma, J. M.,** unpublished data.

65. **Schat, K. A.,** unpublished data.

66. **Gelb, J., Eidson, C. S., Fletcher, O. J., and Kleven, S. H.,** Studies on interferon induction by infectious bursal disease virus (IBDV). II. Interferon production in white leghorn chickens infected with an attenuated or pathogenic isolant of IBDV, *Avian Dis.*, 23, 634, 1979.

67. **Gelb, J., Eidson, C. S., and Kleven, S. H.,** Studies on interferon induction by infectious bursal disease virus (IBDV). I. Interferon production in chicken embryo cell cultures infected with IBDV, *Avian Dis.*, 23, 485, 1979.

68. **Sharma, J. M. and Lee, L. F.,** Effect of infectious bursal disease on natural killer cell activity and mitogenic response of chicken lymphoid cells: role of adherent cells in cellular immune suppression, *Infect. Immun.*, 42, 747, 1983.

69. **Sharma, J. M.,** Natural killer cell activity in chickens exposed to Marek's disease virus: inhibition of activity in susceptible chickens and enhancement of activity in resistant and vaccinated chickens, *Avian Dis.*, 25, 882, 1981.

70. **Sharma, J. M., Lee, L. F., and Wakenell, P. S.,** Comparative viral, immunologic and pathologic responses of chickens inoculated with herpesvirus of turkeys as embryos or at hatch, *Am. J. Vet. Res.*, 45, 1619, 1984.

71. **Hong, C. C. and Sevoian, M.,** Interferon production and host resistance to type II avian (Marek's) leukosis virus (JM strain), *Appl. Microbiol.*, 22, 818, 1971.

72. **Kaleta, E. F. and Bankowski, R. A.,** Production of circulating and cell bound interferon in chickens by type 1 and 2 plaque-producing agents of the Cal-1 strain of Marek's disease herpesvirus and herpesvirus of turkeys, *Am. J. Vet. Res.*, 33, 573, 1972.

73. **Kaleta, E. F. and Bankowski, R. A.,** Production of interferon by the Cal-1 and turkey herpesvirus strains associated with Marek's disease, *Am. J. Vet. Res.*, 33, 567, 1972.

74. **Vengris, V. E. and Mare, C. J.,** Protection of chickens against Marek's disease virus JM-V strain with statolon and exogenous interferon, *Avian Dis.,* 17, 758, 1973.

75. **Sharma, J. M.,** *In situ* production of interferon in tissues of chickens exposed as embryos to turkey herpesvirus and Marek's disease virus, *Am. J. Vet. Res.,* 50, 882, 1989.

76. **Sharma, J. M.,** Interferon production *in vitro* by spleen cells of chickens undergoing early lympholytic phase of Marek's disease virus infection, in *Advances in Marek's Disease Research,* Kato, S., Horiuchi, T., Mikami, T., and Hirai, K., Eds., Proc. 3rd Int. Symp. Marek's Disease, Japanese Association on Marek's Disease, Osaka, 1988, 227.

77. **Calnek, B. W., Carlisle, J. C., Fabricant, J., Murthy, K. K., and Schat, K. A.,** Comparative pathogenesis studies with oncogenic and nononcogenic Marek's disease viruses and turkey herpesvirus, *Am. J. Vet. Res.,* 40, 541, 1979.

78. **Yamada, A., Hayami, M., Yamanouchi, K., and Fujiwara, I.,** Detection of natural killer cells in Japanese quails, *Int. J. Cancer,* 26, 381, 1980.

79. **Uksila, J., Lassila, O., Hirvonen, T., and Toivanen, P.,** Development of natural killer cell function in the human fetus, *J. Immunol.,* 130, 153, 1983.

80. **Boyd, R. and Wick, G.,** Killer cells in the chicken: a microcytoxicity assay using antigen-coated erythrocytes as targets, *J. Immunol. Methods,* 35, 233, 1980.

81. **Boyd, R. L., Cole, R. K., and Wick, G.,** Genetically-controlled severity of autoimmune thyroiditis in obese strain (OS) chickens is expressed at both the humoral and cellular effector mechanism levels, *Immunol. Commun.,* 12, 263, 1983.

82. **Cudkowicz, G. and Hochman, P. S.,** Do natural killer cells engage in regulated reactions against self to ensure homeostasis?, *Immunol. Rev.,* 44, 13, 1979.

83. **Kline, K. and Sanders, B. G.,** Developmental profile of chicken splenic lymphocyte responsiveness to Con A and PHA and studies on chicken splenic and bone marrow cells capable of inhibiting mitogen-stimulated blastogenic responses of adult splenic lymphocytes, *J. Immunol.,* 125, 1792, 1980.

84. **Sharma, J. M.,** Presence of natural suppressor cells in the chicken embryo spleen and the effect of virus infection of the embryo on suppressor cell activity, *Vet. Immunol. Immunopathol.,* 19, 51, 1988.

85. **Ohashi, K., Mikami, T., Kodama, H., and Izawa, H.,** Suppression of NK activity of spleen cells by chicken fetal antigens present on Marek's disease lymphoblastoid cell line cells, *Int. J. Cancer,* 40, 378, 1987.

86. **Ohashi, K., Mikami, T., Higashihara, T., Kodama, H., and Izawa, H.,** Monoclonal antibody to chicken fetal antigen on Marek's disease lymphoblastoid cell line (MDCC-MSB1), *Cancer Res.,* 46, 5858, 1986.

87. **Dietert, R. R.,** Oncodevelopmental antigens in avian species, in *Avian Immunology: Basis and Practice,* Vol. 2, Toivanen, A. and Toivanen, P., Eds., CRC Press, Boca Raton, FL, 1987, 71.

88. **Murthy, K. K., Dietert, R. R., and Calnek, B. W.,** Demonstration of chicken fetal antigen (CFA) on normal splenic lymphocytes, Marek's disease lymphoblastoid cell lines and other neoplasms, *Int. J. Cancer,* 24, 349, 1979.

89. **Powell, P. C., Hartley, K. J., Mastill, B. M., and Rennie, M.,** The occurrence of chicken fetal antigen after infection with Marek's disease virus in three strains of chickens, *Oncodev. Biol. Med.,* 4, 261, 1984.

90. **Trembicki, K. A., Qureshi, M. A., and Dietert, R. R.,** Differentiation properties of avian tumor cell lines: analysis using chicken fetal antigen and other markers, *Cancer Res.,* 44, 2616, 1984.

91. **Yamada, A. and Hayami, M.,** Suppression of natural killer cell activity by chicken a-fetoprotein in Japanese quails, *J. Natl. Cancer Inst.,* 70, 735, 1983.

92. **Yamada, A. and Hayami, M.,** Induction and characterization of splenic suppressor cells directed to natural killer cells in Japanese quail, *Jpn. J. Med. Sci. Biol.,* 34, 95, 1981.

93. **Quéré, P., Dambrine, G., and Bach, M. A.,** Influence of thymic hormone on cell-mediated and humoral immune responses in Marek's disease, *Vet. Microbiol.,* 19, 53, 1989.

94. **Quéré, P. and Dambrine, G.,** Development of anti-tumoral cell-mediated cytotoxicity during the course of Marek's disease in chickens, *Ann. Rech. Vet.,* 19, 193, 1988.

95. **Herberman, R. B., Nunn, M. E., Holden, H. T., and Lavrin, D. H.,** Natural cytotoxic reactivity of mouse lymphoid cells against syngeneic and allogeneic tumors. II. Characterization of effector cells, *Int. J. Cancer,* 16, 230, 1975.

96. **Wolfe, S. A., Tracey, D. E., and Henney, C. S.,** BCG induced murine effector cells. II. Characterization of natural killer cells in peritoneal exudate, *J. Immunol.,* 119, 1152, 1977.

97. **Sevoian, M., Larose, R. N., and Chamberlain, D. M.,** Avian lymphomatosis: increased pathogenicity of JM virus, in Proc. 101st Annu. Meet. AVMA, Chicago, IL, 1964, 342.

98. **Stephens, E. A., Witter, R. L., Lee, L. F., Sharma, J. M., Nazerian, K., and Longenecker, B. M.,** Characteristics of JMV Marek's disease tumor: a non-productively infected transplantable cell lacking in rescuable virus, *J. Natl. Cancer Inst.,* 57, 865, 1976.

99. **Ikuta, K., Nakajima, K., Naito, M., Ann, S. H., Ueda, S., Kato, S., and Hirai, K.,** Identification of Marek's disease virus-specific antigens in Marek's disease lymphoblastoid cell lines using monoclonal antibody against virus-specific phosphorylated polypeptides, *Int. J. Cancer,* 35, 257, 185.

100. **Kenyon, A. J., Sevoian, M., Horwitz, M., Jones, N. D., and Helmboldt, C. F.,** Lymphoproliferative disease of fowl immunologic factors associated with passage of lymphoblastic leukemia (JM-V), *Avian Dis.,* 13, 585, 1969.

101. **Jeurissen, S. H. M., Janse, E. M., Koch, G., and de Boer, G. F.,** The monoclonal antibody CV-CHNL-68.1 recognizes cells of the monocytes macrophage lineage in chickens, *Dev. Comp. Immunol.,* 12, 855, 1988.

102. **Wainberg, M. A., Beiss, B., Fong, H., Beaupre, S., and Menezes, J.,** Involvement of macrophage-like cells in growth of tumors induced by avian sarcoma virus, *Cancer Res.,* 43, 1550, 1983.

103. **Calnek, B. W. and Witter, R. L.,** Marek's disease, in *Diseases of Poultry,* Hofstad, M. S., Barnes, J. H., Calnek, B. W., Reid, W. M., and Yoder, H. E., Eds., Iowa State University Press, Ames, 1984, 326.

104. **Sharma, J. M. and Stone, H. A.,** Genetic resistance to Marek's disease. Delineation of the response of genetically resistant chickens to Marek's disease virus infection, *Avian Dis.,* 16, 894, 1972.

105. **Witter, R. L., Sharma, J. M., Solomon, J. J., and Champion, L. R.,** An age-related resistance of chickens to Marek's disease: some preliminary observations, *Avian Pathol.,* 2, 43, 1973.

106. **Calnek, B. W.,** Influence of age at exposure on the pathogenesis of Marek's disease, *J. Natl. Cancer Inst.,* 51, 929, 1973.

107. **Sharma, J. M., Witter, R. L., and Burmester, B. R.,** Pathogenesis of Marek's disease in old chickens: lesion regression as the basis for age-related resistance, *Infect. Immun.,* 8, 715, 1973.

108. **Witter, R. L.,** Principles of vaccination, in *Marek's Disease,* Payne, L. N., Ed., Martinus Nijhoff, Boston, 1985, 203.

109. **Quinnan, G. V. and Manischewitz, J. E.,** The role of natural killer cells and antibody dependent cell mediated cytotoxicity during murine cytomegalovirus infection, *J. Exp. Med.,* 150, 1549, 197.

110. **Welsh, R. M., Zinkernagel, R. M., and Hallenbeck, L. A.,** Cytotoxic cells induced during lymphocytic choriomeningitis virus infection of mice. II. Specificities of the natural killer cell, *J. Immunol.,* 122, 475, 1979.

111. **Welsh, R. M., Biron, C. A., Bukowski, J. F., McIntyre, K. M., and Yang, H.,** Role of natural killer cells in virus infections of mice, *Surv. Synth. Pathol. Res.,* 3, 409, 1984.

112. **Lopez, C., Kirkpatrick, D., and Fitzgerald, P.,** The role of NK (HSV-1) effector cells in resistance to herpesvirus infection in man, in *NK Cells and Other Natural Effector Cells,* Herberman, R. B., Ed., Academic Press, New York, 1982, 1445.

113. **Stephens, E. A., Witter, R. L., Nazerian, K., and Sharma, J. M.,** Development and characterization of Marek's disease transplantable tumor in inbred line 72 chickens homozygous at the major (B) histocompatibility locus, *Avian Dis.,* 24, 358, 1980.

114. **Payne, L. N. and Roszkowski, J.,** The presence of immunologically uncommitted bursa and thymus dependent lymphoid cells in the lymphomas of Marek's disease, *Avian Pathol.,* 1, 27, 1972.

115. **Lillehoj, H. S. and Ruff, M. D.,** Comparison of disease susceptibility and subclass-specific antibody response in SC and FP chickens experimentally inoculated with *Eimeria tenella, E. acervulina,* or *E. maxima, Avian Dis.,* 31, 112, 1987.

116. **Herberman, R. B.,** Natural killer (NK) cells and their role in resistance against disease, *Clin. Immunol. Rev.,* 1, 1, 1981.

117. **Pearson, G. R.,** *In vitro* and *in vivo* investigations on antibody dependent cellular cytotoxicity, *Curr. Top. Microbiol. Immunol.,* 6, 827, 1977.

118. **Imir, T., Suni, J., Hortling, L., and Vaheri, A.,** Antibody-dependent cell-mediated cytotoxicity in various orders of vertebrates, *Scand. J. Immunol.,* 6, 827, 1977.

119. **Bubenik, J., Perlmann, P., and Hosek, M.,** Induction of cytotoxicity of lymphocytes from tolerant donors by antibodies to target cell alloantigens, *Transplantation,* 10, 290, 1970.

120. **Chi, D. S. and Thorbecke, J.,** Cytotoxicity of allogeneic cells in the chicken. III. Antibody dependent cell-mediated cytotoxicity in normal and agammaglobulinemic chickens, *Cell. Immunol.,* 64, 258, 1981.

121. **Calder, E. A., Aitken, R. M., Penhale, W. J., McLeman, D., and Irvine, W. J.,** Lymphoid cell-mediated antibody-dependent cytotoxicity in untreated and bursectomized chickens, *Clin. Exp. Immunol.,* 16, 137, 1974.

122. **Kodama, H., Sugimoto, C., Inage, F., and Mikami, T.,** Antiviral immunity against Marek's disease virus-infected chicken kidney cells, *Avian Pathol.,* 8, 33, 1979.

123. **Lee, L. F., Powell, P. C., Rennie, M., Ross, L. J. N., and Payne, L. N.,** Nature of genetic resistance to Marek's disease in chickens, *J. Natl. Cancer Inst.,* 66, 789, 1981.

124. **Mandi, Y., Bakay, M., and Beladi, I.,** Effect of human adenovirus on antibody-dependent cellular cytotoxicity (ADCC) in chickens, *Cell. Immunol.,* 69, 395, 1982.

125. **Mandi, Y., Bakay, M., and Beladi, I.,** Effect of interferon on antibody-dependent cellular cytotoxicity (ADCC) in chickens, *Acta Microbiol. Hung.,* 31, 127, 1984.

Chapter 5

THE AVIAN MACROPHAGE IN CELLULAR IMMUNITY

R. R. Dietert, K. A. Golemboski, S. E. Bloom, and M. A. Qureshi

TABLE OF CONTENTS

I. INTRODUCTION

Macrophages are mobile scavenger cells that represent a first line of defense against infectious organisms. These cells arise in the bone marrow and subsequently enter the circulation as blood monocytes, an immature form of tissue macrophages.[1] These macrophage precursors serve as a reservoir for mature macrophages which reside in most tissues of mammalian and avian species. However, these tissue macrophages display considerable differences in morphology and functional capacity depending upon the tissue of residence.[2,3] The interaction of macrophages with the local environment and/or the selective infiltration of tissues by macrophage subpopulations results in the observed functional heterogeneity among tissue macrophages. Comparative analyses of differential gene expression among different sources of macrophages (e.g., Kupffer cells [liver macrophages], bursal macrophages, seminal fluid macrophages) have yet to be made in the avian system. However, a comprehensive analysis of differential gene expression in these distinct macrophage populations should facilitate identification of the underlying base for the complete functional repertoire of avian macrophages. This chapter will describe the identification and characterization of avian macrophages relative to their mammalian counterparts. In addition, the role of macrophages in cellular immunity and some examples of genetic and environmental modulations of macrophage function will be discussed. Because of the limited research that has been conducted using macrophages of non-chicken avian species, discussion within this chapter will emphasize chicken macrophage function.

II. THE DUAL ROLE OF MACROPHAGES

Macrophages play crucial roles in both nonspecific immunity, the surveillance processes leading to direct destruction of microbes and tumor cells, and acquired immunity, the antigen-driven immune response involving T and/or B lymphocytes. In the latter process, macrophages are central players as accessory cells that process antigens and present antigenic fragments to T lymphocytes in the context of class I and class II cell-surface products of the major histocompatibility complex (MHC).[4,5] Because many factors can influence the ability of animals to mount an immune response via the macrophage accessory cell function, knowledge of control of these factors can be particularly relevant to considerations of poultry health. Such factors include the ability of macrophages to accumulate in locations rich in pathogens, the uptake of pathogenic products by macrophages, the level of macrophage catabolism of peptides, the spectrum of proteases utilized by a macrophage population for catabolism, the ability of peptide fragments to bind to macrophage class I and class II molecules, the level of expression of MHC products on the macrophage cell surface, the ability of T-cell clones to recognize and respond to macrophage-presented antigen, and the ability of macrophages to secrete certain cytokines (e.g., interleukin 1 [IL-1] and interleukin 6 [IL-6]) during the course of antigen-specific lymphoid stimulation. Among chicken macrophage populations, any environmental or genetic factors that influence any of these processes could be expected to affect the quality of macrophage-dependent immune responses. As a result, the impact of potential biological response modifiers on these macrophage-dependent factors should represent useful information in strategies designed to optimize vaccine-mediated protection from disease.

Nonspecific immune processes, although not antigen-driven, are dependent upon various specific recognition features of macrophage populations. The role of macrophages in nonspecific immunity can range from clearance processes associated with the reticuloendothelial system (RES) to response to and subsequent regulation of acute and chronic inflammation, to serving as effector cells that provide microbicidal and tumoricidal activities. While nonspecific immunity bypasses the dependency on antigen-specificity, it is incorrect to view such first line processes as lacking specificity. In fact, where investigated, the specificity of these clearance and inflammatory processes is quite exquisite.

For example, it has long been known that autologous clearance of erythrocytes from circulation, as a model for cell aging, is based on subtle changes in cell-surface glycosylation.[6] Species specificity of this RES process is evident since the carbohydrate linkage recognized in clearing human erythrocytes is distinct from that utilized by chickens.[6] Recently, the role of macrophages in the specific recognition of aged RBCs was described.[7] Likewise, a recent finding in the mouse that aged neutrophils are engulfed and destroyed by macrophages at sites of inflammation through an R-Arg-Gly-Asp (RGD)-type ligand interaction has significant implications. The question can now be raised whether the short life of polymorphonuclear neutrophils (PMNs) is, in fact, regulated by the ability of macrophages to recognize and clear these cells based on the time-dependent exposure of a cryptic recognition structure. Therefore, even clearance of debris and aged cells by macrophages may involve the ability of macrophages to survey cells of many lineages and to identify key cell-surface structures that determine life or death of the potential target.

In many instances, the nonspecific and acquired immune roles of macrophages can become intertwined. This occurs in the case of hypersensitivity reactions where both inflammatory macrophage function and antigen-presenting functions influence the ultimate response.[8]

III. REGULATORY ACTIVITY OF MACROPHAGES

While much of the information presented in this chapter concerns macrophages as effector cells, macrophages also serve as important regulatory cells of the immune system. In mammalian systems, these cells can influence the activity of lymphocytes and of target cells through the production of various monokines including growth factors and metabolites of arachidonic acid. Macrophage metabolism of arachidonic acid via the cyclooxygenase pathway can result in the production of prostaglandins (PGs); several of these compounds serve to depress lymphoid function locally. In contrast, the leukotrienes (LT) produced from arachidonic acid by the lipooxygenase pathway are positive regulators of immune function; leukotriene B_4 (LTB_4) serves as a potent lymphoid chemotactic factor. Macrophage-derived cytokines can also produce major changes in lymphoid activity. IL-1, IL-6, and tumor necrosis factor (TNF) have pleiotropic effects on both immune cells and nonhematopoietic cells. These monokines not only regulate the activity of lymphocytes but also serve in feedback loops to influence macrophage populations. Likewise, the growth factors GM-CSF and G-CSF produced by macrophages can regulate, in part, the production of both macrophage and granulocytic leukocyte populations. Macrophages also have regulatory interactions with endothelial cells.

While macrophages are generally thought to represent a primary effector cell against tumor cells, the regulatory aspect of macrophages places them in a position either to inhibit or facilitate tumor cell growth.[9,10] In Balb/c mice, the production of growth factors by macrophages responding to intraperitoneal (i.p.) mineral oil injection is an important component for myeloma (B-cell tumor) formation.[10] The activated macrophage apparently secretes monokines that facilitate tumor cell growth in this strain. Macrophages can regulate the activity of natural killer (NK) cells locally.[11] They are also capable of regulating T-cell growth through cell-cell contact,[12] and they have long been known to play a role in T-cell mitogenesis.[13] Several studies suggest that immune associated antigen (Ia) expression by macrophages is an important consideration in their regulatory capacities.[12,14,15] It is perhaps important that macrophages can self-regulate their Ia expression through the production of endogenous arachidonate metabolites.[16]

Despite the limited number of studies on chicken macrophage function, it is clear that these cells also exert significant regulatory influences on lymphoid function. For example, chicken macrophages are required for certain mitogenic responses of lymphocytes.[17] Fredericksen and Gilmour[18] found that the inbred chicken lines East Lansing 6 and East Lansing 7 differed in mitogenic response to concanavalin A (Con A). They also demonstrated that monocyte/macrophages were responsible for this differential response by T lymphocytes. While monocyte/macrophages are required for effective T-lymphocyte stimulation, Schaefer et al.[19] described the existence of suppressor monocytes capable of depressing the mitogenic response of chicken T lymphocytes. Likewise, Kline and Sanders[20] reported that splenic suppressor macrophages from hereditary muscular dystrophic chickens were capable of irreversibly suppressing the con A mitogenic response with no suppression of the response to phytohemagglutinin (PHA). Suppressor macrophage populations have also been detected in normal chickens,[21] among macrophages in chickens inoculated with Marek's disease virus (MDV),[22] and among adherent leukocytes from chickens infected with infectious bursal disease virus (IBDV).[23]

In mammals, studies suggest that macrophages possessing suppressor activity can be physically separated from those with other functional capacities. In addition, macrophage-defective mouse strains were used to partition macrophage tumoricidal capacity from suppressor activity.[24] Mouse peritoneal macrophages with tumoricidal activities were also separable from those secreting prostaglandin E_2 (PGE_2) and IL-1.[25] This suggests that macrophages with discrete regulatory and/or effector functions may represent distinct populations that can be elicited under different conditions within the animal.

In addition to the apparent ability of macrophages to directly suppress lymphoid function, macrophages have a major role in the generation of T-suppressor (Ts) lymphocytes. Noma et al.[26] described the nature of the accessory cells required for Ts-cell production. Macrophage intervention is required at several stages in this process. Therefore, macrophages can greatly influence overall lymphoid function via their required role in the production of Ts cells.

With the previous examples of the ability of macrophage populations to control the growth, proliferation, and functional activity of both lymphocytes and tumor cells, it is clear that knowledge concerning the induction of macrophage populations with positive *or* negative regulatory capacities is a crucial factor in consideration of immune protection from disease. One need only consider the possibilities arising with tumor-associated macrophages (TA Mφs) to emphasize this point. The maturation status and activation level of these cells are important factors in the ultimate outcome of the tumor. Infiltrated macrophages could down-regulate any lymphoid response via PGE_2 and at the same time secrete monokines facilitating the growth of the tumor. In contrast, these cells could mobilize lymphocytes via the leukotrienes, process and present tumor-associated antigens (TAAs) to T lymphocytes, further activate lymphocytes with selected monokines, and, finally, directly kill the tumor cells via any combination of multiple pathways. As a result, even with diseases where macrophages are not the principal effector cells, the regulatory profile of these cells should be a prime concern relative to the ultimate disposition of the host. A discussion of macrophage monokine autoregulation is presented later in the chapter. Attempts to design appropriate adjuvants for use in new vaccination strategies will likely involve the production of regulatory and effector macrophages that facilitate the destruction of pathogens and tumor cells.

IV. AVIAN MACROPHAGE IDENTIFICATION

The ability to distinguish avian macrophages from other cell types both in free cell preparations and *in situ* is particularly important in understanding the role of these cells in immune processes. Because macrophages can possess such a wide array of functional capacities which reflect underlying phenotypic heterogeneity, identification of cells as macrophages or nonmacrophages is sometimes problematic.

Physical considerations are often important in macrophage identification. Macrophages can be separated from lymphocytes by adherence to substrate. Glass, plastic, Sephadex® G-10 beads, nylon wool, and fibronectin-coated matrices are some of the substrates that have been employed. Whether adherence is equally effective in separating all avian macrophages has not been evaluated in a comprehensive fashion.

Size can also be a distinguishing feature of some macrophages. However, effective separation/identification may be dependent upon the activation state of the macrophages. For example, chicken blood monocytes overlap extensively with lymphocytes in size.[27] Size is not an effective identifying feature of these cells. In contrast, certain inflammatory macrophages are readily distinguishable from lymphocytes based on size as well as other features.[28-30]

The physical capacity of phagocytosis has also been used as a means of either identifying or studying avian macrophages. Examples of targets for phagocytosis include india ink and FITC-conjugated Ficoll®,[31] colloidal carbon,[32] fixed *Escherichia coli*,[33] live *E. coli*,[34] *Eimeria tenella*,[35] heat-inactivated *Candida albicans*,[36] latex beads,[36] and ovalbumin-coated latex beads.[37] In most cases, macrophages engulf targets by recognizing a specific chemical structure on the target or by recognizing specific host components that can coat the particulate target. In the avian system, it is unclear how macrophages recognize such inert particles as carbon or iron. While phagocytic capacity is an extremely useful method of identifying avian macrophages, the targets should be carefully selected to avoid any confounding overlap with nonprofessional phagocyte (e.g., fibroblast) activity.

In addition to physical properties, avian macrophages can often be distinguished based on chemical properties. As in mammals, the enzymatic marker, nonspecific esterase, has been widely used to identify avian macrophages.[36,38-40] Nonspecific esterase activity is a feature of macrophages, but it is not known if it is a characteristic of all chicken macrophages. Among inflammatory macrophage preparations, we have observed considerable cell-to-cell variation in nonspecific esterase activity.[177] Other enzymatic markers reported for chicken macrophages include lysozyme[41] and acid phosphatase.[34] Chicken macrophage secretory products include avidin,[42] IL-1,[43] TNF,[178] and thromboxane.[179]

Avian macrophages possess a variety of cell-surface molecules which can be used in their identification. Most surface markers are shared with other cell types, and any single marker may only be expressed by a subset of all avian macrophages. Some of the most useful cell surface markers are those associated with specific macrophage functions. Chicken macrophages have been reported to express the Fc receptor for immunoglobulin,[44] the B-L (class II) glycoprotein,[45] the transferrin receptor,[46] the C3b receptor for complement,[38] and a mannose receptor.[47] In mammals, expression of the transferrin receptor gene has been associated with macrophage maturation[48] and has been shown to vary with the stage of functional activation.[49] The mannose receptor has also been found to decrease during the latter stages of mouse macrophage activation.[50] At present, the avian homolog of the mammalian Mac-1, LFA-1, P150/95 adhesion protein family has yet to be described despite the fact that the related integrins were initially described in chickens.[51] One important distinction between some mammalian and avian macrophages is in the expression of the CD4 cell surface molecule. Rat[52] and human[53] macrophages express CD4, while this cell surface marker, prominent on T-helper cells, is absent from chicken macrophages.[54] To emphasize the problem of identifying an individual chicken macrophage with a single marker, a majority of early inflammatory macrophages lack cell-surface B-L antigen and the transferrin receptor; however, these same cells are particularly high in respiratory burst activity.[30,55,179]

Specific antibodies and plant lectins have shown excellent promise for the identification of chicken macrophages. Rabbit polyclonal antisera have been prepared that specifically react with chicken macrophages.[33,45] In addition, mouse monoclonal antibodies specific for chicken inflammatory macrophages (CMTD-1, CMTD-2) have been described[56] and used

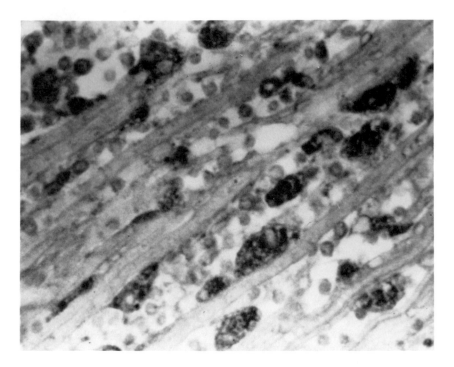

FIGURE 1.   A tissue section of a quail-chicken hybrid heart containing a metastasized tumor is shown. Tumor-associated avian macrophages are evident following reaction with peroxidase-labeled concanavalin A (Con A) (20 μg/ml) and development with substrate. Lectin cytochemistry using low concentrations of Con A provides one means of identifying avian macrophages within tissues. (Magnification × 700.)

to study both the pathogenesis of spontaneous autoimmune thyroiditis[57] and the genetic control of macrophage activation.[58] More recently, additional mouse monoclonal antibodies have been produced that show particular promise in reacting with large populations of chicken macrophages.[31,59] CVI-ChNL-68.1 was found to react specifically with monocytes, tissue macrophages, and antigen-presenting interdigitating cells while CVI-ChNL-68.2 reacted with splenic ellipsoid-associated reticulin cells and Kupffer cells (liver macrophages). Other antimacrophage monoclonal antibodies have been developed, and these are being characterized.[60]

Chicken macrophages can also be distinguished from certain cell types, including lymphocytes, based on the apparent incidence of Con A receptors.[28] Using FITC-labeled Con A under conditions of reduced concentration (20 μg/ml), most chicken macrophages bound more Con A than did bursal lymphocytes. This quantitative difference among free cell preparations translates into a qualitative difference in cytochemical staining applying peroxidase-labeled Con A to a variety of avian tissue sections.[28,61] A similar result was previously described for human macrophages.[62] An example of the use of peroxidase-labeled Con A for identification of avian tumor-associated macrophages is shown in Figure 1.

V. AVIAN MACROPHAGE ISOLATION

Despite the considerable importance of macrophages in host resistance to disease, these cells have not received the attention in the avian system that has been devoted to lymphocytes. At least part of the explanation for the relative dearth of macrophage studies has been the lack of the conventional source of macrophages commonly utilized in mammalian animal models. In mice and rats, significant numbers of peritoneal macrophages can be obtained as resident cells. However, there is evidence that mouse vs. rat resident macrophages differ considerably in their level of activation.[63]

In the chicken, few, if any, harvestable resident peritoneal macrophages are routinely obtained.[64] This has both disadvantages and advantages. A disadvantage of the relative absence of chicken resident peritoneal macrophages has been the lack of an equivalent avian standard source to that commonly used in mammals for macrophages. As a result, avian immunologists have utilized a variety of sources of macrophages. These include bone marrow macrophages (BMM),[45] peripheral blood monocytes (PBM),[40,65] elicited peritoneal macrophages (PM),[32,39,64,66] bursal-derived macrophages (BDM),[45] thymic-derived macrophages,[45] and splenic macrophages (SM).[45,67,68]

While the conventional source of resident macrophages is unavailable to the avian researcher, the chicken provides a system that is ideal for analysis of *in vivo* inflammatory responses. Mammalian scientists have had to contend with the existence of resident vs. elicited peritoneal macrophages that differ greatly in their response to inflammatory agents. For example, mouse resident peritoneal macrophages are relatively refractory to stimulation with interferon (IFN).[69] Harvested peritoneal macrophages, following i.p. stimulation of the mouse, will inevitably contain a mixture of elicited responsive macrophages and resident nonresponsive macrophages. In contrast, the macrophages obtained from the chicken following i.p. stimulation more accurately reflect the actual cellular responses to inflammatory signals. In this way, such processes as *in vivo* chemotaxis and functional activation may be analyzed without confounding factors.

Several procedures utilizing numerous eliciting agents have been used to obtain PM. Early studies described the use of starch to obtain PM for *in vitro* experiments.[64] In 1977, Sephadex® (cross-linked dextran) was shown to elicit a peritoneal exudate cell (PEC) population that was remarkably rich in macrophages.[66] It was later shown that a single i.p. injection of Sephadex® was as effective as multiple injections for eliciting chicken macrophages.[39] Sephadex® is a particularly effective elicitor of chicken macrophages because, in contrast with other agents such as starch and LPS, Sephadex® recruits a predominantly macrophage population of chicken peritoneal exudate cells.[65,70,71] This is in contrast with the much higher heterophil infiltration elicited by Sephadex® in the Japanese quail (*Coturnix coturnix japonica*).[180] In the chicken, Sephadex® has been shown to activate macrophages for bactericidal activity.[72] Sephadex®-elicited mouse macrophages possessed both bactericidal and tumoricidal activity.[73]

It has been suggested that Sephadex® elicits and activates macrophages via the alternative complement pathway.[74] The physicochemical properties of Sephadex® appear to be particularly important in this regard. The nature of the chicken inflammatory cell response could be modulated by altering either size of the cross-linked dextran or the glycosidic linkages themselves.[70] This is compatible with recent results concerning Sephadex® derivatives and the human complement system.[74] It is intriguing that i.p. Sephadex® exposure can produce a dramatic granulocytic mobilization in the circulation of chickens without extensive granulocyte emigration.[29] Other agents used to obtain chicken peritoneal macrophages include glycogen and peptone,[39] supernatant from *Enterobacter cloacae* cultures,[181] iron gluconate,[182] and lipopolysaccharide (LPS).[65]

VI. MACROPHAGE INFLAMMATORY RESPONSES

Macrophages are recruited to sites of infection or tumor-cell growth via a complex process that involves induction of the Mac-1 glycoprotein family of adhesion molecules, chemotaxis toward increasing concentrations of chemoattractants, and diapedesis. In mammals, a system of complementary molecules on macrophages and endothelial cells is upregulated by chemoattractant exposure, permitting inflammatory leukocytes to migrate to extravascular areas of high chemoattractant concentrations.[75] The avian equivalents of the macrophage and endothelial cell adhesion molecules have not yet been described. Once macrophages reach locations where chemoattractants are of sufficiently high concentrations, they stop migrating and undergo a respiratory burst. This process leads to the production of reactive oxygen intermediates (ROIs) such as superoxide anion (O_2^-) that are important in extracellular microbicidal activity.[76] This process of shifting to a respiratory burst only under high chemoattractant concentrations helps ensure that oxidative destruction is focused to areas of high pathogen incidence.[77]

A. CHEMOTAXIS

Chemotaxis represents the initial step of macrophage participation in the inflammatory response. Chicken monocytes and macrophages can undergo chemotaxis in response to a variety of compounds. Occupation of cell-surface receptors by chemotactic agents results in cellular polarization and directed migration. Among the chemoattractants employed for chicken mononuclear leukocytes is the synthetic polypeptide N-formylated-methionyl-leucinyl-phenyalanine (fMet-Leu-Phe).[29] fMet-Leu-Phe is similar to the chemotactic peptides of certain bacteria. Because chicken leukocytes appear to require a higher concentration of fMet-Leu-Phe to stimulate chemotaxis than is needed by human leukocytes, the actual receptors may optimally bind somewhat different polypeptide structures than their mammalian counterparts. It is interesting that turkey leukocytes apparently lack the fMet-Leu-Phe receptor.[78] Other chemoattractants that have been used in avian systems include endotoxin-activated chicken serum[65] and *E. cloacae* culture supernatant.[79]

B. RESPIRATORY BURST

Leukocyte chemotaxis during an inflammatory response will frequently culminate in a respiratory burst. Macrophages can be stimulated to undergo a respiratory burst through a variety of stimuli. These include the occupation of specific membrane receptors by chemoattractants, the phagocytosis of particles, and the interaction of phorbol esters with membrane-triggering components.[80] The respiratory burst that results is a rapid process that consumes oxygen for the production of superoxide anion (O_2^-) and hydrogen peroxide (H_2O_2) and, indirectly, hydroxyl radical (OH^-) and singlet oxygen ($^1O_2$). These metabolites are important in microbicidal activity and can also result in significant oxidative damage of tissues in localized areas of inflammation. Extensive lipid peroxidation can result from this process if free-radical scavenging is not sufficient. Macrophage-mediated diseases resulting from oxygen radical production have been characterized for a variety of target organs including lung[81] and kidney.[82]

Information on the respiratory burst in chicken macrophages and heterophils is limited. However, we recently found that early inflammatory macrophages from young chickens are superior to either blood monocytes or late inflammatory macrophages in the ability to generate superoxide anion upon stimulation with phorbol myristic acid (PMA).[179] As a result, protection of tissues during chicken inflammatory responses is likely to be of greatest concern during the initial wave of infiltration and where chronic inflammation results.

C. MONOKINE PRODUCTION

The stimulation of macrophages that occurs during the early stages of an inflammatory response results in the production and secretion of monokines. These monokines have profound effects on both lymphoid populations and nonleukocytic cells and can feed back to influence macrophages themselves. Macrophage-derived cytokines known to be produced in mammalian systems include IL-1, IL-6, TNF, GM-CSF, G-CSF, IFNs α and β, and transforming growth factor-β (TGF-β). Studies with monokines in the avian system have been limited; however, research with IL-1 has been performed,[43,83,84] and TNF is under current investigation. A chicken myelomonocytic growth factor produced by the macrophage cell line, HD11, has also been described.[85] It is interesting that regulatory loops exist for monokine production and action. The neuroendocrine-immune loops that exist relative to monokine production and action are extensive[86] and beyond the scope of this chapter. However, it is important to consider that macrophages can autoregulate their own monokine action. For example, reactive oxygen species may help stimulate the release of TNF.[87] Likewise, IL-1 and TNF may directly stimulate certain macrophages to produce ROIs.[81] These studies suggest that macrophage populations can push other subpopulations through inflammatory stages in a positive regulatory loop.

Negative regulatory loops also exist. Macrophages are known producers of inhibitors of interleukins.[88] TGF-β, which can be produced by monocytes as well as other leukocytes, inhibits the ability of IL-1 to induce lymphoid proliferation.[89] A major regulatory loop for IL-1 synthesis and secretion involves arachidonic acid metabolism by macrophages. PGE_2, a product of the cyclooxygenase pathway, is a negative endogenous regulator of IL-1 synthesis and secretion.[90] Inhibition of this pathway can result in enhanced production of both IL-1 and TNF.[86]

Knowledge of monokine regulation in the avian system is particularly important when one considers the far ranging effects of these hormone-like products. The previous examples of autoregulatory influences indicate that macrophage secretory products can regulate lymphoid activity, as well as activity among macrophage populations, by controlling the profile of regulatory molecules produced.

D. PHAGOCYTOSIS

The phagocytic function of macrophages is particularly important for four processes: (1) clearance of foreign compounds by the reticuloendothial system (RES), (2) programmed elimination of dead and/or dying cells, (3) the internalization of antigens for subsequent processing and presentation, and (4) the internalization of pathogens for destruction within macrophage phagolysosome vacuoles. As scavengers, macrophages possess the ability to distinguish pathogens from self and to distinguish compromised host cells from those that are fully viable. Interaction with extracellular matrix proteins such as fibronectin and laminin can markedly enhance macrophage phagocytosis.[91] Such interactions occur via specific macrophage receptors for fibronectin[92] and laminin.[93] Phagocytosis is often referred to as specific and nonspecific; however, as more is learned about the diversity of macrophage receptors, it is becoming clear that the term "nonspecific phagocytosis" is frequently misleading. The distinction between "specific" and "nonspecific" phagocytosis is based more on the nature of the macrophage receptor required for particle recognition than on the absence of such a receptor. "Specific" phagocytosis usually involves uptake via the Fc (crystalizable fragment) receptor for immunoglobulin or the C3 (third component of complement) receptor. "Specific" phagocytosis, therefore, can be operationally defined as the phagocytosis of particles coated by soluble components of the immune system that bind to specific macrophage cell surface receptors.

Because macrophages are quite discriminating in what they engulf, most "nonspecific" phagocytosis also occurs via specific receptors. In this case, receptors for glycosylated structures are likely to be involved. For example, the mannose-fucose receptor has been defined on both mouse[94] and chicken macrophages.[47,95] The β-glucan receptor is another example of a functionally important cell-surface receptor on macrophages.[96] Some mammalian macrophages apparently possess a receptor for the recognition of galactose that is important in aged red blood cell (RBC) clearance.[7] It is likely that uptake of many viruses and bacteria occur via such receptors for glycosidic linkages.

Peptide-specific receptors can also be important in "nonspecific" phagocytosis. PMNs in mammals are relatively short-lived cells compared with macrophages. During an inflam-

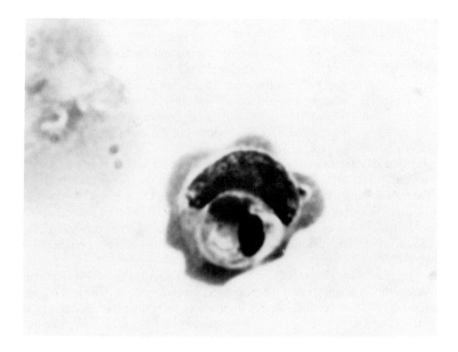

FIGURE 2.   The phagocytosis of an elicited heterophil by an inflammatory chicken macrophage is shown. These cells were isolated from the peritoneal cavity of a Cornell K strain chicken following intraperitoneal Sephadex® injection. (Cytospin preparation; May-Grünwald and Giemsa stain; magnification × 1750.)

matory response, macrophages will frequently phagocytize PMNs. Chicken macrophages also perform this function (Figure 2). It was recently shown that mouse macrophages recognize a tetrapeptide containing the integrin-related Arg-Gly-Asp (RGD) tripeptide[97] on the surface of aging PMNs. The PMN receptor is acquired by macrophages during maturation. These investigators proposed that this "nonspecific" phagocytosis of aged PMNs by macrophages is an integral component in the programmed cell death of the short-lived inflammatory PMN.[98] Elucidation of the specificity of the chicken peptide receptor should be important in understanding avian leukocyte homeostasis.

Phagocytosis of unopsonized sheep red blood cells (SRBCs) by chicken macrophages appears to be an inducible property acquired during the *in vivo* activation of chicken macrophages[70] or the *in vitro* activation of monocytes.[65] Indirect evidence suggests that receptor-mediated recognition of SRBCs is required, since over 30% of early inflammatory chicken macrophages can phagocytize opsonized SRBCs, via the Fc receptor, but not uncoated SRBCs. The association of the capacity to phagocytize SRBCs with the activation of chicken macrophages is consistent with a recent finding in the mouse.[99]

VII. MACROPHAGE ACTIVATION

The process of macrophage activation, including the acquisition of microbicidal and/or tumoricidal activity, has undergone considerable scrutiny in mouse[100] and humans.[101,102] Although it is clear that numerous steps are involved in this process,[103] the murine model is usually presented as a two-signal process of activation. Upon receipt of the first signal, macrophages shift from a responsive state to a primed state. The prototype signal for this step is the lymphokine, gamma interferon (IFN-γ), synthesized by T lymphocytes. IFN-γ induces a wide range of changes in macrophage gene expression following interaction with a specific receptor on the macrophage cell surface. Ribosomal RNA synthesis is affected, and expression of a minimum of four genes is induced by exposure to IFN-γ.[103,104] A shift in macrophages to a primed state also means that these cells can be terminally activated when exposed to minute amounts of the second signal. Prior IFN-γ exposure can reduce the level of the second signal required by at least two orders of magnitude. The prototype second signal has been LPS, the cell-wall component of gram-negative bacteria. In mice, LPS induces the same set of four genes induced by IFN-γ and induces two LPS-exclusive genes.[104] If responsive macrophages are exposed to sufficient amounts of LPS (i.e., microgram quantities) for prolonged periods, the need for the first signal is eliminated.[105] In the murine system, macrophages may develop microbicidal and tumoricidal capacities independently.[25] This has raised the question of whether both functions are acquired during a single pathway of activation or, in contrast, represent distinct pathways of terminal activation.[25] Mammalian macrophage activation has been associated with differential gene expression,[104] including the competence genes *JE* and *KC*.[106,107] Expression of a 120 kDa protein has also been associated with the acquisition of tumoricidal activity by mouse peritoneal macrophages.[104]

Macrophages appear to be capable of killing tumor cells using at least four distinct processes. Production and secretion of the monokine, TNF, occur relatively early in the inflammatory response.[108] TNF is capable of both cytostatic and cytolytic activity against certain tumor cells[109] and also possesses regulatory features for certain leukocytes.[110] Antibody-dependent cellular cytotoxicity (ADCC), a receptor-mediated cytotoxic activity, requires that effector cells have achieved a cytolytic potential; however, specificity of killing is mediated via the Fc receptor for immunoglobulin. Macrophages and other cells that perform ADCC recognize immunoglobulin molecules that are bound to cellular targets. The ability of chicken macrophages to perform ADCC has been previously described.[111,112] Given that normal spleen cells with macrophage characteristics can perform ADCC[111] and that early inflammatory macrophages are very efficient at Fc-mediated binding,[70] it appears likely that ADCC potential is acquired early rather than late in the macrophage activation process.

Two other tumoricidal processes have been described that are associated with the later stages of macrophage activation. Mammalian macrophages have been shown to utilize an arginine-dependent process that is effective against both tumor cells and fungi.[113,114] It has been proposed that the enzyme, arginine deiminase, is induced during macrophage activation,[115] enabling arginine to be converted to citrulline and nitric oxide (NO). The formation of NO has been associated with the ability of macrophages to actively deplete tumor cells of iron-sulfur prosthetic groups.[116] The sensitive target for this action appears to be the aconitase enzyme of Kreb's cycle. As a result, activated mammalian macrophages can block mitochondrial respiration in tumor cells.[116] This process is exquisitely sensitive to local environmental conditions.[117] A further result of this macrophage metabolic pathway is the production of nitrite, nitrate, and, ultimately, nitrosamine compounds.[118] The ability of macrophages to produce carcinogenic nitrosamines during activation also raises questions concerning the balance of positive vs. negative results from this macrophage pathway. Does the production of nitrosamines by macrophages represent a secondary health hazard, or do these compounds, along with NO, facilitate the removal of tumor cells with little carcinogenic impact on normal cells in the involved area?

It is not yet known if avian macrophages can use arginine to produce NO, nitrite, nitrate, and nitrosamines. However, this question is particularly relevant to poultry production because of the known genetic control over arginine utilization.[119] Because different chicken strains would be expected to utilize arginine with different efficiencies for particular metabolic pathways, it is possible that avian macrophage utilization of arginine would be quite heterogeneous among strains. This question is currently under examination.[183]

A fourth pathway for macrophage cytotoxic action is a classic cytolytic process that involves enzymes broadly designated as cytolytic proteases. This capacity does not develop until the terminal stages of macrophage activation.[120] Control over the ability of macrophages to kill targets is based exclusively on integral binding to targets; superficial contact is not sufficient for killing to occur. Binding of tumor cells is thought to proceed through two distinct stages[121] and is receptor-mediated. The induced cell-surface receptor on mouse macrophages that is responsible for binding to complementary tumor-cell surface molecules was recently found to possess a characteristic lectin binding site(s).[122]

Given that macrophages are designed to communicate with various cells including T lymphocytes via cell-cell contact, in addition to killing tumor cells via cell-cell contact, it is particularly important to consider the regulation of cell recognition by the tumoricidal macrophage. If binding to targets is the crucial step in cytolytic action, then it would be necessary to minimize the macrophage-lymphoid interactions that would normally occur with antigen presentation.

The present authors recently found that chicken macrophages exhibit a reduced cell-surface expression of B-L (Ia) molecules during the later stages of activation compared with earlier stages.[55] This finding would be compatible with previous mammalian observations.[120,123] As a result, fully activated macrophages may minimize contact with normal cells by down-regulating the interaction molecules for lymphocytes and endothelial cells while upregulating the receptor which permits binding to a variety of tumor cells.

Activated macrophages appear to be important in several virally induced neoplasias in chickens. Evidence suggests that they can restrict both viral multiplication and the growth of tumor cells in Marek's disease.[124] Macrophage-like adherent cytotoxic leukocytes have been reported to be associated with Marek's disease tumors.[125] In this study, a distinction in the susceptibility of these effector cells to treatment with carbonyl iron and carrageenan was observed when the cells were isolated from progressive vs. regressive tumors. It was also possible to transfer resistance to Rous sarcoma by the transfer of peritoneal macrophages from regressor to progressor sublines.[126]

VIII. MACROPHAGES AND INFECTIOUS AGENTS

Macrophages represent an important focal point for interactions with infectious agents. This is true both for mammalian and avian macrophages. As previously discussed, macrophages can destroy virally transformed cells in a variety of ways and employ both extracellular and intracellular processes to kill bacteria. However, these cells can also serve as important reservoirs for infectious agents. Certain viruses and bacteria can avoid macrophage antipathogen processes to utilize these cells as a protective system for replication and/or dispersal. As a result, it is important to consider the various activation states of macrophage populations and their resulting capacity to control infection in considering the outcome of a host-pathogen interaction.

Intracellular killing of bacteria can occur via ingestion and subsequent digestion within vacuoles. Therefore, a minimum of two independent processes subject to changes during activation are important in successful bactericidal action of macrophages: (1) recognition and phagocytosis with subsequent incorporation into a phagosome vesicle and (2) the development of lysosomal vacuoles containing hydrolytic enzymes. Digestion is accomplished by the fusion of these vacuoles into phagolysosomes.

For particular pathogens, the activation state of the macrophage is an important factor in the capability of the cell to destroy the pathogen. For example, mouse inflammatory macrophages are known to possess superior listericidal activity in comparison with resident macrophages.[127] Likewise, with other facultative intracellular parasites such as *Brucella*, *Leishmania*, and *Salmonella*, activation of the macrophage is an important consideration in resistance. Age of the chicken has also been reported as an important factor for the resistance of chicken splenic macrophages to certain *Salmonella*.[128]

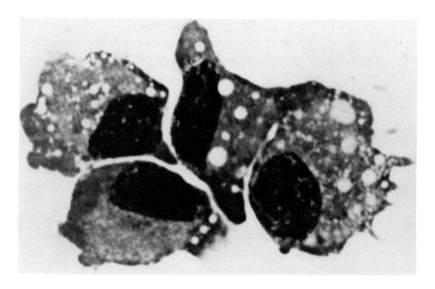

FIGURE 3. A photomicrograph of a recently developed chicken macrophage cell line is illustrated. These cells initially grow as rapidly proliferating clumps of cells with a high incidence of intracytoplasmic phase-lucent granules. Cells which detach from clumps readily adhere to the substrate and spread. This cell line was developed by M. A. Qureshi (Reference 136). (Magnification × 1750.)

The phenotype of the pathogen can also be an important consideration in the pathogen-macrophage interaction. For example, smooth (virulent) strains of *Brucella abortus* were reported to have an increased survival and replicating capacity compared with rough strains when bovine blood monocytes and mammary gland macrophages were employed.[129] Similar differences based on bacterial phenotype have been observed in chickens. Chicken elicited peritoneal macrophages were found to phagocytize the virulent (congo red-positive) phenotype of *E. coli* more efficiently *in vitro* than the avirulent (congo red-negative) phenotype. However, the latter phenotype was cleared more efficiently from circulation than was the virulent phenotype.[130] Differential recognition and killing of bacterial phenotypes by macrophages have been shown to be associated with discrete chemical structures such as sulfatide groups.[131]

Chicken macrophages have been examined for a number of viral interactions. Activated macrophages were shown to restrict the growth of Marek's disease virus-transformed T-lymphoblastoid cell lines.[36] In a parallel study, bone marrow-derived chicken macrophages were reported to be resistant to infection with reticuloendotheliosis virus, infectious virus bronchitis, and serveral strains of MDV. In contrast, several viruses were found to replicate in chicken macrophages producing demonstrable morphological modifications of the macrophages. Such viruses include adenovirus, Newcastle's Disease virus, reovirus, infectious laryngotracheitis virus, and IBDV.[132] Chicken macrophages can be infected with myelocytomatosis virus[133] and transformed by the MC-29 virus.[33,134] The HD11 macrophage cell line was developed from such a transformation.[33] In contrast, *src* gene expression by chicken macrophages failed to result in a transformed cell phenotype.[135] An additional chicken macrophage cell line was recently developed that appears to possess a more activated phenotype compared with that of HD11 cells.[136] However, the responsible etiological agent for this transformation is not yet known. Cells from this line are shown in Figure 3.

Macrophages are also known to function in the resistance to parasites. As with other diseases, macrophages can contribute to host protection via either their antigen-presenting function or their direct action against the parasite. Macrophages can also serve to disseminate parasites and viruses. Sporozoites of several *Eimeria* species have been shown to be transported by macrophages to their sites of development. However, cultured chicken macrophages can limit the growth of *E. tenella*.[35] The relationship between macrophages and *Eimeria* coccidia has been recently reviewed.[137]

IX. GENETIC CONTROL OF MACROPHAGE FUNCTION

One need only consider both the diversity of macrophage functions and the complexity of the inflammatory response to become aware of the many opportunities for genetic influences on macrophage processes. Evidence from both avian and mammalian systems indicates that such functions as chemotaxis, phagocytosis, colony formation, bactericidal activity, tumoricidal activity, superoxide production, antigen presentation, and regulation of mitogenesis can be dramatically influenced by specific genetic differences between strains. Table 1 provides examples of such genetic influences. Several genes have been identified in the mouse that directly or indirectly influence macrophage function. These include the *Lps* gene on chromosome 4[138] and the *Lr-1* (*Hc*) and *Lr-2* genes associated with *Listeria* resistance,[127] the *Ity* gene controlling *Salmonella* resistance,[139,140] and the *Bcg* gene on chromosome 1.[141] The latter two genes are closely linked and may be identical. Biozzi strain mice also possess polygenic factors that determine the level of macrophage catabolic activity and, thereby, influence host resistance to certain bacterial infections.[142] These mouse genes differ in the type of control that is exerted. *Lr-1* affects the extent of macrophage infiltration, while *Bcg* (*Ity*) resistant vs. susceptible animals exhibit comparable numbers of infiltrated macrophages. In additon, *Lr-1* affects macrophages indirectly, probably through influence of C5a levels, while *Lps* and *Bcg* appear to involve intrinsic properties of the macrophage. The contrasting effects of these genes illustrate the multiple opportunities for genetic modulation of macrophage-mediated host resistance.

While inflammatory processes have not been well characterized in the chicken, it is clear that genetic factors can also influence the early stages of the macrophage inflammatory response. The allelic linkage or haplotype of the chicken major histocompatibility (*B*) complex (MHC) and the dosage of the microchromosome bearing the same gene complex were both found to influence blood mononuclear leukocyte chemotaxis to bacterially derived chemoattractants[58,71,79] (Table 1). In contrast, the profile of elicited leukocytes responding to an inflammatory stimulus would appear to be relatively invariant to *B* haplotype differences.[71] Since this parameter does vary greatly between different lines of chickens,[32,67] it is likely to be influenced primarily by non-MHC genes. This is also supported by the observation of Powell et al.[32] that inbred lines carrying the identical B^2 haplotype responded to i.p. starch injection with different inflammatory cell profiles (Table 1).

While the profile of inflammatory cells does not appear to be influenced by B-complex haplotype, the functional activation of elicited chicken macrophages appears to be dramatically affected by the *B*-complex genotype.[65,71,72] The *B*-complex gene controlling macrophage responsiveness appears to act at the level of the monocyte-LPS interaction.[65,71] The MHC is capable of controlling the acquired immune response via the macrophage;[4] however, innate macrophage responses generally have not been associated with mammalian MHC control. One exception to this is a recent report that polymorphism of human class II genes is associated with the level of monocyte response to LPS.[143] Therefore, it is conceivable that classical MHC genes could influence chicken macrophage activation. A second explanation could be based on the particular composition of the chicken MHC. The *B*-complex is known to differ in composition with that of the mouse *H-2* and human *HLA*. Among these differences is the localization of a gene designated *12.3* in the *B*-complex that represents an avian homologue of a human G-protein subunit. The homologous human gene is not *HLA* linked.[144] It is possible that a gene tied to transmembrane signaling, such as this within the *B*-complex, could explain the broad spectrum of differences observed in macrophage responses extending to several receptor triggering systems.

TABLE 1
Examples of Genetic Control of Avian and Mammalian Macrophage Function

Species	Genetic strains	Genetic control	Ref.
		Phagocytosis/Clearance	
Chicken	$15I_5$-*B*-congenics	MHC region	71,72
Chicken	FCT-15 trisomic	MHC dosage	58
Chicken	Iowa state lines	Selected line differences	145
Mouse	A/J and C57BL/10	Strain differences	160
Human		MHC region	161
Chicken	EL 6_1 and 7_2 lines	Non-MHC difference	32
Mouse	C3H/HeJ and other strains	*LPS* gene	162
Chicken	Storrs *Am* mutation and control	Strain difference	163
		Bactericidal Activity	
Chicken	$15I_5$-*B*-congenics	MHC region	72
Mouse	Biozzi strains	Polygeneic control	142
Mouse	Beige strains	*bg* mutation	164
Human		*Ch* mutation	165
Mouse	Inbred strains, congenic lines	*Bcg* gene	141
Mouse	C3H/HeJ and other strains	*Lps* gene	138
Mouse	A/J and other strains	*Lr-1* gene	127
Mouse	Balb/c and other strains	*Lr-2* gene	127
		Lysosomal Function	
Mouse	Beige strains	*bg* mutation	166
		Chemotaxis	
Chicken	$15I_5$-*B*-congenics	MHC region	71,79
Chicken	FCT-15 trisomic	MHC dosage	58
Human		LFA-1 defect	167
Mouse	A/J, C57BL, and others	Two genes	168
		Respiratory Burst	
Chicken	$15I_5$-*B*-congenics	MHC region	71
Mouse	MRL-*lpr/lpr* and control	Single gene	169
		Regulation of Mitogenesis	
Chicken	EL 6_3 and 7_2 lines	Non-MHC alleles	18
Chicken	Storrs *Am* mutation	Non-MHC alleles	20
		Inflammatory Macrophage Accumulation	
Mouse	C3H/HeJ and other strains	*Lps* gene	138
Mouse	A/J and other strains	*Lr-1* gene	127
		Viral Restriction	
Mouse	C3H/HeJ and other strains	*Lps* gene	170
		Colony Formation	
Mouse	Various inbred and congenic lines	Single non-MHC gene	171

TABLE 1 (continued)
Examples of Genetic Control of Avian and Mammalian Macrophage Function

Species	Genetic strains	Genetic control	Ref.
	Antibody-Dependent Cellular Cytotoxicity		
Mouse	MLR-*lpr/lpr* and control	Single gene	169
	Tumoricidal Activity		
Mouse	C57BL/6J, A/J crosses and recombinants	Single gene	172
Mouse	C3H/HeJ and related strains; A/J and related strains	Two distinct genetic controls	173
	Protozoan Cytotoxicity		
Mouse	C3H/HeJ and C3H/HeN	Possibly *Lps* gene or another control	174
	Antigen Presentation		
Mouse	Biozzi	Polygenic control	141
Mouse	*Bcg* congenics	*Bcg* gene	175
	Monokine Production		
Mouse	A/J, C57BL/6J, and other strains	Single non-MHC gene	176

Additional genetic influences on chicken macrophage function have been described. Different specialized lines of chickens possess different blood clearance rates for foreign particles.[145] It is not known whether the genetic effect is manifest predominantly in blood monocytes, heterophils, or thrombocytes. The nature of this genetic difference remains to be determined.

In general, the genes identified thus far in avian and mammalian systems fall into two primary categories: genes that influence the mobilization of macrophages, resulting in a quantitative deficiency of inflammatory macrophages, and genes that permit accumulation of inflammatory macrophages but result in a qualitative difference in macrophage activation. The opportunity would appear to exist to use these categories of genes to optimize both inflammatory responses and macrophage activation within experimental and commercial poultry lines and crosses.

X. ENVIRONMENTAL CONTROL OF MACROPHAGE FUNCTION

With the diverse metabolic pathways employed by macrophages in immune interactions and the many macrophage cell-surface receptors that bind ligand products of the immune and neuroendocrine sytems, it is not surprising that environmental conditions can play a significant role in modulating macrophage function. Significant environmental factors can include the categories of dietary intake, drug interactions, and exposure to toxicants. The investigations of mammalian macrophage modulation by environmental factors are extensive and cover a variety of factors, including dietary lipid intake,[146] arginine availability,[115] and exposure to compounds such as dextran sulfate, carrageenan, diprophytlin dichloride, indomethacin, levamisole, vanillin, propyl gallate, lead acetate, hydrocortisone 21-phosphate,[147] 3-methylcholanthrene,[148] crocidolite asbestos,[149] morpholine,[150] and benzo[*a*]pyrene.[151]

The number of environmental compounds investigated specifically for avian macrophage modulating ability is quite limited. Nevertheless, diverse classes of compounds are represented among the known avian macrophage modulators. The direct-acting mutagen-carcinogen, methylmethane sulfonate (MMS), was found to depress the phagocytic and bactericidal activities of chicken macrophages.[34] Carrageenan[152-154] and silica[155] have been employed as modulators of chicken macrophage function. Aflatoxin-B$_1$, an indirect-acting mutagen-carcinogen, has been reported to depress monocyte phagoctyic capabilities.[156] With regard to nutritional effects, combined deficiencies in selenium and vitamin E result in impaired adherence capabilities of chicken macrophages.[37] Finally, as alluded to in earlier sections, direct or indirect exposure of chicken macrophages to pathogens and/or their products can result in modulation of cellular activity.[79,132,133,157-159] Given improved methodologies for identifying, isolating, and functionally evaluating avian macrophages, the opportunities for employing environmental modifications of macrophage function within poultry management regimes are particularly promising.

XI. SUMMARY AND FUTURE PROSPECTS

In this chapter, the role of the macrophage in three major capacities associated with cellular immunity has been discussed. Macrophages function in innate resistance as effector cells possessing potent microbicidal and tumoricidal activities. These cells are also pivotal in acquired immunity via their ability to process and present antigens to lymphocytes. Finally, macrophages can greatly influence local or systemic immune responses through their capacity as regulatory cells. Production and secretion of immunomodulatory cytokines and metabolites by macrophages can have a profound effect on the ability of a host to overcome a pathogenic challenge. Therefore, knowledge concerning the basic biology of the macrophage and the ability of these cells to be influenced by genetic and environmental variation is particularly relevant to developing new strategies for enhancing the disease resistance of poultry stocks.

While information on the avian macrophage has lagged behind that of analogous mammalian cells, recent progress in the identification, isolation, and analysis of avian macrophages has provided a clearer picture concerning the role of these cells in immune protection processes. As a result, it is now possible to consider the characteristics and properties of a maximally effective avian macrophage population and the steps necessary to achieve the genetic or environmental conditions permitting optimum macrophage function. It is clear that avian macrophages, like their mammalian counterparts, are particularly sensitive to genetic and environmental manipulation. However, with avian species such as the chicken, the functional capacity of the host macrophage population could be enhanced to achieve a positive economic outcome. As a result, it may be desirable in the future to tailor macrophage function within chicken flocks to desired characteristics. This could be accomplished through the combined or separate use of conventional breeding and selection, transgenic applications, and modifications in diet and housing conditions.

On example of macrophage manipulation with possible economic ramifications pertains to the use of new vaccine strategies. If vaccine vehicles (adjuvants) and routes of exposure could be designed to maximize the antigen-presenting capabilities and longevity of presenting capacities of macrophages, then a greater immune protection would likely result from a single vaccine exposure. Dietary intake designed to optimize macrophage function and overall immune function could result in reduced losses among poultry flocks. Likewise, an excellent opportunity would appear to exist in the genetic regulation of macrophage function. Specific disease resistance is greatly influenced by the MHC and can be manifested at the level of the macrophage because of the requirement for antigen presentation using MHC gene products. Therefore, the mammalian and avian MHC can influence acquired immunity. However, recent evidence suggests that a gene or genes within the chicken MHC can affect macrophage innate immune responses. Similar control is apparently unlinked to many mammalian MHCs. This means that in the chicken, both branches of macrophage function (as accessory antigen-presenting cells and as effector cells) would be largely controlled by the same genetic region. Because of this genetic consolidation, the process of optimizing chicken macrophage function through conventional breeding and/or recombinant DNA technology could initially be focused on the *B*-complex region; other non-MHC genes influencing macrophage and overall immune function could then be considered as more information concerning these genes becomes available. Finally, the use of macrophage products, such as the monokines and lipid metabolites, in poultry health management may be important in attempts to optimize induced protection from disease.

ACKNOWLEDGMENTS

The authors thank Diane Colf for her editorial assistance and Forrest Sanders for photomicroscopy. Photographs used in the manuscripts were provided through the asssistance of R. R. Dietert, C. L. Greenfield, B. E. Johnson, H. K. Lin, M. A. Qureshi, and F. S. Sanders. Recent research of the authors described within this chapter was supported in part by National Institute of Environmental Health Services (NIEHS) Grant ESO3499 (SEB,RRD), Cornell Biotechnology grant 1574442 (RRD, KAG), U.S. Department of Agriculture Special Grant 157321 (RRD), and student support from NIEHS Training Grant ESO7052, the People's Republic of China, and the Taiwan Ministry of Education.

REFERENCES

1. **Van Furth, R.,** Cells of the mononuclear phagocyte system. Nomenclature in terms of sites and conditions, in *Mononuclear Phagocytes. Functional Aspects,* Van Furth, R., Ed., Martinus-Nijhoff, The Hague, 1980, 1.

2. **Bersuker, I. and Goldman, R.,** On the origin of macrophage heterogeneity: a hypothesis, *J. Reticuloendothelial Soc.,* 33, 207, 1983.

3. **Gordon, S., Crocker, P. R., Morris, L., Lee, S. H., Perry, V. H., and Hume, D.,** Localization and function of tissue macrophages, in *Biochemistry of Macrophages,* Evered, D., Nugent, J., and O'Connor, M., Eds., Ciba Foundation. Symp. 118, Pitman, London, 1986, 54.

4. **Unanue, E. R.,** Antigen-presenting function of the macrophage, *Annu. Rev. Immunol.,* 2, 395, 1984.

5. **Unanue, E. R., Beller, O. I., Lu, C. Y., and Allen, P. M.,** Antigen presentation: comments on its regulation and mechanism, *J. Immunol.,* 132, 1, 1984.

6. **Bell, W. C., Levy, G. N., Williams, R., and Aminoff, D.,** Effect of galactose oxidase, with and without prior siolidase treatment, on the viability of erythrocytes in circulation, *Proc. Natl. Acad. Sci. U.S.A.,* 74, 4205, 1977.

7. **Schlepper-Schäfer, J. and Kolb-Bachofen, J.,** Red cell aging results in a change of cell surface carbohydrate epitopes allowing for recognition by galactose-specific receptors of rat liver macrophages, *Blood Cells,* 14, 259, 1988.

8. **Wei, Y., Heghinian, K., Bell, R. L., and Jakschik, B. A.,** Contribution of macrophages to immediate hypersensitivity reaction, *J. Immunol.,* 137, 1993, 1986.

9. **DeGroot, J. W., Compier-Spies, P. I., Wilbrink, B., Dullens, H. F. J., DeWeger, R. A., and Rademakers, L. H. P. M.,** Tumor growth stimulatory macrophages induced by a subliminal infection *in vivo, J. Leuk. Biol.,* 40, 433, 1986.

10. **Nordan, R. P. and Potter, M.,** A macrophage-derived factor required by plasinacytomas for survival and proliferation *in vivo, Science,* 233, 566, 1986.

11. **Combe, B., Pope, R., Darnell, B., Kincaid, W., and Tolol, N.,** Regulation of natural killer cell activity by macrophages in the rheumatoid joint and peripheral blood, *J. Immunol.,* 133, 709, 1984.

12. **Kedar, I., Rosenberg, Y. J., and Steinberg, A. D.,** Growth regulation of transformed T cells by non-activated macrophages: the role of Ia expression, *J. Immunol.,* 136, 3166, 1986.

13. **Mills, G., Monticone, V., and Paetkau, V.,** The role of macrophages in thymocyte mitogenesis, *J. Immunol.,* 117, 1325, 1976.

14. **Garner, R. E., Malick, A. P., and Elgert, K. D.,** Variations in macrophage antigen phenotype: a correlation between Ia antigen reduction and immune dysfunction during tumor growth, *J. Leuk. Biol.,* 40, 561, 1986.

15. **Bancroft, G. J., Bosma, M. J., Bosma, G. C., and Unanue, E. R.,** Regulation of macrophage Ia expression in mice with severe combined immunodeficiency: induction of Ia expression by a T cell-independent mechanism, *J. Immunol.,* 137, 4, 1986.

16. **Tripp, C. S., Wyche, A., Unanue, E. R., and Needleman, P.,** The functional significance of the regulation of macrophage Ia expression by endogenous arachidonate metabolites *in vitro, J. Immunol.,* 137, 3915, 1986.

17. **Vainio, O. and Ratcliffe, M. J. H.,** Proliferation of chicken peripheral blood leukocytes in response to pokeweed mitogen is macrophage dependent, *Cell. Immunol.,* 85, 235, 1984.

18. **Fredericksen, T. L. and Gilmour, D. G.,** Ontogeny of conA and PHA responses of chicken blood cells in MHC-compatible lines 6_3 and 7_2, *J. Immunol.,* 130, 2528, 1983.

19. **Schaefer, A. E., Scafuri, A. R., Fredericksen, T. L., and Gilmour, D. G.,** Strong suppression by monocytes of T cell mitogenesis in chicken peripheral blood leukocytes, *J. Immunol.,* 135, 1653, 1985.

20. **Kline, K. and Sanders, B. G.,** Suppression of concanavalin A mitogen-induced proliferation of normal spleen cells by macrophages from chickens with hereditary muscular dystrophy, *J. Immunol.,* 132, 2813, 1984.

21. **Sharma, J. M.,** *In vitro* suppression of T-cell mitogenic response and tumor cell proliferation from normal chickens, *Infect. Immun.,* 28, 914, 1980.

22. **Lee, L. F., Sharma, J. M., Nazerian, K., and Witter, R. L.,** Suppression of mitogen-induced proliferation of normal spleen cells by macrophages from chickens inoculated with Marek's disease virus, *J. Immunol.,* 120, 1554, 1978.

23. **Sharma, J. M. and Lee, L. F.,** Effect of infectious bursal disease on natural killer cell activity and mitogenic response of chicken lymphoid cells: role of adherent cells in cellular immune suppression, *Infect. Immun.,* 42, 747, 1983.

24. **Boraschi, D., Pasqualetto, E., Ghezzi, M., Salmona, G., Bartolani, S., Barbarulli, G., Censini, S., Soldateschi, D., and Tagliabue, A.,** Dissociation between macrophage tumoricidal capacity and suppressive activity: analysis with macrophage-defective mouse strains, *J. Immunol.,* 131, 1707, 1983.

25. **Hopper, K. E. and Cahill, J. M.,** Immunoregulation by macrophages. II. Separation of mouse peritoneal macrophages having tumoricidal and bactericidal activities and those secreting PGE and interleukin 1, *J. Reticuloendothelial Soc.,* 33, 443, 1983.

26. **Noma, T., Usui, M., and Dorf, M. E.,** Characterization of the accessory cells involved in suppressor T cell induction, *J. Immunol.,* 134, 1374, 1985.

27. **Lucas, A. M. and Jamroz, C.,** *Atlas of Avian Hematology,* U.S. Department of Agriculture Agricultural Monogr. 25, U.S.D.A., Washington, D.C., 1961.

28. **Greenfield, C. L., Sanders, F. S., and Dietert, R. R.,** Detection of avian macrophages with concanavalin A, *Avian Pathol.,* 17, 803, 1988.

29. **Golemboski, K. A., Bloom, S. E. and Dietert, R. R.,** Dynamics of the avian inflammatory responses to cross-linked dextran: changes in avian blood leukocyte populations, *Inflammation,* 14, 31, 1990.

30. **Golemboski, K. A., Chu, Y., and Dietert, R. R.,** Cell surface changes in chicken inflammatory macrophages, in *Recent Advances in Avian Immunology Research,* Bhogal, B. S. and Koch, G., Eds., Alan R. Liss, New York, 1989, 159.

31. **Jerissen, S. H. M. and Janse, E. M.,** Distribution and function of non-lymphoid cells in liver and spleen of embryonic and adult chickens, in *Recent Advances in Avian Immunology Research,* Bhogal, B. and Koch, G., Eds., Alan R. Liss, New York, 1989, 149.

32. **Powell, P. C., Harltey, K. J., Mustill, B. M., and Rennie, M.,** Studies on the role of macrophages in Marek's disease of the chicken, *J. Reticuloendothelial Soc.,* 34, 289, 1983.

33. **Beug, H., von Kirchbach, A., Doderlein, G., Conscience, J.-F., and Graf, T.,** Chicken hemotopoietic cells transformed by seven strains of defective avian leukemia viruses display three distinct phenotypes of differentiation, *Cell,* 18, 375, 1979.

34. **Qureshi, M. A., Bloom, S. E., Hamilton, J. W., and Dietert, R. R.,** Toxic effects of methyl methanesulfonate (MMS) on activated macrophages from chickens, *Environ. Mol. Mutagen.,* 13, 253, 1989.

35. **Long, P. L. and Rose, M. E.,** Growth of *Eimeria tenella* in macrophages from chicken peritoneal exudate, *Z. Parasitenkd.,* 48, 291, 1976.

36. **Von Bülow, V. and Klasen, A.,** Growth inhibition of Marek's disease T-lymphoblastoid cell lines by chicken bone marrow-derived macrophages activated *in vitro, Avian Pathol.,* 12, 161, 1983.

37. **Dietert, R. R., Combs, G. F., Jr., Lin, H. K., Puzzi, J. V., Golemboski, K. A., and Marsh, J. A.,** Impact of combined vitamin E and selenium deficiency on chicken macrophage function, *Ann. N.Y. Acad. Sci.,* 587, 281, 1990.

38. **Wainberg, M. A., Beiss, B., Fong, H., Beaupré, S., and Menezes, J.,** Involvement of macrophage-like cells in growth of tumors induced by avian sarcoma virus, *Cancer Res.,* 43, 1550, 1983.

39. **Trembicki, K. A., Qureshi, M. A., and Dietert, R. R.,** Avian peritoneal exudate cells: a comparison of stimulation protocols, *Dev. Comp. Immunol.,* 8, 395, 1984.

40. **Vainio, O., Peck, R., Koch, C., and Toivanen, A.,** Origin of peripheral blood macrophages in bursa-cell-reconstituted chickens, *Scand. J. Immunol.,* 17, 193, 1983.

41. **Hauser, H., Graf, T. H., Beug, H., deWilke, J. C., and Schutz, G.,** The chicken lysozyme gene is expressed under different control in macrophages and in the oviduct, *Eur. J. Cell Biol.,* 22, 51, 1980.

42. **Korpela, J.,** Chicken macrophages synthesize and secrete avidin in culture, *Eur. J. Cell Biol.,* 33, 105, 1984.

43. **Klasing, K. C. and Peng, R. K.,** Influence of cell sources, stimulating agents and incubating conditions on release of interleukin-1 from chicken macrophages, *Dev. Comp. Immunol.,* 11, 385, 1987.

44. **Duncan, R. L., Jr. and McArthur, W. P.,** Partial characterization and the distribution of chicken mononuclear cells bearing the Fc receptor, *J. Immunol.,* 120, 1014, 1978.

45. **Peck, R., Murthy, K. K., and Vanio, O.,** Expression of B-L (Ia-like) antigens on macrophages from chicken lymphoid organs, *J. Immunol.,* 129, 4, 1982.

46. **Schmidt, J. A., Marshall, J., and Hayman, M. J.,** Identification and characterization of the chicken transferrin receptor, *Biochem. J.,* 232, 735, 1985.

47. **Rossi, G. and Himmelhoch, S.,** Binding sites for 2-methyl-mannopyranoside and yeast mannan on chicken bone marrow macrophages, *Immunobiology,* 162, 411, 1982.

48. **Hirata, T., Bitterman, P. B., Mornex, J.-F., and Crystal, R. G.,** Expression of the transferrin receptor gene during the process of mononuclear phagoctye maturation, *J. Immunol.,* 136, 1339, 1986.

49. **Hamilton, T. A., Weiel, J. E., and Adams, D. O.,** Expression of the transferrin receptor is modulated in macrophages in different stages of functional activation, *J. Immunol.,* 132, 2285, 1984.

50. **Imber, M., Pizzo, S. V., Johnson, W. J., and Adams, D. O.,** Selective diminution of the binding of mannose by murine macrophages in the latter stages of activation, *J. Biol. Chem.,* 257, 5129, 1982.

51. **Hynes, R. O.,** Integrins: a family of cell surface receptors, *Cell,* 48, 549, 1987.

52. **Jefferies, W. A., Green, J. R., and Williams, A. F.,** Authentic T helper CD4 (W3/25) antigen on rat peritoneal macrophages, *J. Exp. Med.,* 162, 117, 1985.

53. **Wood, G. S., Warner, N. L., and Warnke, R. A.,** Anti-Leu 3/T4 antibodies react with cells of monocyte/macrophage and Langerhans lineage, *J. Immunol.,* 131, 212, 1983.

54. **Chan, M. M., Chen, C.-L., H., Ager, L. L., and Cooper, M. D.,** Identification of the avian homologues of mammalian CD4 and CD8, *J. Immunol.,* 140, 2133, 1988.

55. **Dietert, R. R., Shaw, S. L., and Golemboski, K. A.,** Cell surface Ia and transferrin receptor have distinct induction patterns on chicken inflammatory macrophages, *Poult. Sci.,* 68(S1), 44, 1989.

56. **Trembicki, K. A., Qureshi, M. A., and Dietert, R. R.,** Monoclonal antibodies reactive with chicken peritoneal macrophages: identification of macrophage heterogeneity, *Pro. Soc. Exp. Biol. Med.,* 183, 28, 1986.

57. **Dietert, R. R., Qureshi, M. A., Gause, W. C., Trembicki, K. A., and Marsh, J. A.,** Detection of a macrophage population in the thyroids of obese strain chickens using monoclonal antibodies, in *Progress in Clinical and Biological Research,* Vol. 238, Weber, W. T. and Ewert, D. L., Eds., Alan R. Liss, New York, 1987, 109.

58. **Qureshi, M. A., Bloom, S. E., and Dietert, R. R.,** Effect of major histocompatibility complex gene dosage on chicken monocyte-macrophage function, *Proc. Soc. Exp. Biol. Med.,* 190, 195, 1989.

59. **Jeurissen, S. H. M., Janse, E. M., Koch, G., and de Boer, G. F.,** The monoclonal antibody CVI-CHNL-68.1 recognizes cells of the monocyte-macrophage lineage in chickens, *Dev. Comp. Immunol.,* 12, 855, 1988.

60. **Greenfield, C. L., Dohms, J. E., and Dietert, R. R.,** Infectious bursal disease virus infection in the quail-chicken hybrid, *Avian Dis.,* 30, 536, 1986.

61. **Chung, K.-S. and Lillehoj, H. S.,** Development and characterization of monoclonal antibodies detecting chicken macrophages and natural killer cells, *Poultry Sci.,* 68(S1), 31, 1989.

62. **Strauchen, J. A.,** Lectin receptors as markers of lymphoid cells. I. Demonstration in tissue sections by peroxidase technique, *Am. J. Pathol.,* 116, 297, 1984.

63. **McCabe, R. E. and Remington, J. S.,** Mechanisms of killing *Toxoplasma gondii* by rat peritoneal macrophages, *Infect. Immunol.,* 52, 151, 1986.

64. **Rose, M. E. and Hesketh, P.,** Fowl peritoneal exudate cells, collection and use for the macrophage migration inhibition test, *Avian Pathol.,* 3, 297, 1974.

65. **Puzzi, J. V., Bacon , L. D., and Dietert, R. R.,** B-Congenic chickens differ in macrophage inflammatory responses, *Vet. Immunol. Immunopathol.,* in press, 1989.

66. **Sabet, T., Hsia, W. C., Stanisz, M., El-Domeiri, A., and VanAlten, P.,** A simple method for obtaining peritoneal macrophages from chickens, *J. Immunol. Methods,* 14, 103, 1977.

67. **Dietert, R. R. and Sanders, B. G.,** Leukocyte cell populations in hereditary muscular dystrophic chickens, *J. Hered.,* 76(4), 285, 1985.

68. **Cummins, T. J. and Smith, R. E.**, Association of persistent synthesis of viral DNA with macrophage accessory cell dysfunction induced by avian retrovirus myeloblastosis-associated virus of subgroup B inducing osteopetrosis in chickens, *Cancer Res.*, 47, 6033, 1987.

69. **Lepay, D. A., Steinman, R. M., Nathan, C. F., Murray, H. W., and Cohn, Z. A.**, Liver macrophages in murine listeriosis. Cell-mediated immunity is correlated with an influx of macrophages capable of generating reactive oxygen intermediates, *J. Exp. Med.*, 161, 1503, 1985.

70. **Chu, Y. and Dietert, R. R.**, The chicken macrophage response to carbohydrate-based irritants: temporal changes in peritoneal cell populations, *Dev. Comp. Immunol.*, 12, 109, 1988.

71. **Puzzi, J. V., Bacon, L. D., and Dietert, R. R.**, A gene controlling macrophage functional activation is linked to the chicken B-complex, *Anim. Biotechnol.*, 1, 33, 1990.

72. **Qureshi, M. A. Dietert, R. R., and Bacon, L. D.**, Genetic variation in the recruitment and activation of chicken peritoneal macrophages, *Proc. Soc. Exp. Biol. Med.*, 181, 560, 1986.

73. **Blanckmeister, C. A. and Sussdorf, D. H.**, Macrophage activation by cross-linked dextran, *J. Leuk. Biol.*, 37, 209, 1984.

74. **Carreno, M. P., Labaree, D., Jozefowicz, M., and Kazatchkine, M. D.**, The ability of Sephadex to activate human complement is suppressed in specifically substituted Sephadex derivatives, *Mol. Immunol.*, 25, 165, 1988.

75. **Doherty, D. E., Haslett, C., Tonnesen, M. G., and Henson, P. M.**, Human monocyte adherence: a primary effect of chemotactic factors on the monocyte to stimulate adherence to human endothelium, *J. Immunol.*, 138, 1762, 1987.

76. **Johnston, R. B., Jr., Godzik, C. A., and Cohn, Z. A.**, Increased superoxide anion production by immunologically activated and chemically elicited macrophages, *J. Exp. Med.*, 148, 115, 1978.

77. **Snyderman, R. and Pike, M. C.**, Chemoattractant receptors on phagocytic cells, *Annu. Rev. Immunol.*, 2, 257, 1984.

78. **Thies, E. S., Nelson, R. D., and Maheswavan, S. K.**, Isolation of the turkey heterophil and measurement of its migratory functions under agarose, *Am. J. Vet. Res.*, 44, 228, 1983.

79. **Qureshi, M. A., Dietert, R. R., and Bacon, L. D.**, Chemotactic activity of chicken blood mononuclear leukocytes from $15I_5$-B-congenic lines to bacterially-derived chemoattractants, *Vet. Immunol. Immunopath.*, 19, 351, 1988.

80. **Babior, B. M.**, The respiratory burst of phagoctyes, *J. Clin. Invest.*, 73, 599, 1984.

81. **Ward, P. A., Johnson, K. J., Warren, J. S., and Kunkel, R. G.**, Immune complexes, oxygen radicals and lung injury, in *Oxygen Radicals and Tissue Injury*, Halliwell, B., Ed., The Upjohn Co.-FASEB Publication, Bethesda, MD, 1988, 107.

82. **Johnson, K. J., Rehan, A., and Ward, P. A.**, The role of oxygen radicals in kidney disease, in *Oxygen Radicals and Tissue Injury*, Halliwell, B., Ed., The Upjohn Co.-FASEB Publication, Bethesda, MD, 1988, 115.

83. **Schauenstein, K., Fassler, R., Dietrich, H., Schwarz, S., Kromer, G., and Wick, G.**, Disturbed immune-endocrine communication in autoimmune disease: lack of corticosterone response to immune signals in Obese strain chickens with spontaneous autoimmune thyroiditis, *J. Immunol.*, 139, 1830, 1987.

84. **Hayari, Y., Schuenstein, K., and Golberson, A.**, Avian lymphokines. II. Interleukin-1 activity in supernatants of stimulated adherent splenocytes of chickens, *Dev. Comp. Immunol.*, 6, 785, 1982.

85. **Leutz, A., Beug, H., Walter, C., and Graf, T.**, Hematopoietic growth factor glycosylation, *J. Biol. Chem.*, 263, 3905, 1988.

86. **Larrick, J. W.**, Native interleukin-1 inhibitors, *Immunol. Today*, 10, 61, 1989.

87. **Clark, J. A., Thumwood, C. M., Chaudhri, G., Cowden, W. B., and Hunt, N. H.**, Tumor necrosis factor and reactive oxygen species: implications for free radical-induced tissue injury, in *Oxygen Radicals and Tissue Injury*, Halliwell, B., Ed., The Upjohn Co.-FASEB Publication, Bethesda, MD, 1988, 122.

88. **Arend, W. P., Joslin, F. G., and Massoni, R. J.**, Effects of immune complexes on production by human monocytes of interleukin-1 or an interleukin-1 inhibitor, *J. Immunol.*, 134, 3868, 1985.

89. **Wahl, S. M., Hunt, D. A., Wong, H. L., Dougherty, S., McCartney-Francis, N., Wahl, L. M., Ellingsworth, L., Schmidt, J. A., Hall, G., Roberts, A. B., and Sporn, M. B.**, Transforming growth factor-B is a potent immunosuppressive agent that inhibits Il-1 dependent lymphocyte proliferation, *J. Immunol.*, 140, 3026, 1988.

90. **Kunkel, S. L., Wiggins, S. W., and Phan, S. H.**, Prostaglandins as endogenous mediators of interleukin-1 production, *J. Immunol.*, 136, 186, 1986.

91. **Brown, E. J.**, The role of extracellular matrix proteins in the control of phagocytosis, *J. Leuk. Biol.*, 39, 579, 1986.

92. **Bevilaequa, M., Amrani, D., Mosesson, M., and Bianco, C.**, Receptors for cold insoluble globulin (plasma fibrinecton) on human monocytes, *J. Exp. Med.*, 153, 42, 1981.

93. **Bohnsack, J. F., Kleinman, H. K., Takahashi, T., O'Shea, J. J., and Brown, E. J.**, Connective tissue proteins for phagocytic cell function. Laminen enhances complement and Fc-mediated phagocytosis by cultural human macrophages, *J. Exp. Med.*, 161, 912, 1985.

94. **Stahl, P., Schlesinger, P. H., Sigardson, E., Rodman, J. S., and Lee, Y. S.,** Receptor-mediated pinocytosis of mannose glycoconjugates by macrophages. Characterization and evidence for membrane recycling, *Cell,* 19, 207, 1980.

95. **Rossi, G. and Hillehoch, S.,** Development of mannose-receptor-mediated endocytosis of chicken bone marrow macrophages, *Immunobiology,* 165, 340, 1983.

96. **Czop, J. K.,** Phagocytosis of particular activators of the alternative complement pathway: effects of fibronectin, *Adv. Immunol.,* 38, 361, 1986.

97. **Savill, J. and Haslett, C.,** Macrophage surface structures with integrin-like properties participate in recognition of aged neutrophils, *FASEB J.,* 3(4), A1103, 1989.

98. **Meagher, L., Savill, J., Baker, A., Fuller, R., and Haslett, C.,** Macrophage responses to ingestion of aged neutrophils, *FASEB. J.,* 3(4), A1102, 1989.

99. **Mantovani, B.,** Phagocytosis of *in vitro*-aged erythrocytes — a sharp distinction between activated and normal macrophages, *Exp. Cell Res.,* 173, 282, 1987.

100. **Adams, D. O. and Hamilton, T. A.,** The cell biology of macrophage activation, *Annu. Rev. Immunol.,* 2, 283, 1984.

101. **Nissen-Meyer, J., Kildahl-Andersen, O., and Austgulen, R.,** Human monocyte-released cytotoxic factor: effect on various cellular functions, and dependency of cytolysis on various metabolic processes, *J. Leuk. Biol.,* 40, 121, 1986.

102. **Kildahl-Andersen, O. and Nissen-Meyer, J.,** Production and characterization of cytostatic protein factors released from human monocytes during exposure to lipopolysaccharide and muramyl dipeptide, *Cell Immunol.,* 93, 375, 1985.

103. **Hamilton, T. A. and Adams, D. O.,** Molecular mechanisms of signal transduction in macrophages, *Immunol. Today,* 8, 151, 1987.

104. **Tannenbaum, C. S., Koerner, T. J., Jansen, M. M., and Hamilton, T. A.,** Characterization of lipopolysaccharide-induced macrophage gene expression, *J. Immunol.,* 140, 3640, 1988.

105. **Johnston, P. A., Somers, S. D., and Hamilton, T. A.,** Expression of a 120 kilodalton protein during tumoricidal activation in murine peritoneal macrophages, *J. Immunol.,* 138, 2739, 1987.

106. **Koerner, T. J., Hamilton, T. A., Introna, M., Tannenbaum, C. S., Bast, R. C., Jr., and Adams, D. O.,** The early competence genes *JE* and *KC* are differentially regulated in murine peritoneal macrophages in response to lipopolysaccharide, *Biochem. Biophys. Res. Commun.,* 149, 969, 1987.

107. **Introna, M., Bast, R. C., Jr., Tannenbaum, C. S., Hamilton, T. A., and Adams, D. O.,** The effect of Lps on expression of the early competence gene *JE* and *KC* in murine peritoneal macrophages, *J. Immunol.,* 138, 3891, 1987.

108. **Beutler, B. A., Milsark, I. W., and Cerami, A.,** Cachetin/tumor necrosis factor: production distribution and metabolic fate *in vivo, J. Immunol.,* 135, 3972, 1985.

109. **Ruggiero, V., Latham, K., and Baglioni, C.,** Cytostatic and cytotoxic activity of tumor necrosis factor on human cancer cells, *J. Immunol.,* 138, 2711, 1987.

110. **Ulich, T. R., del Castillo, J., Ni, R.-X., Bikhazi, N., and Calvin, L.,** Mechanisms of tumor necrosis factor alpha-induced lymphopenia, neutropenia and biophasic neutrophilia: a study of lymphocyte recirculation and hematological interactions of TNF with endogenous mediators of leukocyte trafficking, *J. Leuk. Biol.,* 45, 155, 1989.

111. **Chi, D. S. and Thorbecke, G. J.,** Cytotoxicity to allogeneic cells in the chicken. III. Antibody-dependent cell-mediated cytotoxicity in normal and agammaglobulinemic chickens, *Cell. Immunol.,* 64, 258, 1981.

112. **Chi, D. S., Blyznak, N., Kimura, A., Polladino, M. A., and Thorbecke, G. J.,** Cytotoxicity to allogeneic cells in the chicken. II. Specific cytotoxic T cells and macrophages in the spleens of agammaglobulinemic and normal alloimmune chickens, *Cell. Immunol.,* 64, 246, 1981.

113. **Hibbs, J. B., Jr., Vavrin, Z., and Taintor, R. R.,** L-arginine is required for expression of the activated macrophage effector mechanism causing selective metabolic inhibition in target cells, *J. Immunol.,* 138, 550, 1987.

114. **Granger, D. L., Hibbs, J. B., Jr., Perfect, J. R., and Durack, D. T.,** Specific amino acid requirement for the microbistatic activity of murine macrophages, *J. Clin. Invest.,* 81, 1129, 1988.

115. **Hibbs, J. B., Jr., Taintor, R. R., and Vavrin, Z.,** Macrophage cytotoxicity: role for L-arginine deiminase and immunonitrogenoxidation to nitrite, *Science,* 235, 473, 1987.

116. **Drapier, J.-C. and Hibbs, J. B., Jr.,** Differentiation of murine macrophages to express nonspecific cytotoxicity for tumor cells results in L-arginine-dependent inhibition of mitochondrial iron-sulfur enzymes in the macrophage effector cells, *J. Immunol.,* 140, 2829, 1988.

117. **Hibbs, J. B., Jr., Taintor, R. R., Chapman, H. A., Jr., and Weinberg, J. B.,** Macrophage tumor killing: influence of the local environment, *Science,* 197, 279, 1977.

118. **Stuehr, D. J. and Marletta, M. A.,** Mammalian nitrate biosynthesis: mouse macrophages produce nitrite and nitrate in response to *Escherichia coli* lipopolysaccharide, *Proc. Natl. Acad. Sci. U.S.A.,* 82, 7738, 1985.

119. **Austic, R. E. and Nesheim, M. C.,** Arginine, ornithine and proline metabolism of chicks: influence of diet and heredity, *J. Nutr.*, 101, 1403, 1971.

120. **Adams, D. O. and Hamilton, T. A.,** Molecular transductional mechanisms by which IFN and other signals regulate macrophage development, *Immunol. Rev.*, 97, 5, 1987.

121. **Somers, S. D., Whisnant, C. C., and Adams, D. O.,** Quantification of the strength of cell-cell adhesion: the capture of tumor cells by activated murine macrophages proceeds through two distinct stages, *J. Immunol.*, 136, 1490, 1986.

122. **Takacs, B. and Staehli, C.,** Activated macrophages and antibodies against the plant lectin GSI-B$_4$ recognize the same tumor-associated structure (TAS), *J. Immunol.*, 138, 1999, 1987.

123. **Steeg, P. S., Johnson, H. M., and Oppenheim, J. J.,** Regulation of murine macrophage I-A antigen expression by an immune interferon-like lymphokine: inhibitory effect of endotoxins, *J. Immunol.*, 129, 2402, 1982.

124. **Haffer, K., Sevoian, M., and Wilder, M.,** The role of macrophages in Marek's disease: *in vitro* and *in vivo* studies, *Int. J. Cancer*, 23, 648, 1979.

125. **Sharma, J. M.,** Presence of adherent cytotoxic cells and non-adherent natural killer cells in progressive and regressive Marek's disease tumors, *Vet. Immunol. Immunopathol.*, 5, 125, 1983.

126. **Whitfill, C. E., Akbar, W., and Gyles, N. R.,** *In vitro* transfer of chicken peritoneal macrophages between histocompatibility regressor and progressor chicken sublines, *Poult. Sci.*, 61, 1568, 1982.

127. **Kongshavn, P. A. L.,** Genetic control of resistance to *Listeria* infection, *Curr. Top. Microbiol. Immunol.*, 124, 67, 1986.

128. **Kodama, H., Sato, G., and Mikami, T.,** Age-dependent resistance to Salmonella *in vitro:* phagocytic and bactericidal activities of splenic phagocytes, *Am. J. Vet. Res.*, 37, 1091, 1976.

129. **Harmon, B. G., Adams, L. D., and Frey, M.,** Survival of rough and smooth strains of *Brucella abortus* in bovine mammary gland macrophages, *Am. J. Vet. Res.*, 49, 1092, 1988.

130. **Miller, L., Qureshi, M. A., and Berkhoff, H. A.,** Interaction of *Escherichia coli* variants with chicken mononuclear phagocytic system cells, *Dev. Comp. Immunol.*, in press, 1989.

131. **Pabst, M. J., Gross, J. M., Bronza, J. P., and Goren, M. B.,** Inhibition of macrophage activation by sulfatide from *Mycobacterium tuberculosis, J. Immunol.*, 140, 634, 1988.

132. **Von Bülow, V. and Klasen, A.,** Effects of avian viruses on cultured chicken bone-marrow-derived macrophages, *Avian Pathol.*, 12, 179, 1983.

133. **Durban, E. M. and Bottiger, D.,** Differential effects of transforming RNA tumor viruses on avian macrophages, *Proc. Natl. Acad. Sci. U.S.A.*, 78, 3600, 1981.

134. **Durban, E. M. and Boettinger, D.,** Replicating differential macrophages can serve as *in vitro* targets for transformation by avian myeloblastosis virus, *J. Virol.*, 37, 488, 1981.

135. **Lipsich, L., Brugge, J. S., and Bottiger, D.,** Expression of the Rous sarcoma virus *src* gene in avian macrophages fails to elicit transformed cell phenotype, *Mol. Cell. Biol.*, 4, 1420, 1984.

136. **Qureshi, M. A., Muller, L., Lillehoj, H. S., and Ficken, M. D.,** Establishment and characterization of a chicken macrophage cell line, *Vet. Immunol. Immunopathol.*, in press, 1990.

137. **Long, P. L.,** Coccidiosis in poultry, *Crit. Rev. Poult. Biol.*, 1, 25, 1987.

138. **Colwell, D. E., Michalek, S. M., and McGee, J. R.,** *Lps* gene regulation of mucosal immunity and susceptibility to *Salmonella* infection in mice, *Curr. Top. Microbiol. Immunol.*, 124, 121, 1986.

139. **O'Brien, A. D.,** Influence of host genes on resistance of inbred mice to lethal infection with *Salmonella typhimurium, Curr. Top. Microbiol. Immunol.*, 124, 37, 1986.

140. **Lissner, C. R., Swanson, R. N., and O'Brien, A. D.,** Genetic control of the innate resistance of mice to *Salmonella typhimurium:* expression of the *Ity* gene *in vitro, J. Immunol.*, 131, 3006, 1983.

141. **Skamene, E.,** Genetic control of resistance to mycobacterial infection, *Curr. Top. Microbiol. Immunol.*, 124, 49, 1986.

142. **Biozzi, G., Mouton, D., Stiffel, C., and Bouthillier, Y.,** A major role of the macrophage in quantitative genetic regulation of immunoresponsiveness and antiinfectious immunity, *Adv. Immunol.*, 36, 189, 1984.

143. **Santamaria, P., Gehrz, R. C., Bryan, M. K., and Barbosa, J. J.,** Involvement of class II MHC molecules in the LPS-induction of IL-1/TNF secretions by human monocytes. Quantitative differences at the polymorphic level, *J. Immunol.*, 143, 913, 1989.

144. **Guillemot, F. and Auffray, G.,** Molecular biology of the chicken major histocompatibility complex, *Crit. Rev. Poult. Biol.*, 2, 255, 1989.

145. **Lamont, S. J.,** Genetic associations of reticuloendothelial activity in chickens, in *Proc. 2nd World Congr. Genetics Applied to Livestock Production. XI. Genetics of Reproduction, Lactation, Growth, Adaptation, Disease and Parasite Resistance*, Dickenson, G. E. and Johnson, R. K., Eds., Agricultural Communication, University of Nebraska, Lincoln, 1986, 643.

146. **Lokesh, B. R., Hsieh, H. L., and Kinsela, J. E.,** Peritoneal macrophages from mice fed dietary (n-3) polyunsaturated fatty acids secrete low levels of prostaglandins, *J. Nutr.*, 116, 2547, 1986.

147. **Tam, P. E. and Hinsdill, R. D.,** Evaluation of immunomodulatory chemicals: alteration of macrophage function *in vitro, Toxicol. Appl. Pharmacol.*, 76, 183, 1984.

148. **Johnson, B. E., Bell, R. G., and Dietert, R. R.,** 3-Methylcholanthrene-induced immunosuppression in mice to *Trichinella spiralis* antigens, *FASEB J.,* 2(4), 698, 1988.

149. **Miller, K. and Kagan, E.,** Immune adherence reactivity of rat alveolar macrophages following inhalation of crocidolite asbestos, *Clin. Exp. Immunol.,* 29, 152, 1977.

150. **Tombropoulos, E. G., Koo, J. O., Gibson, W., and Hook, G. E. R.,** Induction by morpholine of lysosomal α-mannosidase and acid phosphotase in rabbit alveolar macrophages *in vivo* and *in vitro, Toxicol. Appl. Pharmacol.,* 70, 1, 1983.

151. **Myers, M. J., Schook, L. B., and Bick, P. H.,** Mechanisms of benzo(a)pyrene-induced modulation of antigen presentation, *J. Pharmacol. Exp. Ther.,* 242, 399, 1987.

152. **Murthy, K. K. and Ragland, W. L.,** Modification of humoral immune response in chickens following treatment with carrageenan, *Vet. Immunol. Immunopathol.,* 7, 347, 1984.

153. **Murthy, K. K. and Ragland, W. L.,** Carrageevan induced suppression of chicken lymphocyte proliferation, *Dev. Comp. Immunol.,* 8, 387, 1984.

154. **Lee, E.-H. and Al-Izzi, S. A.,** Selective killing of macrophages in the peritoneal cavity by carrageenan and its effect on normal infection of *Eimeria tenella* in chickens, *Avian Dis.,* 25, 503, 1982.

155. **Higgins, D. A. and Calnek, B. W.,** Some effects of silica treatment on Marek's diseases, *Infect. Immun.,* 13, 1054, 1976.

156. **Chang, C. F. and Hamilton, P. B.,** Impairment of phagocytosis in chicken monocytes during aflatoxicosis, *Poult. Sci.,* 58, 562, 1979.

157. **Onaga, H. and Tajima, M.,** Activation of macrophages by culture fluid of antigen-stimulated spleen cells collected from chickens immunized with *Eimeria tenella, Vet. Parasitol.,* 13, 1, 1983.

158. **Von Bülow, V., Weiler, H., and Klasen, A.,** Activating effects of interferon, lymphokines and viruses on cultured chicken macrophages, *Avian Pathol.,* 13, 621, 1984.

159. **Gazzola, L., Moscovici, M. G., and Moscovici, C.,** Susceptibility and resistance of chicken macrophages to avian RNA tumor viruses, *Virology,* 67, 553, 1975.

160. **Vetvicka, V., Fornusek, L., Blanka, R., and Kopecek, J.,** Properties of macrophages from low- and high-responder strains of mice. I. Effect of antigen stimulation, *Folia Biol. (Prague),* 31, 20, 1985.

161. **Legrand, L., Rivat-Perran, L., Huttin, C., and Dausset, J.,** HLA- and Gm-linked genes affecting the degradation rate of antigens (sheep red blood cells) endocytized by macrophages, *Hum. Immunol.,* 4, 1, 1982.

162. **Vogel, S. N., Weedon, L. L., Oppenheim, J. J., and Rosenstreich, D. L.,** Defective Fc-mediated phagocytosis by LPS-hyporesponsive (LPS^d) C3H/HeJ macrophages: correction by agents that elevated intracellular cyclic AMP, in *Genetic Control of Natural Resistance to Infection and Malignancy,* Skamene, E., Kongshavn, P. A. L., and Landy, M., Eds., Academic Press, New York, 1980, 583.

163. **Chu, Y. and Dietert, R. R.,** Monocyte function in chickens with hereditary muscular dystrophy, *Poultry Sci.,* 68, 226, 1989.

164. **Elin, R. J., Edelin, J. B., and Wolff, S. M.,** Infection and immunoglobulin concentrations in Chediak-Higashi mice, *Infect. Immun.,* 10, 88, 1974.

165. **Wolff, S. M., Dole, D. C., Clark, R. A., Root, R. K., and Kimball, H. R.,** The Chediak-Higashi syndrome: studies of host defenses, *Ann. Int. Med.,* 76, 293, 1972.

166. **Morahan, P. S., Morse, S. S., and Mahoney, K. H.,** The beige (Chediak-Higashi Syndrome) mouse as a model for macrophage functional studies, in *Genetic Control of Natural Resistance to Infection and Malignancy,* Skamene, E., Kongshavn, P. A. L., and Landy, M., Eds., Academic Press, New York, 1980, 575.

167. **Springer, T. A. and Anderson, D. C.,** The importance of the Mac-1, LFA-1 glycoprotein family in monocyte and granulocyte adherence, chemotaxis, and migration into inflammatory sites: insights from an experiment of nature, in *Biochemistry of Macrophages,* Ciba Foundation Symposium 118, Evered, D., Nugent, J., and O'Connor, M., Eds., Pitman, London, England, 1986, 102.

168. **Stevenson, M. M., Skamene, E., and McCall, R. D.,** Macrophage chemotactic response in mice is controlled by two genetic loci, *Immunogenetics,* 23, 11, 1986.

169. **Dang-Vu, A., Pisetsky, D. S., and Weinberg, J. B.,** Functional alterations of macrophages in autoimmune MRL-1pr/1pr mice, *J. Immunol.,* 138, 1757, 1987.

170. **Vogel, S. N. and Fultz, M. J.,** Lps gene-associated functions, *Curr. Top. Microbiol. Immunol.,* 137, 165, 1988.

171. **Stewart, C. C., Skamene, E., and Kongshavn, P. A. L.,** The genetic basis of macrophage colony formation, in *Genetic Control of Natural Resistance to Infection and Malignancy,* Skamene, E., Kongshavn, P. A. L., and Landy, M., Eds., Academic Press, New York, 1980, 499.

172. **Skamene, E., James, S. L., Meltzer, M. S., and Nesbitt, M. N.,** Genetic control of macrophage activation for killing of extracellular targets, *J. Leuk. Biol.,* 35, 65, 1984.

173. **Meltzer, M. S., Ruco, L. P., Boraschi, D., Mannel, D. N., and Edelstein, M. C.,** Macrophage activation for tumor cytotoxicity: genetic influences on development of macrophages with nonspecific tumoricidal activity, in *Genetic Control of Natural Resistance to Infection and Malignancy,* Skamene, E., Kongshavn, P. A. L., and Landy, M., Eds., Academic Press, New York, 1980, 537.

174. **Smith, P. D., Keister, D. B., Wahl, S. M., and Meltzer, M. S.,** Defective spontaneous but normal antibody-dependent cytotoxicity for an extracellular protozoan parasite, *Giardia lamblia,* by C3H/HeJ mouse macrophages, *Cell. Immunol.,* 85, 244, 1984.

175. **Denis, M., Forget, A., Pelletier, M., and Skamene, E.,** Pleiotropic effects of the *Bcg* gene. I. Antigen presentation in genetically susceptible and resistant congenic mouse strains, *J. Immunol.,* 140, 2395, 1988.

176. **Brandwein, S. R., Skamene, E., Aubut, J. A., Gervus, C. E., and Nesbitt, M. N.,** Genetic regulation of lipopolysaccharide-induced interleukin 1 production by murine peritoneal macrophages, *J. Immunol.,* 138, 4263, 1987.

177. **Dietert, R. R. and Golemboski, K. A.,** unpublished observation.

178. **Qureshi, M. A.,** unpublished data.

179. **Golemboski, K. A. et al.,** in preparation.

180. **Greenfield, C. L. and Dietert, R. R.,** unpublished observation.

181. **Puzzi, J. V. and Dietert, R. R.,** unpublished data.

182. **Fleet, J. C. et al.,** submitted for publication.

183. **Austic, R. E., Sung, Y.-J., Hotchkiss, J., and Dietert, R. R.,** unpublished observations.

Chapter 6

CELLULAR IMMUNE SUPPRESSION

David S. Chi, Pascale Quéré, and G. Jeanette Thorbecke

TABLE OF CONTENTS

I. INTRODUCTION

Although the phenomenon of immune suppression is clearly reproducible in certain experimental systems, the existence of "suppressor cells" as a separate functional T-cell subpopulation is not generally accepted. Suppression may be the result of the production of suppressive cytokines or of the negative interaction between two cytokines, in which case the "suppressor" cells are the T cells and/or macrophages producing the factor with inhibitory effects. In other experimental designs, suppression may be associated with the killing of antigen-presenting cells or with so-called Veto cells, i.e., cells that kill upon contact with any other cell which specifically recognizes antigen on the Veto cells.[1] In the mammalian systems studied, suppressor cells were originally thought to belong to the CD8[+] T-cell subpopulation and to exhibit a phenotype distinct from cytotoxic CD8[+] T cells.[2-9] In many cases they appeared to require induction by suppressor-inducer CD4[+] T cells, which also exhibited phenotypic markers different from CD4[+] helper T cells.[8,10-18] However, it has since been shown that some immune suppression effects appear mediated directly by CD4[+] T cells[19] and/or activated macrophages.[20-24]

As in mammals, suppression of antibody production and cellular immunity is observed in chickens. Suppressive activity has been found associated with thymocytes injected *in vivo*[25-27] and with spleen and bone marrow cells in the developing embryo or newly hatched chickens assayed *in vitro* on mitogen-induced proliferative responses.[28] Such activity is reminiscent of the suppressor activity associated with neonatal T cells in mammals.[29] Virus infections, such as Marek's disease[30] and reticuloendotheliosis,[31] have been shown to induce the appearance of cells which suppress mitogen-induced T-cell responses. Again, this is similar to the situation in mammals, where suppression is frequently associated with virally induced lymphoproliferative disorders.[32,33]

Since induction of agammaglobulinemia (Aγ) is easily achieved in the chicken, T-cell function in this species can be studied in the total absence of antibody formation or B cells. Prominent suppressor T cells which appear directed at antibody-forming cells can be activated in such animals by the injection of bursa cells. Here again, a similarity with mammals is suggested by the occurrence of suppressor T cell in Aγ patients[34-36] and by the phenomenon of allotype suppression in mice.[37-39]

Antigen-specific suppressor T cells have been demonstrated after an intravenous (i.v.) injection of antigen, in normal and Aγ chickens, by both cell transfer or *in vitro* cultures. Suppressor cells can also be induced by mitogens as will be discussed in detail below.

Recently, monoclonal antibodies to chicken T-cell antigens have been developed[40] and used to characterize chicken T cells.[41-44] The chicken T-cell differentiation antigens appear to be the homologues of human CD3, CD4, and CD8. As will be discussed below, in most suppressor T-cell-mediated phenomenon studied so far in the chicken, the suppressor cells appear to be CT8[+] CT4[-]. In addition, in several of these systems chicken suppressor cells also bear histamine type 2 receptors (H2R).[45]

II. EXPERIMENTAL *IN VITRO* MODELS OF SUPPRESSION

A. ANTIGEN-INDUCED SUPPRESSOR CELLS

Using SRBC as the antigen, we have demonstrated the presence of both antigen-specific helper and suppressor T cells in both normal and Aγ chickens after a single i.v. antigen injection.[46] The method of detection for these helper and suppressor activities was an *in vitro* culture system, using the plaque-forming cell (PFC) assay to enumerate antibody-producing cells at the end of the culture period. The response of primed spleen cells, taken 2 to 4 d after an i.v. injection of sheep red blood cells (SRBC), was low when antigen was

TABLE 1
In Vitro Anti-SRBC Response of SRBC-
Primed Chicken Spleen Cells[46]

Culture period	Day SRBC added to culture	Mean $\log_{10}$ PFC/culture
4 d	Day 0	3.15
	Day 2	4.95
5 d	Day 0	3.20
	Day 2	5.40
6 d	Day 0	3.10
	Day 2	5.20

Note: 10^7 Spleen cells/dish taken from an SC chicken 4 d after i.v. injection of 0.2 ml 2% sheep red blood cells (SRBC). Dose of antigen *in vitro* was 50 μl 2% SRBC/dish.

added at the beginning of the culture. However, a higher response was observed when antigen addition was delayed until day 2 of culture. A striking feature of this higher responsiveness upon delayed antigen addition was the extreme rapidity of the responses. PFC per dish assayed on day 4 of culture, i.e. 2 d after exposure to SRBC on day 2, were higher than PFC per dish 4 d after exposure to SRBC on day 0 of culture. This phenomenon of the higher response of the culture with delayed addition of antigen was independent of the culture period (Table 1). PFC determined after 4, 5, or 6 d of culture were always much higher in the dishes receiving SRBC on day 2 of culture than in the dishes receiving SRBC on day 0.

Evidence for suppressor cell activity was obtained from cell mixing experiments in which the primed cells reexposed to SRBC immediately upon explantation were found to be suppressive for added antibody-forming spleen cells *in vitro*.[46] Unrelated antigen such as human gamma globulin (HGG) could not induce suppressor activity in SRBC-primed cells, suggesting that the induction of suppression by SRBC in SRBC-primed cells, but not in normal spleen cells, was antigen-specific, at least with respect to *induction* of the suppressor activity (Table 2). The suppressor cells which were activated by exposure to SRBC on day 0 of the culture were resistant to mitomycin C treatment or γ-irradiation and, thus, apparently did not need to proliferate in order to exert their effect (Table 3).

Pretreatment with anti-T antiserum and complement abolished the suppressor activity suggesting that either T cells alone or a cell interaction requiring T cells was needed for the suppressor activity (Table 3). Moreover, spleen cells from Aγ chickens injected i.v. with SRBC exhibited a similar ability to suppress antibody production by normal immune spleen cells. This suppression was again much stronger when the cells had been precultured with SRBC than when they had been precultured without SRBC.[46] In addition, when the primed spleen cells were depleted of CT8$^+$ cells, they would no longer be induced to exert suppressor activity by exposure to antigen on day 0 of culture (Table 4).[43] However, sham-depleted or CT4$^+$ cell-depleted populations still did exhibit suppression of the anti-SRBC response of cocultured cells. The effect of cimetidine, an H2R antagonist, on suppression of the secondary anti-SRBC response, induced by addition of antigen on day 0 of culture, was also investigated. Addition of 2×10^{-4} M cimetidine at the initiation of culture diminished the suppression of the anti-SRBC response (Table 5).

The effect of temperature on these suppressor T cells in SRBC-primed spleen cell cultures was also studied.[47] The response of cultures kept at 40°C was low regardless of the time of antigen addition. In cell mixing experiments, cells from SRBC-primed chickens, cultured at 37°C with antigen for 2 d or at 40°C with or without antigen, suppressed the PFC responses

TABLE 2
Specificity of Suppressor Cell Induction *In*
***Vitro*[46]**

Suppressor cells		% Suppression of control anti-SRBC response[b]
Immune to	Precultured with[a]	
SRBC	SRBC	45.8
None	SRBC	11.0
SRBC	HGG	4.5
None	HGG	−12.5

[a] 10^7 Spleen cells/dish precultured with sheep red blood cells (SRBC) (50 µl 2%) or human gamma globulin (HGG) (10 µg) for 2 d.

[b] Response of target cells (10^7 cells/dish) taken from SRBC-injected donor (day − 4, i.v., 0.2 ml of 2% SRBC) and precultured for 2 d without antigen. Control response (100%) is that obtained with cells to which on day 2 were added "suppressor cells" precultured without antigen. SRBC (50 µl 2%) were added to all cultures on day 2. Plaque-forming cells (PFC) were determined on day 4.

TABLE 3
Characterization of the Antigen-Induced Suppressor Cells[46]

Suppressor cells precultured with SRBC[a]	% Suppression of control anti-SRBC response (mean ± S.E.M.)[b]
Nontreated	80.4 ± 4.8 (n = 8)
γ-Irradiated	77.1 ± 7.4 (n = 4)
Mitomycin C treated	85.2 ± 3.7 (n = 5)
Anti-T + C treated and irradiated	9.3 ± 10.4 (n = 2)

[a] 10^7 Spleen cells/dish taken from sheep red blood cells (SRBC)-injected chickens (day − 4, i.v., 0.2 ml 2% SRBC) and precultured with SRBC (50 µl 2%) for 2 d, then added to target cells on day 2 with antigen.

[b] Response of target cells (10^7 cells/dish) taken from SRBC-injected chickens and precultured for 2 d without antigen. Control response (100%) is that obtained with cells to which on day 2 were added "suppressor cells" also precultured without antigen. SRBC (50 µl 2%) were added to all cultures on day 2. Plaque-forming cells (PFC) were determined on day 4.

of target cells which were precultured without antigen. However, primed spleen cells cultured at 37°C without antigen did not show this suppressor effect, but instead enhanced the PFC response.[47] These results suggest that the disappearance of suppressor cell activity in culture without addition of the antigen is temperature dependent.[47]

Recently, Bhogal et al.[48] have generated T-cell clones from splenic lymphocytes of immunized chickens, reacting specifically with antigenic components of *Eimeria tenella*. Functionally, 19% of the T-cell clones obtained from immune normal chickens and 7% of those obtained from immune Aγ chickens showed suppression of *in vitro* antibody production. Since the suppression induced by some clones required the presence of syngeneic T cells, these cloned T cells perhaps represent suppressor-inducer T cells. Unfortunately, the phenotype of these T-cell clones is not yet studied.

TABLE 4
Effect of Depletion of CT8 or CT4 Positive Spleen Cells on Secondary Responsiveness to SRBC *In Vitro*[43]

| Cells cultured[a] | % of control anti-SRBC response[b] (ag added on day 2) mean ± S.E.M. | | |
	Ag on day 0	Ag on day 2	Ratio (day 0/day 2)
Unfractionated	29.3 ± 9.1	100	0.29 ($n = 7$)
Sham-depleted	44.0 ± 9.0	83.1 ± 9.2	0.52 ($n = 2$)
CT4$^+$ cell-depleted	13.4 ± 9.1	58.3 ± 8.6	0.25 ($n = 2$)
CT8$^+$ cell-depleted	92.8 ± 13.9	103.3 ± 10.0	0.92 ($n = 5$)

Note: Spleen cells taken from 4- to 6-month-old SC chickens 4 d after i.v. injection of 0.25 ml 5% sheep red blood cells (SRBC). Antigen in culture (50 μl 2% SRBC) added at initiation of culture (day 0) or 2 d later (day 2).

a   Spleen cells depleted of CT8- or CT4-positive cells by indirect panning using incubation at 0°C with the relevant monoclonal mouse anti-chicken cell surface antigen followed by incubation of the washed cells in goat anti-mouse Ig-coated Petri dishes.
b   Plaque-forming cells (PFC) developed with rabbit anti-chicken Ig plus guinea pig C. PFC represented as increments in culture due to addition of antigen (ag); PFC present in cultures without SRBC were subtracted.

TABLE 5
Effect of Cimetidine on Suppression of the Secondary Anti-SRBC Response Induced by Addition of Antigen on Day 0[43]

| Cimetidine ($2 \times 10^{-4} M$)[a] | % of control anti-SRBC response (mean ± S.E.M.) | |
	Ag added on day 0	Ag added on day 2
−	20.2 ± 7.6 (n = 5)	100 (n = 4)
+	40.4 ± 11.2 (n = 5)	61.5 ± 10.7 (n = 4)

Note: Spleen cells taken from 4- to 6-month-old SC chickens 4 d after i.v. injection of 0.25 ml 5% sheep red blood cells (SRBC). Antigen (ag) in culture (50 μl 2% SRBC) added at the initiation of culture (day 0) or 2 d later (day 2). Plaque-forming cells (PFC) were determined on day 4.

a   Cimetidine ($2 \times 10^{-4} M$) added at the initiation of culture.

B. MITOGEN-INDUCED SUPPRESSOR CELLS

With cells taken from chickens injected with SRBC 2 to 4 d earlier, the addition of lectins such as pokeweed mitogen (PWM)[46] and concanavalin A (Con A)[47] on day 0 of culture could, even in the absence of SRBC, maintain the suppressor cell activity for the *in vitro* anti-SRBC response. Table 6 shows that SRBC-primed spleen cells, precultured with either the antigen or PWM for 2 d, caused a suppression of the anti-SRBC response. Furthermore, PWM induced suppressor activity in spleen cells from unprimed chickens when added on day 0, but not when added on day 2 of culture. This suggested that the induction

TABLE 6
Induction of Suppressor-Cell Activity by Pokeweed
Mitogen in SRBC-Immune Spleen Cells[46]

Suppressor cells[a] precultured with	% Suppression of control anti-SRBC[b] response (mean ± S.E.M.)
SRBC	58.0 ± 13.8 (n = 3)
PWM (50 μg)	48.0 ± 10.0 (n = 3)

[a] Suppressor cells were taken 2 d after i.v. injection of sheep red blood cells (SRBC) and precultured for 2 d with SRBC (50 μl 2%) or pokeweed mitogen (PWM) (50 μg).

[b] Target cells (10^7 cells/dish) from spleen of immunized chicken, precultured without antigen, and mixed with equal numbers of "suppressor" cells and SRBC (50 μl 2%) on day 2. Control response (100%) is that obtained after mixing with "suppressor cells" precultured without antigen or mitogen. Plaque-forming cells (PFC) were determined on day 4.

TABLE 7
Summary of Properties of Con A-Induced Suppressor Cells as
Assayed on the Secondary Anti-SRBC Response *In Vitro*[44]

T cells added	% Suppression[a] (mean ± S.E.M.)
Normal	12.6 ± 5.2 (*n* = 2)
Con A-induced	62.0 ± 7.7 (*n* = 7)[b,c,d,e]
Con A-induced, CT8[+] cell-depleted	11.8 ± 10.2 (*n* = 3)[c]
Con A-induced + cimetidine (2×10^{-4} *M*)[f]	−28.4 ± 18.7 (*n* = 3)[d]
Con A-induced	
Cimetidine-BSA nonadherent	13.9 ± 26.7 (*n* = 3)[b]
Cimetidine-BSA adherent	65.4 ± 16.6 (*n* = 3)[e]
BSA nonadherent	51.6 ± 17.6 (*n* = 3)

[a] % Suppression as compared to the control anti-SRBC responses obtained in absence of added T cells. Similarly footnoted values compared.

[b] $p = 0.04$.

[c] $p = 0.006$.

[d] $p = 0.005$.

[e] Not significant.

[f] Compared to control anti-SRBC response in absence of added T cells and in presence of 2×10^{-4} *M* cimetidine.

of nonspecific suppressor cell activity by lectins followed the same pattern as that of antigen-specific suppressor cells.[46]

In experiments aimed at studying the properties of Con A-induced nonspecific suppressor cells, CT8[+] cell depletion abolished the suppression of the anti-SRBC response *in vitro* (Table 7).[44] Addition of cimetidine to the culture also abolished the suppression. The results show that cimetidine-bovine serum albumin (BSA) adherent, but not nonadherent, cells exerted suppressor activity, suggesting that lectin-induced nonspecific suppressor T cells also bear histamine type 2 receptors. It is likely that lectins such as phytohemagglutinin (PHA) and Con A also induce suppressor cell activity in chickens *in vivo*, since both of these lectins have been shown to inhibit immune responses *in vivo*.[49,50]

III. ALLOTYPE AND IDIOTYPE SUPPRESSION

Chronic allotype suppression has been achieved in allotypes M-1 and G-1 heterozygous B14-line chickens by the injection of anti-M-1a or anti-M-1b antisera on day 13 of embryonation.[51] Injected chickens have undetectable serum levels of the suppressed IgM-1 and low levels of the linked IgG-1 allotype. This correlates with a complete depletion of cells bearing the relevant IgM-1 allotype and a compensatory increase in the alternative nonsuppressed IgM-1 allotype-bearing cells in the spleen, peripheral blood, and bursa. However, in cell transfers, no suppressor cells could be demonstrated in such chronically allotype-suppressed chickens. Thus, chronic allotype suppression in chickens appeared to be due to a complete depletion of B cells bearing the relevant allotype rather than to allotype-specific suppressor cells. These findings are in agreement with those on allotype suppression in rabbits,[52,53] but they differ from the murine model of allotype suppression, where the presence of allotype-specific suppressor T cells plays an important role, at least in some mouse strains.[37-39]

T-dependent autoantiidiotypic antibody production has been demonstrated in the chicken as early as 4 d after immunization with TNP-Ficoll® or TNP-BA.[54,55] However, no attempts at regulation of the immune response by idiotype specific T cells in the chicken have been reported.

IV. ROLE OF SUPPRESSOR CELLS IN DISEASE MODELS

A. SUPPRESSOR CELLS IN BURSA IMMUNE AGAMMAGLOBULINEMIC CHICKENS

Aγ can be induced in the chicken by either chemical[49,56,57] or surgical[58] bursectomy or by treatment with anti-IgM antiserum.[59] Transfer of lymphoid cells from Aγ donor chickens into irradiated normal recipients causes either agammaglobulinemia in the recipients or specific disappearance of one of the Ig classes.[58,60] This phenomenon has been studied in detail in these authors' laboratory.[49,56,57,61] As shown in Figure 1, injection of B cells into Aγ chickens induced the appearance of suppressor T cells that inhibited adoptive antibody production by simultaneously transferred B cells.[61] Anti-*Brucella abortus* (anti-BA) agglutinin titers determined in sera taken on day 7 were significantly ($p < 0.001$) decreased in the group receiving bursa cells plus suppressor T cells obtained from Aγ chickens that had been injected twice with bursa cells as compared to the group receiving T cells from noninjected Aγ donors. The adoptive antibody production, as judged by sera taken on day 14, was decreased in recipients receiving suppressor T cells from donor chickens injected with bursa cells either once or twice. The agglutinin titers after incubation of sera with 2-mercaptoethanol also showed a significant decrease in both groups receiving suppressor cells ($p < 0.01$). The results indicated that both 19S and 7S anti-BA antibody formation were suppressed.

The cell type that provokes suppressor activity in Aγ chicken spleen cells was studied by comparing spleen cells from Aγ donors injected with a variety of cell types, including peritoneal exudate, thymus, bone marrow, spleen, and bursa cells.[49] Figure 2 shows that bursa cells were far more capable of inducing suppressor activity in spleens of Aγ chickens than any of the other cell types tested. Spleen cells also induced statistically significant suppressor activity, while peritoneal exudate, bone marrow, and thymus cells failed to "immunize". These results indicated that the immunizing cell was of the B-cell lineage.

Various surface components of bursa cells could be responsible for this immunization. Bursa cells from chickens with identical or different major histocompatibility locus possessed the same ability to induce suppressor activity, suggesting that the major histocompatibility complex did not control this induction of suppressor T cells.[49] Despite the indication that

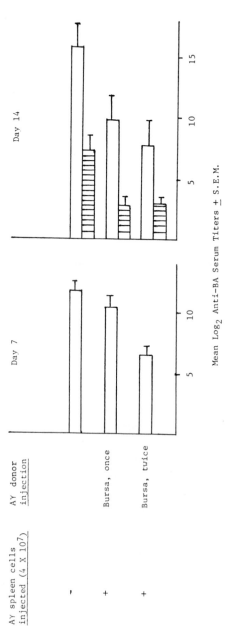

FIGURE 1.   Induction of suppressive activity in spleen cells from Aγ SC chickens by injection of bursa cells.[61] On day 0, 1- to 2-week-old irradiated recipients were injected i.v. with bursa cells from 6- to 9-week-old donors and *Brucella abortus* (2×10^8), with or without spleen cells from Aγ chickens (3 to 6 months old). Aγ donors were immunized with 2×10^7 bursa cells in CFA subcutaneously on day −7 (once) and 2×10^7 cells i.v. on day −52 (twice). ▢ = anti-BA agglutinin titer and ▤ = titer remaining after incubation for 3 h with 0.1 *M* 2-mercaptoethanol. Recipients receiving *B. abortus* alone showed no detectable antibody.

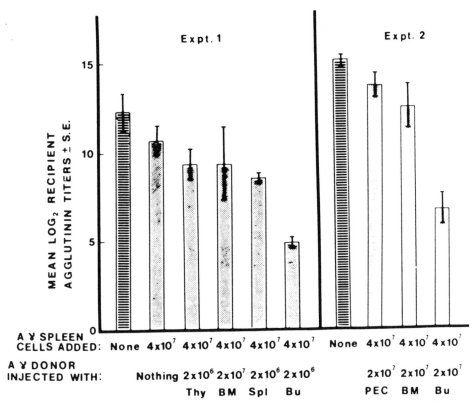

FIGURE 2.   Relative "immunizing" capacity of different cell populations in Aγ FP chickens. Bars represent log₂ anti-*B. abortus* agglutinin titers ± S.E.M. in sera of 1- to 2-week-old irradiated recipient animals receiving *B. abortus*, 4 × 10⁷ normal bursa cells, and, in all but the bars with horizontal cross-hatching, 4 × 10⁷ spleen cells from an Aγ donor injected i.v. previously with the cells noted. Thy = thymus cells, BM = bone marrow cells, Spl = spleen cells, Bu = bursa cells, and PEC = peritoneal exudate cells. Bu and Spl induced suppressor activity (*p* <0.001). Thy, PEC, and BM induced marginal or no suppressor activity (Thy: 0.02 < *p* < 0.05; PEC and BM: not significant). In additional experiment (not shown) neither Thy nor BM induced suppressor activity. (From Grebenau, M. D., Lerman, S. P., Chi, D. S., and Thorbecke, G. J., *Cell Immunol.*, 51, 92, 1980. With permission.)

the immunizing cell was one which displayed Ig on its surface,[49] neither i.v.-administered serum Ig, nor serum Ig in complete Freund's adjuvant (CFA), nor chicken IgM-coated SRBC were capable of provoking suppressor activity in Aγ donors (Experiment 2, Figure 3). The results suggest a surface B-cell antigen other than Ig as the stimulating agent. The fact that both γ-irradiated bursa cells and cell membranes from frozen and thawed bursa cells were quite capable of "immunizing" Aγ donors (Figure 3) further suggested that determinants already present on bursa cells were sufficient for the induction of suppressor-cell activity.

The suppressor activity could be attributed to suppressor T cells.[49] Removal of macrophages from the bursa immune Aγ donor spleen-cell preparation by treatment with carbonyl iron, followed by a passage through a magnet, did not prevent the suppression of the antibody response (Experiment 1, Table 8). On the other hand, treatment of bursa-immune Aγ spleen cells with rabbit anti-chicken thymus antiserum plus complement *in vitro*, prior to transfer, abolished the suppression of the immune response (Experiment 2, Table 8). While γ-irradiation or mitomycin C treatment did not affect the suppression, disruption of the cells removed the suppressor activity of the Aγ spleen cells (Experiment 3, Table 8). This suggests that during the first week after transfer, live cells, but not cell proliferation, were required for suppression. The suppressor T cells were nylon wool nonadherent and were partially

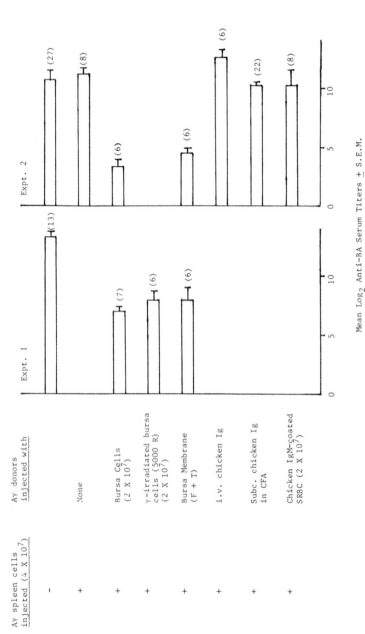

FIGURE 3.   Characteristics of the induction of suppressor cells in Aγ FP chickens.[49] Irradiated (1- to 2-week-old) recipients received i.v. 4×10^7 bursa cells + *B. abortus* ± Aγ spleen cells on day 0. Aγ chickens in Experiment 1 were injected with 2×10^7 bursa cells, normal, or γ-irradiated with 5000 rads *in vitro*, or cell membranes from the equivalent of 10^8 FP bursa cells after repeated freezing and thawing (F + T). Donors used were 12 to 14 d after bursa injection and were 13 to 15 weeks old. In Experiment 2, donors were injected i.v. at least 1 week prior to transfer. Multiple doses of chicken Ig were administered i.v. Chicken IgM-SRBC were prepared by incubating 1% SRBC with an equal volume of a subagglutinating dilution of chicken anti-sheep erythrocyte IgM.

TABLE 8
Characteristics of the Suppressor Cells from Agammaglobulinemic FP Chicken Spleens[49]

Experiment no.	Bursa "immune" Aγ spleen cells	In Vitro pretreatment of Aγ spleen cells	Mean log$_2$ agglutinin serum titer ± S.E.M. in recipients (day 7)[a]
1	None		16.2 ± 0.40 (6)[b]
	4 × 10^7	Sham carbonyl iron treated[c]	11.5 ± 0.72 (6)
	4 × 10^7	Carbonyl iron treated	12.8 ± 1.25 (6)[b]
2	None		14.4 ± 0.80 (8)[d]
	4 × 10^7	None	0.3 ± 0.00 (9)
	4 × 10^7	NRS + C[e]	0.0 ± 0.00 (8)
	4 × 10^7	Anti-T + C[e]	11.8 ± 1.30 (8)[d]
3	None		10.3 ± 1.30 (9)[d,f]
	4 × 10^7	None	4.4 ± 0.50 (9)
	4 × 10^7	Irradiated or mitomycin C-treated[g]	4.4 ± 0.55 (16)[f]
	3.4 × 10^8	Frozen-thawed-sonicated[h,i]	9.8 ± 1.17 (16)[d]

[a]   On day 0, recipients injected i.v. with 4 × 10^7 bursa cells and 0.1 ml 1:12 BA with or without agammaglobulinemic (Aγ) spleen cells. Aγ spleen-cell donors (13 to 15 weeks old) were injected i.v. with 2 × 10^7 bursa cells 7 to 13 d prior to transfer (bursa "immune").

[b]   Similar footnoted values compared, p <0.05.

[c]   Incubation with lymphocyte-separating reagent with or without carbonyl iron and passage over magnet.

[d]   Not significant.

[e]   NRS or rabbit anti-chicken thymus antiserum (anti-T) (1:90) and complement (C) (1:18) for 1 h at 37°C.

[f] p <0.001.

[g]   Not significant.

[h]   Mitomycin C (50 μg/ml) for 45 min at 37°C.

[i]   Cells frozen and thawed repeatedly and sonicated for 3 min. The extract so prepared was injected into recipient in small amounts distributed over day 0 (i.v. and i.p.) and days 1, 3, and 5 (i.p.).

depleted by removal of FcR$^+$ cells.[62] Depletion of CT8$^+$ cells, but not CT4$^+$ cells, from the suppressor T-cell preparation abolished the suppressor activity for adoptive anti-BA antibody production (Figure 4). Suppression of in vitro secondary anti-SRBC response was also abolished by depletion of CT8$^+$ cells from bursa cell immune Aγ chicken spleen cells (Table 9). Furthermore, addition of cimetidine (2 × 10^{-4} M) to the cultures diminished the suppressor activity of spleen cells from bursa-cell immune Aγ chickens, suggesting that some of the suppressor cells may possess H2R (Table 10). However, in vivo treatment of recipients of suppressor cells with cimetidine did not prevent the suppression of the anti-BA response.[42]

Since the injection of bursa cells leads to an increase in the number of these suppressor T cells, it is likely that suppression is directed at B cells. Indeed, the notion of B-cell lineage as the target of suppressor T cells was supported by the observations that the thymus-independent immune response to BA antigen was suppressed and that plasma cells in recipients disappeared within 1 to 2 weeks after the transfer of suppressor cells.[56] Bursas in recipients, however, were not destroyed by transferred suppressor cells, and peripheral B cells, as well as primed memory B cells, did not appear to be decreased to the same extent as were plasma cells and Ig secretion.[49,56] The results suggest a direct effect of suppressor cells on antibody-forming cells with a less marked effect on their precursors.

Recipients of Bursa Cells +

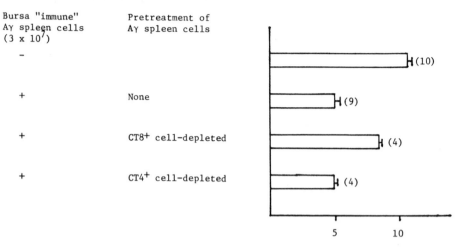

FIGURE 4.   Phenotype of suppressor cells in bursa-"immune" Aγ SC chicken spleen.[42] Irradiated 1- to 2-week-old recipients received i.v. 4 × 10⁷ bursa cells + *B. abortus* ± Aγ spleen cells on day 0. Anti-*B. abortus* serum agglutinin titers were determined 7 d later. Aγ donors of spleen cells were injected twice with SC bursa cells i.v. On the day of transfer, the Aγ spleen cells were preincubated to remove CT4⁺ or CT8⁺ cells by indirect panning.

TABLE 9
Effect of CT8⁺ Cell-Depletion on Suppression by Bursa Cell-Immune Agammaglobulinemic Chicken Spleen Cells of Secondary Anti-SRBC Plaque-Forming Cell Responses *In Vitro*[a]

Suppressor cells added[b]	% Suppression of control anti-SRBC response (mean ± S.E.M.)	
	Experiment 1	Experiment 2
Bursa cell-immune Aγ chicken spleen cells:		
Unfractioned	66.1	68.8
CT8⁺ cell-depleted[c,d]	23.0	43.0
Sham-depleted	60.4	62.0

[a] Response of splenic target cells (10⁷ cells/dish) taken from sheep red blood cell (SRBC)-injected chickens. SRBC (50 μl 2%) were added on day 2 of culture and plaque-forming cells (PFC) determined on day 4.

[b] Suppressor cells from spleen of agammaglobulinemic (Aγ) chicken that has received 2 injections of 4 × 10⁷ bursa cells, the last one on day −7, were added at the initiation of the culture.

[c] Suppressor cells were depleted of CT8⁺ cells by indirect panning.

[d] Data taken from Reference 42.

TABLE 10

**Partial Reversal by Cimetidine of the Suppressive
Activity of Spleen Cells from Bursa Cell-Immune
Agammaglobulinemic Chickens on the Secondary
Anti-SRBC PFC Response *In Vitro*[a]**

Cimetidine	% Suppression of control anti-SRBC response[b,c] (mean ± S.E.M.)
—	58.5 ± 7.3 (*n* = 5)
10^{-4} *M*	45.4 ± 4.8 (*n* = 5)
2×10^{-4} *M*	30.4 ± 5.6 (*n* = 5)

[a] Suppressor cells from spleen of agammaglobulinemic (Aγ) chickens that have received 2 or 3 injections of 4×10^7 bursa cells, the last one on day -7, and added at the initiation of the culture.

[b] Response of splenic target cells (10^7 cells/dish) taken from sheep red blood cell (SRBC)-injected chickens. SRBC (50 μl 2%) were added on day 2 of culture and plaque-forming cells (PFC) determined on day 4. 100% control values without cimetidine ranged from 1148 to 9549 PFC/dish and with cimetidine from 928 to 8197 PFC/dish.

[c] Data taken from Reference 42.

In the transfer of Aγ isotype-specific suppression has sometimes been demonstrated;[60] some recipient chickens were found to have isolated IgA deficiency.[63] The spontaneous occurrence of T cells that are specifically suppressive for IgG production has been reported in a White Leghorn strain (UCD line 140) of chickens with a high incidence of inherited IgG deficiency accompanied by greatly increased levels of IgM.[64] This type of abnormality is apparently not rare in chickens since an independently derived line with similar abnormalities has also been documented.[65,66]

B-cell-specific suppressor T cells from Aγ chickens can inhibit the *in vitro* and *in vivo* growth of a B-cell lymphoma.[67] A B-cell lymphoma, RP6, induced by avian leukosis virus (RAV-2) in $15I_5 \times 7_1$ chickens,[68] could be transplanted by i.v. injection of the tumor cells and grown throughout the spleen and liver of recipients. This tumor growth was inhibited in Aγ chicken, as indicated by a lower tumor mass in both spleen and liver of Aγ than of normal chickens.[67] The inhibition of the growth of the B-cell lymphoma was specific, since the growth of RP11, a T-cell tumor, was not suppressed in Aγ chickens. The suppressor effect could also be shown in a culture system in which spleen cells from bursa immune $15I_5 \times 7_1$ Aγ chickens inhibited the *in vitro* growth of tumor cells as indicated by a decrease in ^{3}H-thymidine incorporation.[69]

B. SUPPRESSOR CELLS IN VIRUS INFECTIONS

Sharma[70] has reported marked suppression of *in vitro* proliferative responses of spleen cells to mitogens by spleen macrophages from normal chickens. This activity was enhanced during the early stages of infection by infectious bursal disease virus.[71-76] The mitogenic hyporesponsiveness was due to the presence of suppressor cells since addition of spleen cells from infected chickens prevented normal spleen cells from responding to mitogen.[30] The suppressor activity could be removed by pretreatment of suppressor cells with carbonyl iron/magnet or Cytodex-3® microcarrier beads. The suppressor effect appeared to be mediated by soluble factor(s) released by the suppressor cells, since cell-cell contact between suppressor and responder cells was not necessary for suppression to occur.[30] Soluble suppressor factors have also been demonstrated in conditioned media from Con A-stimulated peripheral blood suppressor monocytes; those factors inhibited Con A stimulation of peripheral blood lymphocytes (PBL).[77] Suppression of the mitogenic response by spleen cells from avian retrovirus MAV-2-0-infected chickens has also been demonstrated. This suppressed mitogenic responsiveness could be restored by the addition of conditioned media rich in T-cell growth factor activity.[78]

Spleen cells from chickens infected with reticuloendotheliosis viruses (REV) have also been shown to depress mixed lymphocyte and mitogen responses *in vitro*.[31] Furthermore, Rup et al.[79] have reported a rapid induction of splenic suppressor cells in chickens injected with nonproducer REV-transformed cells. The induction of suppressor cells was dependent on the number of transformed cells injected and on the development of tumor foci in the infected chickens. The suppressor cells could not be removed by adherence to plastic,[80] but they could by lysed by antibody to the major envelope viral glycoprotein, suggesting that they exhibit this protein on their surface.[79]

Theis[81] has studied the induction of suppressor cells in chickens by injection of transplantable JM-V leukemia, derived from Marek's disease virus-infected chickens. Three distinct subpopulations of cells with suppressor activity for mitogenic responses were identified by Ficoll® density gradient centrifugation of the spleen cells from 3- to 4-week-old chickens injected with cultured lymphoblastoid cells (JC-VLC). One subpopulation consisted of nylon-wool-nonadherent cells and was located in the T-cell-rich intermediate gradient fraction. The second subpopulation consisted of phagocytic cells (macrophages), the most effective suppressor cells of responses to mitogens. The third subpopulation was identified as the JM-VLC cells themselves, found in the buoyant gradient fractions of leukemic chicken spleens.

Thus, it appears that injection of leukemia cells in chickens results not only in the induction of suppressor T cells but also of suppressor macrophages. However, in all these examples of suppressor cell induction by virally induced lymphomas, it is difficult to exclude a direct effect of the virus in mediating suppression.

C. SUPPRESSOR MACROPHAGES IN CHICKENS WITH HEREDITARY MUSCULAR DYSTROPHY

Kline and Sanders[82] have shown that spleen cells from chickens with hereditary muscular dystrophy give low proliferative responses to Con A, but not to PHA. The addition of spleen cells from muscular dystrophy chickens caused a marked suppression of the Con A response of normal spleen cells, while responses to PHA were not affected. The suppressive activity was attributed to the presence of suppressor macrophages. The suppressor activity was not affected by the treatment of anti-T- or anti-B-cell antiserum plus complement, but it was abolished by treatment with carrageenan or carbonyl iron/magnet, by passage through a Sephadex® G-10 column, or by adherence to plastic petri dishes or glass beads. The suppressive activity by the spleen cells from muscular dystrophy chickens required viable cells and was contact mediated.

D. SUPPRESSOR CELLS IN TUMOR IMMUNITY

The transplantable chemically induced fibrosarcoma model in SC chickens has also been used to study tumor-induced suppressor T cells.[45] Progressive growth of tumors can, under certain experimental conditions, be prevented by pretreatment of the host with a low dose of cyclophosphamide suggesting the existence of suppressor cells in the animal.[45] Immunity to a local (wing web) challenge with transplantable, chemically induced tumors, such as CHCT-NYU-4, can be transferred to histocompatible SC chickens with intravenously injected splenic T cells from tumor-immune chickens.[45] This system has been utilized for testing the presence of suppressor cells in the spleens from chickens bearing progressively growing tumors. Indeed, suppression of i.v. transferred immunity could be accomplished by simul-

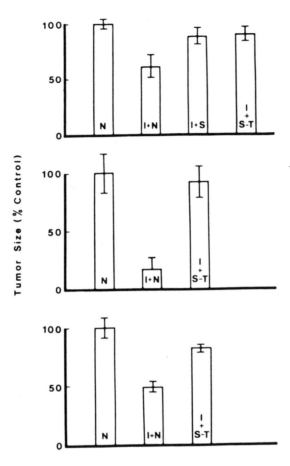

FIGURE 5. Three experiments showing the systemic transfer of immunity and suppression by i.v. injection of 10^8 spleen cells from NYU-4-immune syngeneic SC chickens (I), SC chickens bearing progressively growing NYU-4 tumors (S), or with both (I + S). Control animals received 10^8 spleen cells from normal chickens (N). In one group of each experiment, animals received T-cell-enriched spleen cells (nylon wool nonadherent = NWNA) from the suppressor cell donors (S-T) along with the immune spleen cells (I + S-T). Tumor sizes are reported as percentages of the average tumor sizes in the control group (N) at 3 weeks after challenge with 10^5 NYU-4 tumor cells subcutaneously. Tumor sizes in the I + N group are significantly smaller than in any other group ($p < 0.05$) in each experiment. (From Edelman, A. S., Robinson, M. E., Sanchez, P., and Thorbecke, G. J., *Cell. Immunol.*, 110, 321, 1987. With permission.)

taneous transfer of spleen cells from progressively growing tumor-bearing animals (Figure 5). In the three experiments shown, the cotransfer of immune and normal spleen cells significantly inhibited tumor-cell growth as compared with control animals receiving normal spleen cells alone. The transfer of immune spleen cells with suppressor cells, either as unfractionated or as nylon-wool-nonadherent spleen cells, inhibited the effect of the immune spleen cells. Cells responsible for the inhibition of tumor immunity were characterized as nylon-wool-nonadherent T cells bearing H2R and surface immune associated antigen (Ia).[45] In the experiments illustrated in Figure 6, nylon-wool-nonadherent suppressor cells com-

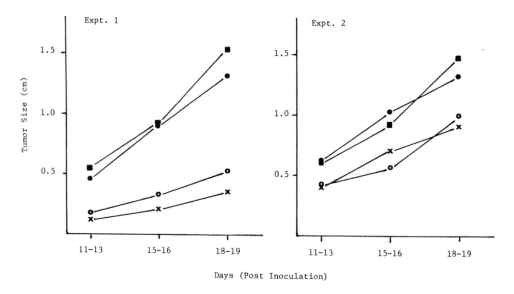

FIGURE 6.   Tumor growth in recipients of 10^5 NYU-4 tumor cells (subcutaneously) plus immune spleen cells (i.v.) and H2R$^+$ or H2R$^-$ suppressor (SU) T cells (i.v.) from spleen of chickens with progressively growing fibrosarcoma.[45] Normal control spleen cells, ×; unfractioned SU-T cells (nylon wool nonadherent), ■; cimetidine nonadherent SU-T cells (H2R$^-$), ○; cimetidine adherent SU-T cells (H2R$^+$), ●.

pletely inhibited the effect of the immune cells at all time points observed. The splenic T cells adherent to dishes coated with cimetidine-protein conjugate, but not the nonadherent cells, inhibited the adoptive tumor immunity, suggesting that the suppressor cells were H2R$^+$ (Figure 6). Moreover, treatment with anti-chicken Ia antigen and complement abolished the suppressor activity.[45]

E. ROLE OF SUPPRESSOR CELLS IN TOLERANCE

Tolerance has been demonstrated in chickens to allogeneic cells[83,84,89] and to protein antigens.[85-88] Hraba et al.[90] were unable to demonstrate suppressor activity in spleen cells from chickens that had been tolerized to human serum albumin (HSA) at hatching, as shown by their inability to suppress the anti-HSA antibody production of simultaneously transferred HSA-immune spleen cells.

In contrast to the above, Morgan et al.[91,92] showed two soluble suppressor factors in the sera of BSA-tolerant chickens. These factors suppressed, nonspecifically, both *in vitro* and *in vivo* responses of normal spleen cells to SRBC. Recently, they have further demonstrated the presence of suppressor T cells in chickens neonatally rendered tolerant to BSA.[93] Transfer of BSA-tolerant spleen cells without or with specifically primed adult spleen cells into normal recipients, followed by BSA challenge, prevented any significant primary or secondary anti-BSA response. The suppression was antigen specific, since BSA-tolerant spleen cells were unable to suppress either primary or secondary responses of B cells to SRBC. The reasons for the conflicting results between the BSA and HSA systems are not apparent. They may be due to differences in chicken strains or the time at which suppressor activity was assayed.

Thymus cells from immature and young normal adult donors were shown to suppress antibody formation and skin graft rejection in normal or irradiated recipients nonspecifically.[25-27] A few weeks after the thymus cell transfers, the response to an unrelated antigen or graft returned to normal, but the response to the original antigen remained depressed. These suppressor cells were found more prevalent in thymus from chickens with intact bursas than from bursectomized chickens.[27]

We have studied the induction of T-cell tolerance in adult chickens after a single i.v. injection of either SRBC[62] or HGG.[94,95] After i.v. injection of antigen, both Aγ and normal chickens are very rapidly rendered unable to respond with a delayed-type hypersensitivity (DH) to that antigen, and this effect is antigen-specific. The susceptibility to the induction of tolerance at the T-cell level is greater in the Aγ than in normal chickens suggesting the relatively greater effectiveness of the toleragenic dose in the absence of antibody production.[94] Using HGG as the toleragen, we also examined the tolerant chickens for the presence of suppressor cells. Since suppressor cells could not be demonstrated, the T-cell tolerance in these chickens appeared to be primarily due to deletion of antigen-responsive cells. Cell transfer studies showed that spleen cells from tolerant chickens, injected either with HGG intravenously or first with HGG intravenously and then with HGG plus CFA intramuscularly, were deficient in T-helper activity for the response to TNP-HGG of TNP-primed B cells.[95] However, they failed to suppress the helper activity of HGG plus CFA-primed cells from control chickens or the induction of DH in normal recipients.[95] Furthermore, pretreatment of the chickens with a low dose of cyclophosphamide, a toxic agent to suppressor cells, did not affect the induction of antigen-specific tolerance.[62] While the mechanism of deletion of T-helper and T_{DH} cells in this system is unknown, a role for suppressor cells in mediating this event could not be excluded. Presumably, for suppressor cells to be detected in cell transfer studies, a much more expanded population of such cells is needed than for a deletion process in the lymphoid tissue of the tolerized host. Moreover, it should be noted that, in contrast to our findings, Higgins et al.[96] showed that isolated HGG-binding T cells, obtained from Aγ SC (B2/B2) chickens after repeated i.v. injections of deaggregated HGG, were able to suppress the adoptive antibody production of a mixture of TNP-primed B cells and HGG plus CFA-primed T cells in irradiated recipients.

F. DEFECT IN NONSPECIFIC SUPPRESSION AS A CAUSE OF AUTOIMMUNITY

Genetically controlled spontaneous autoimmune thyroiditis has been reported in the Obese strain (OS) of chickens.[97-99] This disease is B-cell dependent, since neonatal bursectomy reduces the disease severity, whereas neonatal thymectomy increases it.[99] In contrast to systemic spontaneous autoimmunity in mammals,[100,101] spontaneous autoimmune thyroiditis (SAT) of OS chickens is associated with a deficiency in thymic nurse cells[102] and a marked T-cell hyperreactivity evidenced by enhanced mitogen responses and increased production of interleukin 2 (IL-2).[103] This T-cell mitogen hyperreactivity has been attributed to a defect in nonspecific suppressor mechanism.[104] This defect can be related to a deficiency, in conditioned media prepared from Con A-stimulated OS splenocytes, of dialyzable inhibitory factors that regulate IL-2 production and IL-2 function of normal lymphocytes *in vitro*. This IL-2 inhibitory activity was also present in serum of normal chickens, but deficient in OS chickens. The cellular origin of IL-2 inhibitory activity in the chicken has been identified to be nonlymphoid, plastic adherent cells (macrophages).[105] The defective IL-2 inhibitory factor production in autoimmune chickens has been shown to be due to a functional, but not numeric, defect of macrophages.[105]

V. CONCLUSIONS

In this chapter conclusive evidence has been presented to show the existence of both nonspecific and antigen-specific cellular immune suppression in the chicken. The cellular effectors of suppression include suppressor T cells and macrophages in peripheral blood, spleen, thymus, or bone marrow. The most prominent CT4$^-$ CT8$^+$ suppressor T cells, which directly affect antibody-forming cells, have been described in Aγ chickens. CT4$^-$ CT8$^+$ histamine type 2 receptor-bearing suppressor T cells can be induced by antigens, such as SRBC, or by mitogens, such as Con A. Suppressor T-cell clones reacting specifically with antigenic components of *E. tenella* have been generated from splenic lymphocytes of immunized chickens. Suppressor macrophages have been shown to be associated with virally induced lymphoproliferative disorders. The suppression of tumor immunity in chickens with progressively growing chemically induced tumors appears to be associated with histamine type 2 receptor-bearing Ia$^+$ T cells.

Soluble suppressor factors have been demonstrated in the supernatants of Con A-stimulated peripheral blood monocytes, but evidence that T-cell mediated suppression is due to soluble factors is lacking in the chicken system.

Since Aγ chickens have a total lack of both antibody formation and B cells, they represent a good model to study the mechanisms of putative T-T cell interactions in induction of suppressor T-cell activities. More advantage should be taken of this model for the evaluation of the existence of the equivalence of a B-cell idiotype network at the level of the T-cell receptor.

ACKNOWLEDGMENTS

This work was supported by U.S. Public Health Service Grants CA-43536, CA-32801, and AG-04980 from the National Cancer Institute; the National Institute of Aging, U.S. Department of Health and Human Services; and by the Ruth R. Harris Endowment, East Tennessee State University. The authors would like to thank Dr. Max D. Cooper of the University of Alabama, Birmingham, for his generous gifts of the monoclonal antibodies.

REFERENCES

1. **Fink, P. J.,** *Annu. Rev. Immunol.,* 6, 115, 1988.
2. **Green, D., Flood, P., and Gershon, R.,** Immunoregulatory T-cell pathways, *Annu. Rev. Immunol.,* 1, 439, 1983.
3. **Reinherz, E. L. and Schlossman, S. F.,** The differentiation and function of human T lymphocytes, *Cell,* 19, 821, 1980.
4. **Reinherz, E. L. and Schlossman, S. F.,** Regulation of the immune response-inducer and suppressor T lymphocyte subsets in human beings, *N. Engl. J. Med.,* 303, 370, 1980.
5. **Reinherz, E. L., Moretta, L., Roper, M., Breard, J. M., Mingari, M. C., Cooper, M. D., and Schlossman, S. F.,** Human T lymphocyte subpopulations defined by Fc receptors and monoclonal antibodies: a comparison, *J. Exp. Med.,* 151, 969, 1980.
6. **Ledbetter, J. A., Evans, R. L., Lipinski, M., Cunningham-Rundles, C., Good, R. A., and Herzenberg, L. A.,** Evolutionary conservation of surface molecules that distinguish T lymphocyte helper/inducer and cytotoxic/suppressor subpopulations in mouse and man, *J. Exp. Med.,* 153, 310, 1981.
7. **Catenby, P. A., Kansas, G. S., Xian, C. Y., Evans, R. L., and Engleman, E. G.,** Dissection of immunoregulatory subpopulations of T lymphocytes within the helper and suppressor sublineages in man, *J. Immunol.,* 129, 1997, 1982.
8. **Thomas, Y, Rogozinski, L., Rothman, P., Rabbani, L. E., Andrews, S., Irigoyen, O. H., and Chess, L.,** Further dissection of the functional heterogeneity within the OKT4$^+$ and OKT8$^+$ human T cell subsets, *J. Clin. Immunol.,* 2, 8S, 1982.
9. **Thomas, Y., Rogozinski, L., and Chess, L.,** Relationship between human T cell functional heterogeneity and human T cell surface molecules, *Immunol. Rev.,* 74, 113, 1983.
10. **Reinherz, E. L., Kung, P. C., Goldstein, G., and Schlossman, S. F.,** Further characterization of the human inducer T cell subset defined by monoclonal antibody, *J. Immunol.,* 123, 2894, 1979.
11. **Thomas, Y., Rogozinski, L., Irigoyen, O. H., Friedman, S. M., Kung, P. C., Goldstein, G., and Chess, L.,** Functional analysis of human T cell subsets defined by monoclonal antibodies. IV. Induction of suppressor cells within the OKT4$^+$ population, *J. Exp. Med.,* 154, 459, 1981.
12. **Thomas, Y., Rogozinski, L., Irigoyen, O. H., Sher, H. H., Talle, M. A., Goldstein, G., and Chess, L.,** Functional analysis of human T cell subsets defined by monoclonal antibodies. V. Suppressor cells within the activated OKT4$^+$ population belong to a distinct subset, *J. Immunol.,* 128, 1386, 1982.

13. **Reinherz, E. L., Morimoto, C., Fitzgerald, K. A., Hussey, R. E., Daley, J. F., and Schlossman, S. F.,** Heterogeneity of human T4$^+$ inducer T cells defined by a monoclonal antibody that delineates two functional subpopulations, *J. Immunol.,* 128, 463, 1982.
14. **Heijnen, C. J., Pot, K. H., and Ballieux, R. E.,** Characterization of human T suppressor-inducer, -precursor and -effector lymphocytes in the antigen-specific plaque-forming cell response, *Eur. J. Immunol.,* 12, 860, 1982.
15. **Morimoto, C., Distaso, J. A., Borel, Y., Schlossman, S. F., and Reinherz, E. L.,** Communicative interactions between subpopulations of human T lymphocytes required for generation of suppressor effector function in a primary antibody response, *J. Immunol.,* 128, 1645, 1982.
16. **Morimoto, C., Reinherz, E. L., Borel, Y., and Schlossman, S. F.,** Direct demonstration of the human suppressor inducer subset by anti-T cell antibodies, *J. Immunol.,* 130, 157, 1983.
17. **Ballieux, R. E. and Heijnen, C. J.,** Immunoregulatory T cell subpopulations in man: dissection by monoclonal antibodies and Fc-receptors, *Immunol. Rev.,* 74, 5, 1983.
18. **Rao, P. E., Talle, M. A., Kung, P., and Goldstein, G.,** Five epitopes of a differentiation antigen on human inducer T cells distinguished by monoclonal antibodies, *Cell. Immunol.,* 80, 310, 1983.
19. **Awwad, M. and North, R. J.,** Immunologically mediated regression of a murine lymphoma after treatment with anti-L3T4 antibody. A consequence of removing L3T4 suppressor T cell from a host generating predominantly Lyt2$^+$ T cell-mediated immunity, *J. Exp. Med.,* 168, 2193, 1988.
20. **Stadecker, M J., Calderon, J., Karnovsky, M. L., and Unanue, E. R.,** Synthesis and release of thymidine by macrophages, *J. Immunol.,* 119, 1738, 1977.
21. **Allison, A. C.,** Mechanisms by which activated macrophages inhibit lymphocyte responses, *Immunol. Rev.,* 40, 3, 1978.
22. **Boraschi, D., Soldateschi, D., and Tagliabue, A.,** Macrophage activation by interferon: dissociation betweem tumoricidal capacity and suppressive activity, *Eur. J. Immunol.,* 12, 320, 1982.
23. **Phipps, R. P. and Scott, D. W.,** A novel role for macrophages: the ability of macrophages to tolerize B cells, *J. Immunol.,* 131, 2122, 1983.
24. **Stout, R. D.,** Cytostatic activity of *in vitro* generated macrophages: evidence for a prostaglandin-independent reversible cytostatic mechanism, *Cell. Immunol.,* 96, 83, 1985.
25. **Droege, W.,** Comparison of the suppressive effect of thymus cells and the suppression by neonatal application antigen, *Eur. J. Immunol.,* 3, 804, 1973.
26. **Droege, W.,** Immunosuppressive effect of syngeneic thymus cells on allograft rejection, *Proc. Natl. Acad. Sci. U.S.A.,* 72, 2371, 1975.
27. **Moticka, E. J.,** The presence of immunoregulatory cells in chicken thymus: function in B and T cell responses, *J. Immunol.,* 119, 987, 1977.
28. **Kline, K. and Sanders, B. G.,** Developmental profile of chicken splenic lymphocyte responsiveness to Con A and PHA and studies on chicken splenic and bone marrow cells capable of inhibiting mitogen-stimulated blastogenic responses of adult splenic lymphocytes, *J. Immunol.,* 125, 1792, 1980.
29. **Murgita, R. A., Hooper, D. C., Stegagno, M., Delovitch, T. L., and Wigzell, H.,** Characterization of murine newborn inhibitory T lymphocytes: functional and phenotypic comparison with an adult T cell subset activated *in vitro* by alpha-fetoprotein, *Eur. J. Immunol.,* 11, 957, 1981.
30. **Sharma, J. M. and Fredericksen, T. L.,** Mechanism of T cell immunosuppression by infectious bursal disease virus of chickens, in *Avian Immunology,* Vol. 2, Weber, W. T. and Ewert, D. L., Eds., Alan R. Liss, New York, 1987, 283.
31. **Walker, M. H., Rup, B. J., Rubin, A. S., and Bose, H. R., Jr.,** Specificity in the immunosuppression induced by avian reticuloendotheliosis virus, *Infect. Immun.,* 40, 225, 1983.
32. **Perryman, L. E., Hoover, E. A., and Yohn, D. S.,** Immunologic reactivity of the cat: immunosuppression in experimental feline leukemia, *J. Natl. Cancer Inst.,* 49, 1357, 1972.
33. **Cimprich, R. S., Specter, S., and Friedman, H.,** Murine lymphoma-induced immunosuppression: requirement for direct tumor cell contact, *Science,* 200, 60, 1978.
34. **Waldmann, T. A., Broder, S., Blaese, R. M., Durm, M., Blackwell, M., and Strober, W.,** Role of suppressor T cells in pathogenesis of common variable hypogammaglobulinemia, *Lancet,* 2, 609, 1974.
35. **Siegal, F. P., Siegal, M., and Good, R. A.,** Suppression of B-cell differentiation by leukocytes from hypogammaglobulinemic patients, *J. Clin. Invest.,* 58, 109, 1976.
36. **Litwin, S. A. and Zanjani, E. D.,** Lymphocytes suppressing both immunoglobulin production and erythroid differentiation in hypogammaglobulinemia, *Nature (London),* 266, 57, 1977.
37. **Jacobson, E. B., Herzenberg, L. A., Riblet, R., and Herzenberg, L. A.,** Active suppression of immunoglobulin allotype synthesis. Transfer of suppressing factor with spleen cells, *J. Exp. Med.,* 135, 1163, 1972.
38. **Jacobson, E. B.,** *In vitro* studies of allotype suppression in mice, *Eur. J. Immunol.,* 3, 619, 1973.
39. **Jacobson, E. B.,** Adoptive transfer of allotype-specific suppressor cells inhibits thymus-independent immunoglobulin production in syngeneic athymic mice, *J. Exp. Med.,* 148, 607, 1978.

40. **Chan, M. M., Chen, C.-L. H., Ager, L. L., and Cooper, M. D.,** Identification of the avian homologues of mammalian CD4 and CD8 antigens, *J. Immunol.,* 140, 2133, 1988.

41. **Quéré, P., Cooper, M. D., and Thorbecke, G. J.,** Suppressor cell properties in the chicken, *FASEB J.,* 3, A807, 1989.

42. **Quéré, P. and Thorbecke, G. J.,** Suppressor cells for antibody production *in vivo,* induced by bursa cell injection into agammaglobulinemic chickens, belong to a CT4⁻, CT8⁺, TCR1⁻ subset of T cells, *Dev. Comp. Immunol.,* in press, 1990.

43. **Quéré, P., Cooper, M. D., and Thorbecke, G. J.,** Characterization of suppressor T cells for antibody production by chicken spleen cells. I. Antigen induced suppressor cells are CT8⁺, TCR1⁺ (γδ) T cells, *Immunology,* in press, 1990.

44. **Quéré, P., Bhogal, B. S., and Thorbecke, G. J.,** Characterization of suppressor T cells for antibody production by chicken spleen cells. II. Comparison of CT8⁺ cells from concanavalin A injected normal and bursa cell injected agammaglobulinemic chickens, in preparation, 1989.

45. **Edelman, A. S., Robinson, M. E., Sanchez, P., and Thorbecke, G. J.,** Suppressor T cells with histamine type II receptors in chickens bearing chemically induced fibrosarcomas, *Cell. Immunol.,* 110, 321, 1987.

46. **Chi, D. S., Grebenau, M. D., and Thorbecke, G. J.,** Antigen-induced helper and suppressor T-cells in normal and agammaglobulinemic chickens, *Eur. J. Immunol.,* 10, 203, 1980.

47. **Bhogal, B. S., Chi, D. S., and Thorbecke, G. J.,** Effect of temperature on suppressor cells in chicken spleen cell cultures, *Proc. Soc. Exp. Biol. Med.,* 176, 414, 1984.

48. **Bhogal, B. S., Tse, H. Y., Jacobson, E. B., and Schmatz, D. M.,** Chicken T lymphocyte clones with specificity for *Eimeria tenella.* I. Generation and functional characterization, *J. Immunol.,* 137, 3318, 1986.

49. **Grebenau, M. D., Lerman, S. P., Chi, D. S., and Thorbecke, G. J.,** Transfer of agammaglobulinemia in the chicken. I. Generation of suppressor activity by injection of bursa cells, *Cell. Immunol.,* 51, 92, 1980.

50. **Rao, D. S. V. S. and Glick, B.,** Antibody and cell-mediated immunity in phytohemagglutinin-treated chickens, *Int. Arch. Allergy Appl. Immunol.,* 48, 30, 1975.

51. **Ratcliffe, M. J. H. and Ivanyi, J.,** Allotype suppression in the chicken. IV. Deletion of B cells and lack of suppressor cells during chronic suppression, *Eur. J. Immunol.,* 11, 306, 1981.

52. **Alder, L. T.,** Studies on allotype suppression and its abrogation in cultured rabbit spleen cells, *Transpl. Rev.,* 27, 3, 1975.

53. **Adler, L. T., Adler, F. L., Cohen, C., and Tissot, R. G.,** Induction of lymphoid cell chimerism in noninbred, histocompatible rabbits. A new model for studying allotype suppression in the rabbit, *J. Exp. Med.,* 154, 1085, 1981.

54. **Bhogal, B. S., Edelman, A., Gibbons, J. J., Jacobson, E. B., Siskind, G. W., and Thorbecke, G. J.,** Production of auto-anti-idiotype antibody during the normal immune response. X. Responses to TNP-Ficoll in the chicken, *Cell. Immunol.,* 91, 159, 1985.

55. **Bhogal, B. S., Goidl, E. A., Jacobson, E. B., Gibbons, J. J., Thorbecke, G. J., and Siskind, G. W.,** Production of auto-anti-idiotype antibody during the normal immune response. XI. Ficoll-induced variations in auto-anti-idiotype production during the response to 2,4,6,-trinitrophenyl-Ficoll, *Cell. Immunol.,* 91, 168, 1985.

56. **Lerman, S. P., Grebenau, M. D., Chi, D. S., Palladino, M. A., Galton, J., and Thorbecke, G. J.,** Transfer of agammaglobulinemia in the chicken. II. Characterization of the target of suppression, *Cell. Immunol.,* 51, 109, 1980.

57. **Palladino, M. A., Lerman, S. P., and Thorbecke, G. J.,** Transfer of hypogammaglobulinemia in two inbred chicken strains by spleen cell from bursectomized donors, *J. Immunol.,* 116, 1673, 1976.

58. **Blaese, R. M., Weiden, R. P., Koski, T., and Dooley, N. J.,** Infectious agammaglobulinemia: transmission of immunodeficiency with grafts of agammaglobulinemic cells, *J. Exp. Med.,* 140, 1097, 1974.

59. **Kermani-Arab, V. and Leslie, G. A.,** Suppression of immunoglobulin synthesis by transplantation of T-cells from anti-μ bursectomized chickens into normal recipients, *J. Immunol.,* 119, 530, 1977.

60. **Blaese, R. M., Muchmore, A. V., Koski, J., and Dooley, N. J.,** Infectious agammaglobulinemia: suppressor T-cells with specificity for individual immunoglobulin classes, *Adv. Exp. Med. Biol.,* 88, 155, 1977.

61. **Grebenau, M. D., Lerman, S. P., Palladino, M. A., and Thorbecke, G. J.,** Suppression of adoptive antibody responses by addition of spleen cells from agammaglobulinemic chickens "immunized" with histocompatible bursa cells, *Nature (London),* 260, 46, 1976.

62. **Chi, D. S., Galton, J. E., and Thorbecke, G. J.,** Role of T-cells in immune responses of the chicken, in *Proc. 16th Poultry Sci. Symp. Avian Immunology,* Rose, M. E., Payne, L. N., and Freeman, B. M., Eds., British Poultry Science, Edinburgh, Scotland, 1981, 103.

63. **Lawrence, E. C., Arnaud-Battancier, F., Koski, I. R., Dooley, N. J., Muchmore, A. V., and Blaese, R. M.,** Tissue distribution of immunoglobulin-secreting cells in normal and IgA-deficient chickens, *J. Immunol.,* 123, 1767, 1979.

64. **Chanh, T. C., Benedict, A. A., Tam. L. W., Abplanalp, H., and Gershwin, M. E.,** Inherited 7S immunoglobulin deficiency in chickens: presence of suppressor T-cells that suppress synthesis of 7S immunoglobulin but not IgM, *J. Immunol.,* 125, 108, 1980.

65. **Bruggeman, J., Merkenschlager, M., Kirchner, B., and Losch, U.,** Eine erbliche Hypo-Bzw Dysgammaglobulinamie beim Haushuhn, *Naturwissenschaften,* 54, 97, 1967.

66. **Fiedler, H., Losch, U., and Hala, K.,** Establishment of a B-compatible chicken line with normogammaglobulinemia and dysgammaglobulinemia, *Folia Biol. (Prague),* 26, 17, 1980.

67. **Chi, D. S. and Sharma, J. M.,** Inhibition of avian B-cell lymphoma by suppressor cells from agammaglobulinemic chicken, *Fed. Proc.,* 44, 1864, 1985.

68. **Okazaki, W., Witter, R. L., Romero, C., Nazerian, K., Sharma, J. M., Fadly, A., and Ewert, D.,** Induction of lymphoid leukosis transplantable tumors and the establishment of lymphoblastoid cell lines, *Avian Pathol.,* 9, 311, 1980.

69. **Chi, D. S. and Sharma, J. M.,** Inhibition of a chicken B-cell lymphoma by suppressor T-cells from agammaglobulinemic chickens, *Anticancer Res.,* in press, 1990.

70. **Sharma, J. M.,** *In vitro* suppression of T-cell mitogenic response and tumor cell proliferation by spleen macrophages from normal chickens, *Infect. Immun.,* 28, 914, 1980.

71. **Theis, G. A., McBride, R. A., and Schierman, L. W.,** Depression of *in vitro* responsiveness to phytohemagglutinin in spleen cells cultured from chickens with Marek's disease, *J. Immunol.,* 115, 848, 1975.

72. **Theis, G. A.,** Effects of lymphocytes from Marek's disease infected chickens on mitogen responses of syngeneic normal chicken spleen cells, *J. Immunol.,* 118, 887, 1977.

73. **Confer, A. W., Springer, W. T., Shane, S. M., and Donovian, J. F.,** Sequential mitogenic stimulation of peripheral blood lymphocytes from chickens inoculated with infectious bursal disease virus, *Am J. Vet. Res.,* 452, 2109, 1981.

74. **Sivanandan, V. and Maheswaran, S. K.,** Immune profile of infectious bursal disease. III. Effect of infectious bursal disease on the lymphocyte responses to phytomitogens and on mixed lymphocyte reaction of chickens, *Avian Dis.,* 25, 112, 1981.

75. **Confer, A. and MacWilliams, P. S.,** Correlation of hematological changes and serum monocyte inhibition with the early suppression of phytohemagglutinin stimulation of lymphocytes in experimental infectious bursal disease, *Can. J. Comp. Med.,* 46, 169, 1982.

76. **Sharma, J. M. and Lee, L. F.,** Effect of infectious bursal disease on natural killer cell activity and mitogenic response of chicken lymphoid cells: role of adherent cells in cellular immune suppression, *Infect. Immun.,* 42, 747, 1983.

77. **Schaefer, A. E., Scafuri, A. R., Fredericksen, T. L., and Gilmour, D. G.,** Strong suppression by monocytes of T cell mitogenesis in chicken peripheral blood leukocytes, *J. Immunol.,* 135, 1652, 1985.

78. **Boni-Schnetzier, M., Boni, J., and Franklin, R. M.,** Reversal of T-cell unresponsiveness by T-cell-conditioned medium in retrovirus MAV-2-O-induced immunosuppression in chickens, *Cancer Res.,* 45, 4871, 1985.

79. **Rup, B. J., Spence, J. L., Hoelzer, J. D., Lewis, R. B., Carpenter, C. R., Rubin, A. S., and Bose, H. R.,** Immunosuppression induced by avian reticuloendotheliosis virus: mechanism of induction of the suppressor cell, *J. Immunol.,* 123, 1362, 1979.

80. **Carpenter, C. R., Bose, H. R., and Rubin, A. S.,** Contact-mediated suppression of mitogen-induced responsiveness by spleen cells in reticuloendotheliosis virus-induced tumorigenesis, *Cell. Immunol.,* 33, 392, 1977.

81. **Theis, G. A.,** Subpopulations of suppressor cells in chickens infected with cells of a transplantable lymphoblastic leukemia, *Infect. Immun.,* 34, 526, 1981.

82. **Kline, K. and Sanders, B. G.,** Suppression of Con A mitogen-induced proliferation of normal spleen cells by macrophage from chickens with hereditary muscular dystrophy, *J. Immunol.,* 132, 2813, 1984.

83. **Crone, M.,** Tolerance to allogenic cells induced in bursectomized chickens, *Scand. J. Immunol.,* 2, 349, 1973.

84. **Szenberg, A. and Warner, N. L.,** Immunological function of thymus and bursa of Fabricius. Dissociation of immunological responsiveness in fowls with a hormonally arrested development of lymphoid tissue, *Nature (London),* 194, 146, 1962.

85. **Mueller, A. P. and Wolfe, H. R.,** Precipitin production following massive injection of BSA in adult chickens, *Int. Arch. Allergy Appl. Immunol.,* 19, 321, 1961.

86. **Salerno, A., Byfield, P., Borsellino, A., Albano, S., Bellavia, A., and Caruso, C.,** Regulation of antibody-formation in chickens escaping from tolerance to human-serum albumin, *Int. Arch. Allergy Appl. Immunol.,* 49, 530, 1975.

87. **Hraba, T., Karakoz, I., and Madar, J.,** Termination of tolerance to HSA in chickens, *Folia Biol. (Prague),* 24, 206, 1978.

88. **Ivanyi, J. and Salerno, A.,** Cellular mechanism of escape from immunological tolerance, *Immunology,* 22, 247, 1972.

89. **Havele, C., Wegmann, T. G., and Longenecker, B. M.,** Tolerance and autoimmunity to erythroid differentiation (B-G) major histocompatibility complex alloantigens of the chicken, *J. Exp. Med.,* 156, 321, 1982.
90. **Hraba, T., Karakoz, I., Nemeckova, S., and Madar, J.,** Persistence of immunological-tolerance to HSA in chickens after cell transfer to immunosuppressed hosts, *Folia Biol. (Prague),* 24, 173, 1978.
91. **Morgan, E. L., Rodrick, M. L., and Tempelis, C. H.,** Immunologic tolerance in the chicken. I. Isolation of two suppressive fractions from serum of chickens tolerant to bovine serum albumin, *J. Immunol.,* 121, 225, 1978.
92. **Morgan, E. L., Rodrick, M. L., and Tempelis, C. H.,** Immunologic tolerance in the chicken. II. Isolation and characterization of a soluble factor from a macrophage-like cell from chickens tolerant to bovine serum albumin, *Cell. Immunol.,* 45, 428, 1979.
93. **Morgan, A. S. and Tempelis, C. H.,** Neonatal splenic suppressor cells in the chicken. I. *In vivo* suppression of the immune response to bovine serum albumin by normal and tolerized neonatal spleen cells, *Cell. Immunol.,* 82, 370, 1983.
94. **Grebenau, M. D. and Thorbecke, G. J.,** T-cell tolerance in the chicken. I. Parameters affecting tolerance induction to human gamma-globulin in agammaglobulinemic and normal chickens, *J. Immunol.,* 120, 1046, 1978.
95. **Grebenau, M. D., Chi, D. S., and Thorbecke, G. J.,** T-cell tolerance in the chicken. II. Lack of evidence for suppressor cells in tolerant agammaglobulinemic and normal chickens, *Eur. J. Immunol.,* 9, 477, 1979.
96. **Higgins, G., McDermott, C., and Choi, Y. S.,** Avian antigen-binding cells. II. Enrichment of antigen-binding B- and T-cells, *J. Immunol.,* 123, 2076, 1979.
97. **Cole, R. K., Kite, J. H., and Witebsbky, E.,** Hereditary autoimmune thyroiditis in the fowl, *Science,* 160, 1357, 1968.
98. **Wick, G., Sundick, R. S., and Albini, B.,** The Obese strain (OS) of chickens: an animal model with spontaneous autoimmune thyroiditis, *Clin. Immunol. Immunopathol.,* 3, 272, 1974.
99. **Rose, N. R., Bacon, L. D., and Sundick, R. S.,** Genetic determinants of thyroiditis in the OS chicken, *Transplant. Rev.,* 31, 264, 1976.
100. **Altman, A., Theofilopoulos, A. N., Weiner, R., Katz, D. H., and Dixon, F. J.,** Analysis of T cell functions in autoimmune murine strains. Defects in production of and responsiveness to interleukin 2, *J. Exp. Med.,* 154, 791, 1981.
101. **Smith, J. B. and Talal, N.,** Significance of self-recognition and IL-2 for immunoregulation, autoimmunity and cancer (Editorial), *Scand. J. Immunol.,* 16, 269, 1982.
102. **Boyd, R. L., Oberhuber, G., Hala, K., and Wick, G.,** Obese strain (OS) chickens with spontaneous autoimmune thyroiditis have a deficiency in thymic nurse cells, *J. Immunol.,* 132, 718, 1984.
103. **Schauenstein, K., Kromer, G., Sundick, R. S., and Wick, G.,** Enchanced response to Con A and production of TCGF by lymphocytes of Obese strain (OS) chickens with spontaneous autoimmune thyroiditis, *J. Immunol.,* 134, 872, 1985.
104. **Kromer, G., Schauenstein, K., Neu, N., Stricker, K., and Wick, G.,** *In vitro* T cell hyperreactivity in Obese strain (OS) chickens is due to a defect in nonspecific suppressor mechanism(s), *J. Immunol.,* 135, 2458, 1985.
105. **Kromer, G., Schauenstein, K., Dietrich, H., Fassler, R., and Wick, G.,** Mechanisms of T cell hyperreactivity in obese strain (OS) chickens with spontaneous autoimmune thyroiditis: lack in nonspecific suppression is due to a primary adherent cell defect, *J. Immunol.,* 138, 2104, 1987.

Chapter 7

CELLULAR IMMUNE TOLERANCE

Constantine H. Tempelis

TABLE OF CONTENTS

I. INTRODUCTION

Immunological tolerance has been studied extensively since Burnet and Fenner[1] predicted that an animal exposed to an antigen prior to the onset of immunological maturity would recognize the antigen as self. Countless model systems have been used in an attempt to determine the mechanism(s) by which an animal is able to distinguish self from nonself. A better understanding of this discrimination, from the practical side, would assist immunologists, physicians, and veterinarians in providing more successful methods of treatment of such immunological events as autoimmune disease, allergy, and transplantation rejection.

The events that take place in the host which give the immune system the ability to discriminate self from nonself are still not well understood. Recent reports are beginning to give us a clearer picture of many of these events. It has been over forty years since the Burnet and Fenner hypothesis, and the accumulation of experimental information now suggests that immunological tolerance, whether established naturally or experimentally, requires multiple participants to initiate and maintain it.

This chapter will review the work in which the chicken has been used as the experimental model in order to address the cell-mediated mechanisms that may be involved in immunological tolerance. There is considerable evidence that some forms of experimentally induced tolerance are reversible and that the temporary "shutdown" of the specific immune response involves, in many, but not all cases, T-suppressor (T_s) cells and their products. The participation of T_s cells in immunological tolerance will not be discussed as this represents what is called peripheral inhibition and is usually temporary. The review will be restricted to those experiments that demonstrate a failure to respond to an antigen (tolerogen) because of an inability of any specific cell that is part of the immune system to react to that antigen. A phenomenon that has been called irreversible tolerance[2] or central unresponsiveness[3] will be emphasized. At various times this has also been called clonal deletion, clonal elimination, clonal abortion, and clonal anergy.[4,5]

Many, but not all, studies on immunological tolerance using the chicken have been modeled after earlier work using mammalian models. Progress has been rapid in these later studies, and it seems appropriate that this review mention some of this work, with the intent of stimulating additional research where the chicken may provide some unique experimental approaches to the study of immunological tolerance.

II. HISTORICAL DEVELOPMENT

In 1949 Burnet and Fenner[1] postulated that contact with an antigen prior to the animal reaching immunological maturity would result in the recognition of the antigen by the animal as self. This is still the accepted basis for the development of immunological tolerance. Two previous observations, both experiments of nature, were the basis of this hypothesis.

The first of these observations was the recognition that mice infected *in utero* with the lymphocytic choriomeningitis virus remained chronically infected throughout life without a recognizable immune response to the virus. However, mice infected postnatally mounted a significant response.[6] The second report was the recognition by Owen[7] that cattle twins which shared a common placenta became seeded with each other's erythrocytes during fetal development. This erythrocyte chimerism was maintained throughout life. The critical feature of this event was the interchange of erythrocyte precursor cells which colonized and continued to provide a source of cells. Although Burnet was unsuccessful in providing experimental evidence for his postulate, it has stimulated 40 years of active research.

The first successful experiments on the induction of immunological tolerance were reported by Billingham et al.[8] They inoculated living cells *in utero* into one strain of mouse from the adult of another. The recipient mouse was subsequently challenged with a skin graft from the donor strain. It was established that the recipient mouse was tolerant or partially tolerant to the skin graft of the donor strain. Along with the experiments with mice, they also reported in the same publication the successful induction of immunological tolerance in chickens. This is a rarely cited aspect of this original work. They inoculated whole blood from Rhode Island Red chickens intravenously into 11- to 12-d white Leghorn embryos. The recipient animals were challenged with skin grafts from the specific blood donors, and graft survival was prolonged. Strict pairing of donor and recipient was necessary for the persistence of the graft. These experiments not only demonstrated that it is possible to induce in an animal immunological tolerance to foreign tissue, but they also showed the specificity of immunological tolerance.

Confirmation of the specificity of immunological tolerance in transplantation and the importance of age of the recipient animal were demonstrated by experiments of Hašek and Hašková.[9] They injected bone marrow and spleen cells from newborn donor ducklings into newly hatched ducklings. The cells were obtained from 1, 20, or 60 donors. The ducklings were challenged at 21 d or later with skin grafts obtained from one of the original cell donors. All of the ducklings tolerant to a single donor retained the graft longer than 30 d, the rejection time of the controls. In those animals that received a mixture of cells from 20 or 60 donors, about 50% of the skin grafts were retained longer than 30 d. This confirmed the strict specificity previously observed.[8] In the same report[9] it was shown that the age of the animal was important in the induction of tolerance in avian species. Homografts made prior to 5 d posthatching were permanently retained. If the homografts were transplanted onto 7-d-old animals, only 50% had a long survival time, and no graft survived if transplanted on to a duck that was 10 d or older.

The key mechanism involved in the discrimination of self from nonself was originally hypothesized to be clonal deletion. To accept this concept, one must also examine another of Burnet's theories, the "clonal selection theory".[10] In this postulate it is stated that there exists "multiple clones", each responsible for one genetically determined antibody. In the clonal deletion theory, if, during the early development of the immunological system, a clone arises that produces an antibody that reacts to self, this clone would be eliminated. No autoreactive clones should escape this selection process.

However, the clonal deletion theory has been challenged and/or revised several times in the intervening years. One of the revisions, called the clonal abortion theory, predicted that a lymphocyte at a particular stage of differentiation could be permanently prevented from maturing into an immunocompetent cell.[11] The characteristic of the susceptible cells was hypothesized to be the initial expression of a receptor for an antigen. This was shown with B lymphocytes in the pre-B-cell stage as the immunoglobulin (Ig) receptor emerged. Therefore, B cells at this stage of differentiation have a unique sensitivity to tolerance induction.

A further evaluation of the theory was the proposal that B cells susceptible to a negative signal develop a form of clonal anergy.[12] With the use of the fluorescence-activated cell sorter, it was observed that after tolerization there was a reduction of specific antigen-binding cells. Within 6 weeks this population returned to control values. Therefore, in a relatively short period of time the specific antigen-binding cells returned to normal levels. In this experiment, even though these cells expressed the full complement of receptors, they were incapable of being stimulated with either antigen or mitogen. With this new data, Nossal[11] considered that "clonal anergy" was a better description of these events.

The clonal abortion and clonal anergy theories evolved out of studies using isolated single or small populations of B cells. These two events may be restricted to B cells. However, clonal deletion may be the mechanism of immunological tolerance to major histocompatibility complex (MHC) antigens.[13] Newborn mice rendered tolerant to H-2^d antigens exhibited a long-lasting deficit of specific cytotoxic T-lymphoctye precursors (CTL-P). Greater than 95% of these expected precursor cells were undetectable at 6 weeks of age. It was suggested that "clonal silencing or elimination" takes place during the process of T-cell differentiation in the thymus or at a prethymic stage. Others who have studied tolerance to histocompatibility antigens have arrived at the same conclusion.[14] Suppressor T cells were not detectable.

Several other important observations have contributed to our knowledge of immunological tolerance or have provided a basis for further experimentation in this area. Dresser[15] noted that the induction in mice of tolerance to foreign proteins was enhanced if the tolerogen was free of "particulate" material. This "particulate" material functioned as an adjuvant, favored antibody production instead of tolerance, and was easily removed by centrifugation. Many investigators in this field who have used purified proteins as tolerogens have centrifuged their preparations prior to use.

A significant series of experiments by Chiller et al.[16-18] demonstrated the relative susceptibilities of the T- and B-cell populations in the induction of immunological tolerance. The initial observations showed that tolerance to a soluble protein antigen involved a functional defect in either or both the T- and B-cell populations. In these experiments they were unable to demonstrate a response when either the T or the B cells from tolerant animals were combined with their counterpart from a normal syngeneic animal. In a continuation of these studies, these investigators found that there was a distinct kinetic pattern for both the induction and loss of the tolerant state.[17] Following the injection of the tolerogen (deaggregated human gamma globulin, DHGG), T cells became tolerant within 48 h and continued to be fully tolerant for the duration of the experiment (49 d). Further studies showed full tolerance remained for 120 to 130 d, but at 155 d tolerance was only 50% of normal.[19] The kinetics were slower in B cells. Complete tolerance was found 3 to 11 d after injection, but was lost by 49 d, with splenic B cells being more susceptible to the initial tolerogenic signal than bone marrow cells. These studies clearly show that there is a distinct connection in tolerance susceptibility between T and B cells. Tolerance can be exhibited in the intact animal if one of the cell types is tolerant.

Tolerance can be terminated if the animal is challenged with a closely related protein or if the tolerogen is combined with a hapten.[20] The specificity of the antibody produced is directed to common determinants or has a higher affinity to the hapten. The data has implications for autoimmune disease. Injection of altered homologous thyroglobulin or certain heterologous thyroglobulins into rabbits resulted in the development of thyroid lesions and autoantibodies to thyroglobulin.[3] Upon cessation of these injections, both lesions and autoantibodies disappeared. A transient reappearance of the disease resulted from a single injection of heterologous thyroglobulin. Continued injections returned the animal to its tolerant state. This phenomenon was explained by the presence of tolerant T cells and the ability of immunocompetent B cells to produce antithyroglobulin.

The discovery of T_s cells opened a new era in the study of immunological tolerance. Their discovery presented a significant challenge to the concept of clonal deletion. Thymic-derived cells were shown to be important in the induction of tolerance.[21] It was suggested that these cells produced a factor with "infectious capability" and that it was this factor that rendered the animal unresponsive. Droege[22] demonstrated suppressor effects produced by thymocytes in the chicken. He showed that T_s cells were separable from T-helper (T_H) cells and that the tolerant state could not be overcome by injection of normal immunocompetent cells.

Considerable controversy developed between those who believed that T_s cells were the major instruments of immunological tolerance and those investigators who continued to support the concept of clonal deletion (central failure). Weigle[3] stated in his 1980 review of the subject that "T_s cells may be concomitant with tolerance but not responsible for it". At about the same time Cinader[23] stated that "there are relatively few situations in which central tolerance may be regarded as definitely established''. As we consider some of the more recent data on the mechanism(s) operational in natural and experimental tolerance, it will be evident that some form of central failure is responsible.

III. ROLE OF THE THYMUS IN SELF TOLERANCE

The central role of the thymus in the discrimination of self from nonself has been shown in both birds and mammals. How the thymus implements the elimination of self-reactive cells is still controversial.[24-26] Several cell populations within the thymus have been shown to play a role. These include the endothelial component of the thymic stroma, macrophages, dendritic cells, and the epithelium. Much of the controversy is related to the varied experimental approaches used to study this phenomenon.

One of the strongest sets of experiments suggesting that the thymic epithelium plays the key role in the (education and/or elimination) development of self-tolerance has used the chicken model. Le Douarin and colleagues[27] have developed an interesting grafting technique in which they can successfully transfer quail pharyngeal endoderm at the 15- to 30-somite stage to the chick embryo (3 to 3.5 d) somatopleura or vice versa. From the endodermal tissue a normal thymus develops in the recipient in an ectopic location. With this technique, extensive and significant studies of the development of the primary lymphoid organs of the chicken and quail have been possible. The cells of these two closely related species are easily distinguishable.[27] The quail cell has the hematochromatin and the nucleoli intimately associated, and upon staining with a DNA dye, the quail and chick cells are easily separated.

In studies of the ontogeny of the quail and chicken immune systems, it has been found that both quail and chick thymuses are populated in three separate waves.[28,29] The first wave in the chick commences at day 6.5 of embryonation (E) and lasts for 36 h, while the second wave starts at day 12E and lasts about 48 h. Prior to day 6.5E, the thymic primordium is devoid of hemopoietic stem cells. It is this important observation that is the basis for much of the work to be discussed on the role of the thymus in the establishment of immune tolerance in the chicken.

Implantation of quail wing buds into 4-d embryonic chicks gave rise to chicks possessing quail limbs.[30-32] The wing grafts were rejected within 2 weeks of hatching — at the onset of immunological maturity. In allogeneic transplants, the foreign wings were tolerated for over a month. A chronic rejection process then developed, but the grafts were never totally rejected. Removal of both the thymic-epithelial analage and wing bud from one donor and subsequent transplantation of these two developing tissues into one 4-d developing chick embryo, along with partial removal of the recipient's own thymic tissue, resulted in tolerance to the quail wing. Only in those chicks in which at least one third of the thymic lobes became chimeric was permanent tolerance established to the grafted wing. In all surviving chimeric chickens, the limb buds remained healthy for several months. One retained a healthy graft until sacrificed at 16 months of age. The wings of the long-term surviving chickens were somewhat stunted, but showed no inflammation, nor was there an impairment of the immune response to the recipients.

In four birds that showed relatively early rejection, two produced antibodies to quail antigens and two did not. The thymuses of tolerant chickens at 1.5 to 3.0 months of age were smaller than those of the controls. In some of the chick thymic lobes, no quail cells were found. However, in other lobes, typical quail major histocompatibility complex (MHC), B-L antigens were observed in the epithelial network. In those lobes in which both chick and quail epithelia were present, zones of these respective cell populations were evident. The investigators also observed that chick host lymphocytes differentiated in an environment provided by the quail epithelial graft. In all lobes, the macrophages and dendritic cells were of host origin.

Using essentially the same protocol as just described, Belo et al.[33] showed that the bursa of Fabricius can be successfully exchanged between quail and chick. Bursal grafts are normally rejected within 1 to 2 weeks posthatching if transplanted early in embryonation, indicating that early exposure to an animal to foreign tissue is in itself insufficient to bring about tolerance. The transplantation of thymic epithelial stroma, in these experiments, was done prior to the initial invasion of hematopoietic tissue (4.5E). In two of the birds in which complete removal of the chick host thymus was accomplished, the host B and T cells developed in a completely xenogenic environment.

However, it has been shown that embryonating chicks tolerant to MHC antigens as the result of the transplantation of semiallogeneic and allogeneic thymic epithelium responded with a graft vs. host reaction.[34] These chickens were tolerant, as demonstrated by the failure to reject allogeneic skin grafts. The reason for the development of this split tolerance is difficult to explain.

Further support for the importance of the thymic epithelium in the induction of tolerance has been demonstrated in transgenic mice.[35] In one group of transgenic mice, the cortical cells expressed the MHC class II I-E gene, whereas almost all of the cells in the medulla were I-E negative. Tests for tolerance were done using the mixed lymphocyte reaction (MLR) and the determination of the frequency of a specific T-cell receptor gene product (Vβ17a). Tolerance was demonstrated in the MLR, and very few mature thymocytes or peripheral T cells displayed Vβ17a.

An additional study in mice supports the hypothesis that thymic epithelium is essential for the elimination of autoreactive cells.[36] Culture-derived thymic epithelium allografted to athymic nude mice resulted in transplantation tolerance. Host-derived lymphocytes taken from the epithelial graft or recipient spleen were unresponsive to the MHC antigens of the donor. Tolerance may reside in the T_H cell and be restricted to class II MHC antigens, because the thymic graft contained CTL-P to class I MHC antigens.

Although several reports cited suggest that recognition of self MHC occurs by the interaction of developing thymocytes with cortical epithelial cells, recent additional data provides evidence that other thymic cells play a significant role in mice. There are experiments that make a strong case for hematopoietic cells being involved in the establishment of self tolerance. The transfer of fetal thymuses depleted of all except epithelium by treatment with deoxyguanosine to allogeneic, athymic nude mice provided an environment for the development of CTL-P. Upon maturation, these CTL responded to MHC antigens of the recipient. Therefore, tolerance to MHC antigens was not demonstrated. However, these cells were shown to be tolerant to minor histocompatibility antigens. It was concluded that hematopoietic rather than epithelial cells tolerize the CTL-P, and only the minor histocompatibility antigens and not the MHC antigens are seen in tolerogenic form.[37]

Using much the same model of depleting thymuses with deoxyguanosine, two groups, one using an *in vivo*[38] and the other an *in vitro* system,[39] came to the same conclusion: that thymic hematopoietic cells rather than epithelium provided the essential message for self tolerance. One group transferred the hematopoietic cell-deprived thymic epithelium into histoincompatible mice. Even though these thymuses expressed both class I and II MHC antigens, they were not rejected, but neither did they induce tolerance. It was suggested that the thymic dendritic cell was the key player in the induction of tolerance.[38] The *in vitro* model depended on the establishment of thymic chimeras in organ culture. Embryonic thymuses depleted of lymphoid stem cells by treatment with deoxyguanosine were recolonized with hematopoietic cells from a MHC dissimilar early thymic rudiment. The resulting lymphocytes were exclusively of the donor type. These lymphocytes, in the presence of cells expressing the same MHC antigens as the epithelium, reacted strongly in a MLR. However, these cells were tolerant to cells of their same genotype.[39] Additional evidence for lack of epithelial cell participation in the induction of tolerance to self-MHC in thymocytes has been provided.[40]

Is the deoxyguanosine-treated thymic rudiment transplanted to a nude mouse a suitable model for the study of self tolerance? Providing a satisfactory resolution of the controversy about the relative importance of the thymic epithelium vs. the hematopoietic cells in the issuing of the negative signal to potentially autoreactive cells would be greatly assisted by the answer to this question. van Ewijk et al.[35] states that the discrepancy may be that deoxyguanosine-treated explants do not fully reconstitute in the nude mouse and, therefore, are unable to induce tolerance. It appears that additional experiments using several different experimental approaches will be necessary to resolve this controversy. Nevertheless, the experiments with chickens strongly implicate the thymic epithelium as the major cell population involved in the elimination of autoreactive cells, at least in chickens.[30,31]

Natural tolerance to autologous protein antigens also appears to be dependent on the thymus.[41] Mice deficient in complement component 5 (C5) that were grafted with thymus from C5-producing mice and immunized with C5 did not make antibody to C5. This data suggests that the thymuses of mice capable of producing C5 had deleted the cells involved in antibody production to C5, whereas in the C5-deficient mice these cells were not eliminated or suppressed. This experiment demonstrates the major role of the thymus in the establishment of tolerance to C5. Boguniewicz et al.[41] postulate that bone-marrow-derived cells in the thymus are involved and that this phenomenon is most likely explained by functional T-cell inactivation by tolerogen without physical deletion.

IV. EXPERIMENTAL CHIMERAS AND IMMUNE TOLERANCE

The use of quail-chick embryonic chimeras has been extended to the study of the development of the nervous system. When parts of the central and peripheral nervous system in the developing chick embryo were replaced by their quail counterparts at day 2E, the grafts, under favorable conditions, were retained for 15 to 70 d.[32,42,43] During this retention period, the quail-chick chimeras appeared to exhibit normal motor behavior. The gross anatomy, histology, and cytology of the peripheral and central nervous systems were normal. All grafts were subsequently rejected. Therefore, complete immunological tolerance was never established. For example, when quail neural tube was grafted to a chick embryo at the brachial level, as the graft was being rejected a flaccid paralysis of the wings developed, followed by a paralysis of the legs. Selected nervous tissue that developed from the neural tube showed a hypertrophy of the blood vessels and massive infiltration of inflammatory cells (T cells, macrophages, plasmocytes). Rupture of the blood-brain barrier resulted from the accumulation of inflammatory cells.

The success of these experiments is interesting. Graft rejection began several weeks after the maturation of the immune system (at about 2 weeks of age). The failure of the immune system to reject these grafts until after 2 months of age may have been due to the special relationship that exists between the nervous and immune systems, with the blood-brain barrier protecting the nervous tissue from immune cells.[32,43] Also, the brain has a low expression of class I MHC antigens. Nevertheless, the initiation of rejection was probably precipitated by an undefined antigen that brought about the rupture of the blood-brain barrier.[43]

In allogeneic combinations, neural implants were made between outbred populations of Rhode Island Red and white Leghorn chickens.[42] To insure maximum genetic disparity between these two groups, B-locus antigens of randomly selected white Leghorns were tested with antisera used to characterize the B locus of the Rhode Island Red population. None of the antisera cross-reacted with the white Leghorn red cells. In these allogeneic combinations, the neural implants were permanently tolerated.

Reconstitution experiments concerned with the ontogeny of the bursa of Fabricius have provided some interesting data on the development of the B-lymphoid system in the chicken and also on immunological tolerance. Allogeneic and semi-allogeneic bursal stem cells from 3-d-old chicks transplanted into cyclophosphamide (CY)-treated, B-cell-depleted chicks of the same age successfully colonized.[44,45] The recipient animals failed to reject skin grafts from the allogeneic donor strain and no graft vs. host disease developed. Full immunocompetence was restored in those animals that received the semi-allogeneic grafts but not in the animals that were recipients of allogeneic grafts. Nevertheless, the allogeneic cells survived, and 4 weeks later were transferred back into the original donor strain. It was clear from these original experiments that the recipient animals became tolerant to the allogeneic bursal stem cells, and stable lymphoid chimeras were established.

This B-cell lymphoid model was used to analyze the mechanism(s) of the transplantation tolerance existent in these chickens. Cyclophosphamide-treated 4-d-old chicks were recipients of either allogeneic stem cells (4-d-old) or postbursal cells from 4-d-old and 8- to 10-week-old donors, respectively. All cell populations survived, were detected in various lymphoid organs, and induced a stable B-cell chimera.[46] Transplantation tolerance to the donor line was established; skin grafts were accepted, graft vs. host disease and the MLR were significantly reduced. The operational mechanism in this system was shown to result from the inactivation or deletion of T_H cells.[47]

Confirmation for the inactivation of the T_H population was forthcoming.[48] T_H-cell depletion was shown to result in tolerance to "total" MHC in chicken chimeras. However, tolerance to class I MHC antigens only was the result of cells within the T-cell compartment, suggesting the action of T_s cells.

Successful induction of transplantation tolerance provided a valuable model for the study of clonal seeding of bursal follicles. Chimeras created by either parabiotic union or by transplantation of allogeneic bursal cells (Bu^+ or Bu^-) into CY-treated animals established the nature of clonal diversity within a single follicle.[49,50]

Many of the experiments detailed in this section demonstrate that although the understanding of the mechanism(s) involved in immunological tolerance is important and interesting in its own right, it has also served as a useful model to study other immunological phenomena. In addition, it has provided valuable data on embryological development.

V. ROLE OF INTERLEUKINS IN IMMUNE TOLERANCE

In 1984, Malkovský and Medawar[51] postulated that the ease with which immunological tolerance (self-recognition) could be induced in the neonate was due to the inability of the young animal to produce interleukin 2 (IL-2). They were able to provide evidence to support their hypothesis with the following experiments. They injected a tolerogenic dose of spleen cells either by the intravenous or intraperitoneal route into newborn mice. Tolerance was demonstrated by the inability of the animals when challenged with donor-strain skin grafts to reject these grafts.[52,53] The solid state of tolerance induced by the spleen cells was brought to an end when the animals were given *in vivo* administration of exogenous IL-2 (either the crude or the recombinant form) or fed a diet of enriched vitamin A acetate. The injection of concanavalin A (Con A), which is known to produce endogenous IL-2, also terminated the tolerant state. The investigators concluded that neonatal tolerance is the result of the exposure to an antigen in the "relative" absence of IL-2.[51,52]

Other experimental evidence has demonstrated the importance of the absence of IL-2 in the establishment and maintenance of immunological tolerance. Neonatal tolerance established in mice to alloantigens resulted not only in a significant reduction or deletion of alloantigen-specific cells, but also in a loss of cells capable of producing IL-2.[54,55] Failure of tolerant cells to respond in an MLR, to induce CTL generation, or to produce IL-2 was used to assess the functional abilities of the respective cell populations. The addition of IL-2 to an MLR culture system that contained tolerant cells as the responder population enhanced the response of this population. Further *in vivo* confirmation has been reported by Jian and Qiuzhao.[56] These investigators showed that adult mice that received allogeneic spleen cells at birth retained donor-strain heart grafts significantly longer than animals similarly treated that received IL-2 24 h later. The MLR with tolerant cells as the responder population was also significantly reduced, and the addition of IL-2 to the culture system enhanced the response.

Donor-strain skin grafts transplanted to tolerant mice at 12 weeks of age were retained in a healthy state for 18 months. Donor spleen cells incubated for 24 h in the presence of IL-2 and then injected into the grafted animals induced the rejection of the long-retained skin grafts. In addition, CTL specific for the allograft appeared in the animal after tolerance was broken.[57]

Essery et al.[58] were able to show that human T-cell clones unresponsive to a peptide antigen reversed the established tolerance in the presence of IL-2. IL-2 was also shown to inhibit the induction of unresponsiveness in a dose-dependent manner. Low doses of IL-2 were able to block induction, whereas high concentrations were required to reverse established tolerance.

In a related experiment, H.B15 (Turku University) homozygous CY-treated chickens received H.B2 bursal cells at 4 d of age. Several weeks later, peripheral blood lymphocytes (PBL) from these B-cell chimeras failed to respond when cocultured with H.B2 stimulator PBL in a MLR.[47] When exogenous IL-2 was added to culture, the response of H.B15 tolerant cells to H.B2 stimulator cells was significantly increased. This study, along with those involving mice, would strongly suggest that IL-2 alters the responsive ability of tolerant cells. However, contradictory data has been reported.

There are a series of experiments that have failed to demonstrate the effects of IL-2 and the reversal of immunological tolerance. Chickens tolerant to both MHC and minor histocompatibility antigens induced by the injection of X-irradiated red blood cells of the B[4] haplotype into B[12] recipients and simultaneously grafted with skin from a congenic line retained these grafts for an extended period.[59] The injection of crude IL-2 and/or Con A simultaneously with transplantation or, in some cases, several days after transplantation failed to enhance graft rejection. IL-2 in and around the surviving grafts also failed to alter the course of graft survival.

An additional failure to reverse tolerance with IL-2 has been demonstrated in mice made neonatally tolerant to alloantigens.[60] In these mice there was a loss of CTL-P- and IL-2-producing cells. In the MLR there was a reduction of the proliferative response and a depressed production of IL-2 very similar to that seen in experiments cited previously.

An interesting aspect of this subject is that experiments from the same laboratory have produced conflicting data. As mentioned previously in this section, Wood et al.[55] reported that a deficit in IL-2 production was, in part, responsible for the maintenance of neonatally induced H-2 tolerance. However, in a more recent study, they reported that lymphocytes from tolerant mice produce large quantities of IL-2 in an MLR in response to the tolerogen.[61]

In summary, there are data that both support and contradict the hypothesis of Malkovský and Medawar.[51] It is difficult to explain these positive and negative effects of IL-2 on tolerance induction and maintenance. Further experimentation will be required to resolve these contradictions.

Interleukin 1 (IL-1) has been shown to interfere with tolerance induction. This effect has been suggested to result from the release of IL-1 by the macrophage, when tolerance induction was being induced *in vitro*.[62] Both human IL-1 containing supernatants and purified IL-1 were shown to interfere with B-cell tolerance.

It has been demonstrated by a number of investigators that a deaggregated protein induces tolerance, whereas an aggregated protein is a good immunogen. The deaggregated protein fails to induce IL-1 production by the macrophage, unlike the aggregated protein which stimulates high levels of IL-1 production by the macrophage.[63,64] The absence of IL-1 has been postulated to deliver a tolerogenic rather than an immunogenic signal to the T_H cell and the B cell. Therefore, the lack of a second nonspecific signal (IL-1) has been hypothesized as the means of tolerance induction.[65] Other experiments, both *in vitro* and *in vivo*, have confirmed that the presence of IL-1 interferes with tolerance induction. DHGG did not stimulate IL-2 production *in vitro*, and therefore, the T_H cell was tolerant. In later experiments, the *in vivo* administration of small amounts of lipopolysaccaride (LPS; inducer of IL-1) for ten consecutive days so as to desensitize mice did not interfere with the induction of tolerance to DHGG. Large doses of LPS given simultaneously with DHGG inhibited tolerance induction.[66] The inability of the LPS to prevent tolerance induction to DHGG in the desensitized animal may be due to the lack of IL-1 production by these animals.

VI. MECHANISMS OF SELF TOLERANCE

This author believes a review of this kind should provide avian immunologists with a brief overview of some of the current research not previously covered that relates to the mechanism(s) of self-tolerance. The role of the thymus in the elimination of self-reactive clones has been discussed. In this section, consideration will be given to the roles of the antigen-presenting cell (APC) and extrathymic sites in the induction of immunological tolerance. Additional information provided by the use of transgenic animals will be presented.

APC can process self-antigens.[67] Therefore, self-discrimination does not depend on the APC. If a processed self-peptide is able to bind to a class II MHC molecule, interaction with the appropriate T cell can be prevented only if the specific T-cell clone is functionally or physically deleted.

Currently, there appears to be little conflict that the thymus is the major center, but not the exclusive site, in the development of self-nonself discrimination.[25] Self-reactive T-cell receptors (TCR) are expressed on cells present in the thymic cortex and at the thymic corticomedullary junction.[68] Negative selection in the thymus is most likely at the CD4[+] CD8[+] differentiation stage following the interaction with class I or class II MHC-expressing nonlymphoid cells.[69-72] The elimination of these autoreactive cells expressing specific TCR genotypes in the thymus has been reported.[70-74]

Although this review has emphasized clonal deletion as the likely mechanism for the removal of self-reactive clones, autologous MLR and autoreactive clones can be demonstrated.[75,76] In some cases, autoreactive T cells have been shown to have immunoregulatory activity.[77] It has been recently reported that neonatal mice tolerant to transplantation antigens by the injection of semi-allogeneic cells contained large numbers of activated T and B cells in the spleen.[78] This lymphoid "hyperactivity" correlated with the tolerant state. Such data would suggest that another pathway of tolerance induction and maintenance has been observed. In addition, tolerance to class II MHC has been shown to be maintained by a mechanism which does not require clonal deletion.[61] Such data reemphasizes the concept that there is no single exclusive series of mechanisms that results in the induction and maintenance of immunological tolerance and that other selective processes may be operational.

How do cells become tolerant to self-antigens that do not encounter the thymus? Using transgenic mice, Miller et al.[79] were able to direct the expression of a class I MHC molecule ($H-2K^b$) on pancreatic islet β cells. It was shown that these mice were tolerant of the transgenic product, $H-2B^K$. Additional data has shown that extrathymic tolerance can be established and may differ from that which operates in the thymus.[80] These reports establish that tolerance in the T-cell population can be established extrathymically.

Other experiments using transgenic mice have provided valuable information for the understanding of immunological tolerance. In mice constructed of α- and β-TCR transgenes derived from CTL clones that were specific for the male antigen H-Y, only the females transcribed and expressed both α and β transgenes.[72] Analysis of male cells revealed the deletion of transgenic α and β sequences. Additional studies using transgenic animals have been done.[79] This new technology provides the opportunity to study immunological tolerance to specific and genuine self antigens generated with the cells of an animal.[26]

VII. SUMMARY

Since the original clonal deletion hypothesis was proposed about 40 years ago, a number of mechanisms have been proposed to explain how the immunological system is able to discriminate self from nonself. Current research suggests that the autoreactive cells are primarily eliminated in the thymus. Whether such elimination is dependent on the ability of the thymic epithelium or the hematopoietic cells to deliver the negative signal remains controversial. Nevertheless, in the chicken, because of the ability to produce quail-chick chimeras so early in embryological development, it has been shown that the thymic epithelium plays a significant role in the establishment of immunological tolerance.

The ability to establish experimental immunological tolerance in the chicken either by the transplantation of xenogeneic or allogeneic grafts into the developing or newly hatched chick or by parabiotic union or chemical treatment has provided a model to study a number of biological events including those that are immunological. Study of embryological development of the nervous system in the chicken has been made possible through the establishment of stable chimeras. Also, an understanding of the clonal seeding of bursal follicles has been made possible by the establishment of immunological tolerance.

Interleukins 1 and 2 (IL-1 and IL-2) have been suggested to interfere with the establishment of immunological tolerance. IL-1 has been shown to be essential for the delivery of the second signal for the induction of the immune response. The lack of IL-1 appears to result in the development of immunological tolerance. Experimental evidence suggests this to be true. The situation with IL-2 is not as clear. It was originally hypothesized that in the presence of IL-2 immunological tolerance could not be induced or maintained. This has been confirmed by a number of experiments. Nevertheless, several investigators have provided data that immunological tolerance can be established and maintained in the presence of IL-2. Both effects have been shown in the chickens. This controversy continues.

New techniques, such as the ability to produce transgenic animals, are providing us with insight into immunological phenomena not previously available for study. This ability allows us to study the fate of self antigens generated within the animal. Although several mechanisms have been postulated as providing the animal with protection against immunological attack on itself, the clonal deletion hypothesis is the prevalent view, and clonal elimination is observed to take place primarily, although not exclusively, in the thymus.

ACKNOWLEDGMENTS

The author would like to thank Dr. Mary Rodrick and Marian Simpson for their constructive comments on this manuscript.

REFERENCES

1. **Burnet, F. M. and Fenner, F.,** *The Production of Antibodies,* 2nd ed., Macmillan, London, 1949, 142.
2. **Howard, J. G. and Mitchison, N. A.,** Immunological tolerance, *Prog. Allergy,* 18, 43, 1975.
3. **Weigle, W. O.,** Analysis of autoimmunity through experimental models of thyroiditis and allergic encephalomyelitis, *Adv. Immunol.,* 30, 159, 1980.

4. **Hraba, T. and Hašek, M., Eds.,** *Cellular and Molecular Mechanisms of Immunologic Tolerance,* Vol. 16, Marcell Dekker, New York, 1981, 570.

5. **Nossal, G. J. V.,** Cellular mechanisms of immunologic tolerance, *Annu. Rev. Immunol.,* 1, 33, 1983.

6. **Traub, E.,** Factors influencing the persistence of choriomeningitis virus in the blood of mice after clinical recovery, *J. Exp. Med.,* 68, 299, 1938.

7. **Owen, R. D.,** Immunogenetic consequences of vascular anastomoses between bovine twins, *Science,* 102, 400, 1945.

8. **Billingham, R. E., Brent, L., and Medawar, P. B.,** Actively acquired tolerance of foreign cells, *Nature (London),* 173, 603, 1953.

9. **Hašek, M. and Hašková, V.,** A contribution to the significance of individual antigenic specificity in homografting, *Tranplant. Bull.,* 5, 69, 1958.

10. **Burnet, M.,** *The Clonal Selection Theory of Acquired Immunity,* Vanderbilt University Press, Nashville, TN, 1959, 209.

11. **Nossal, G. J. V. and Pike, B. L.,** Evidence for the clonal abortion theory of B-lymphocyte tolerance, *J. Exp. Med.,* 141, 904, 1975.

12. **Nossal, G. J. V. and Pike, B. L.,** Clonal anergy: persistence in tolerant mice of antigen-binding B lymphocytes incapable of responding to antigen or mitogen, *Proc. Natl. Acad. Sci. U.S.A.,* 77, 1602, 1980.

13. **Nossal, G. J. V. and Pike, B. L.,** Functional clonal deletion in immunological tolerance to major histocompatibility complex antigens, *Proc. Natl. Acad. Sci. U.S.A.,* 78, 3844, 1981.

14. **von Boehmer, H., Sprent, J., and Nabholz, M.,** Tolerance to histocompatibility determinants in tetraparental bone marrow chimeras, *J. Exp. Med.,* 141, 322, 1975.

15. **Dresser, D. W.,** Specific inhibition of antibody production. II. Paralysis induced in adult mice by small quantities of protein antigen, *Immunology,* 5, 378, 1962.

16. **Chiller, J. M., Habicht, G. S., and Weigle, W. O.,** Cellular sites of immunologic unresponsiveness, *Proc. Natl. Acad. Sci. U.S.A.,* 65, 551, 1970.

17. **Chiller, J. M., Habicht, G. S., and Weigle, W. O.,** Kinetic differences in unresponsiveness of thymus and bone marrow cells, *Science,* 171, 813, 1971.

18. **Chiller, J. M. and Weigle, W. O.,** Restoration of immunocompetency in tolerant lymphoid cell populations by cellular supplementation, *J. Immunol.,* 110, 1051, 1973.

19. **Weigle, W. O.,** Immunological unresponsiveness, *Adv. Immunol.,* 16, 61, 1973.

20. **Linscott, W. E. and Weigle, W. O.,** Anti-bovine serum albumin specificity and binding affinity after termination of tolerance to bovine serum albumin, *J. Immunol.,* 95, 546, 1965.

21. **Gershon, R. K. and Kondo, K.,** Cell interactions in the induction of tolerance: the role of thymic lymphocytes, *Immunology,* 18, 723, 1970.

22. **Droege, W.,** Comparison of the suppressive effect of thymus cells and the suppression by neonatal application of antigen, *Eur. J. Immunol.,* 3, 804, 1973.

23. **Cinader, B.,** Tolerance as a facet of immune regulation — the trail from the past into the future, in *Cellular and Molecular Mechanisms of Immunologic Tolerance,* Vol. 16, Hraba, T. and Hasek, M., Eds., Marcell Dekker, New York, 1981, 570.

24. **Nossal, G. J. V.,** Immunologic tolerance: collaboration between antigen and lymphokines, *Science,* 245, 147, 1989.

25. **Hall, B. M.,** Transplantation tolerance: a 1988 perspective, *Transplant. Proc.,* 21, 816, 1988.

26. **Miller, J. F. A. P., Morahan, G., and Allison, J.,** Immunological tolerance: new approaches using transgenic mice, *Immunol. Today,* 10, 53, 1989.

27. **Le Douarin, N. M., Jotereau, F. V., Houssaint, E., and Thiery, J.-P.,** Primary lymphoid organ ontogeny in birds, in *Chimeras in Developmental Biology,* Le Douarin, N. and McLaren, A., Eds., Academic Press, New York, 1984, chap. 8.

28. **Jotereau, F. V. and Le Douarin, N. M.,** Demonstration of a cyclic renewal of the lymphocyte precursor cells in the quail thymus during embryonic and perinatal life, *J. Immunol.,* 129, 1869, 1982.

29. **Coltey, M., Jotereau, F. V., and Le Douarin, N. M.,** Evidence for a cyclic renewal of lymphocyte precursor cells in the embryonic chick thymus, *Cell Diff.,* 22, 71, 1987.

30. **Ohki, H., Martin, C., Coltey, M., and Le Douarin, N. M.,** Implants of quail thymic epithelium generate permanent tolerance in embryonically constructed quail/chick chimeras, *Development,* 104, 619, 1988.

31. **Ohki, H., Martin, C., Corbel, C., Coltey, M., and Le Douarin, N. M.,** Tolerance induced by thymic epithelial grafts in birds, *Science,* 237, 1032, 1987.

32. **Le Douarin, N. M.,** The Claude Bernard lecture, 1987. Embryonic chimeras: a tool for studying the development of the nervous and immune systems, *Proc. R. Soc. London Ser. B,* 235, 1, 1988.

33. **Belo, M., Corbel, C., Martin, C., and Le Douarin, N. M.,** Thymic epithelium tolerizes chickens to embryonic grafts of quail bursa of Fabricius, *Int. Immunol.,* 1, 105, 1989.

34. **Houssaint, E., Torano, A., and Ivanyi, J.,** Split tolerance induced by chick embryo thymic epithelium allografted to embryonic recipients, *J. Immunol.,* 136, 3155, 1986.

35. **van Ewijk, W., Ron, Y., Monaco, J., Kappler, J., Marrack, P., Le Meur, M., Gerlinger, P., Durand, B., Benoist, C., and Mathis, D.,** Compartmentalization of MHC class II gene expression in transgenic mice, *Cell*, 53, 357, 1988.

36. **Jordan, R. K., Robinson, J. H., Hopkinson, N. A., House, K. C., and Bentley, A. L.,** Thymic epithelium and the induction of transplantation tolerance in nude mice, *Nature (London)*, 314, 454, 1985.

37. **von Boehmer, H. and Hafen, K.,** Minor but not major histocompatibility antigens of thymus epithelium tolerize precursors of cytolytic T cells, *Nature (London)*, 320, 626, 1986.

38. **Ready, A. R., Jenkinson, E. J., Kingston, R., and Owen, J. J. T.,** Successful transplantation across major histocompatibility barrier of deoxyguanosine-treated embryonic thymus expressing class II antigens, *Nature (London)*, 310, 231, 1984.

39. **Jenkinson, E. J., Jhittay, P., Kingston, R., and Owen, J. J. T.,** Studies of the role of the thymic environment in the induction of tolerance to MHC antigens, *Transplantation*, 39, 331, 1985.

40. **Blackman, M. A., Kappler, J. W., and Marrack, P.,** T cell specificity and repertoire, *Immunol. Rev.*, 101, 5, 1988.

41. **Boguniewicz, M., Sunshine, G. H., and Borel, Y.,** Role of the thymus in natural tolerance to an autologous protein antigen, *J. Exp. Med.*, 169, 285, 1989.

42. **Kinutani, M. and Le Douarin, N. M.,** Avian spinal cord chimeras. I. Hatching ability and posthatching survival in homo- and heterospecific chimeras, *Dev. Biol.*, 111, 243, 1985.

43. **Kinutani, M., Coltey, M., and Le Douarin, N. M.,** Postnatal development of a demyelinating disease in avian spinal cord chimeras, *Cell*, 45, 307, 1986.

44. **Toivanen, P., Toivanen, A., and Vainio, O.,** Complete restoration of bursa-dependent immune system after transplantation of semiallogeneic stem cells into immunodeficient chicks, *J. Exp. Med.*, 139, 1344, 1974.

45. **Toivanen, P., Toivanen, A., and Sorvari, T.,** Incomplete restoration of the bursa-dependent immune system after transplantation of allogeneic stem cells into immunodeficient chicks, *Proc. Natl. Acad. Sci. U.S.A.*, 71, 957, 1974.

46. **Lehtonen, L., Vainio, O., Eerola, E., and Toivanen, P.,** Lymphoid cell chimerism and transplantation tolerance induced by bursal and post bursal cells, *Transplantation*, 40, 398, 1985.

47. **Lehtonen, L., Vainio, O., and Toivanen, P.,** Mechanisms of transplantation tolerance in B-cell chimeric chickens. Impairment of tolerance by T cell growth factor, *Transplantation*, 42, 184, 1986.

48. **Lehtonen, L., Vainio, O., Veromaa, T., and Toivanen, P.,** Tolerance to class I major histocompatibility complex antigens in chicken B cell chimeras. Effect of B cell depletion on transferability of tolerance, *Eur. J. Immunol.*, 19, 425, 1989.

49. **Pink, J. R., Vainio, O., and Rijnbeek, A.-M.,** Clones of B lymphocytes in individual follicles of the bursa of Fabricius, *Eur. J. Immunol.*, 15, 83, 1985.

50. **Ratcliffe, M. J. H.,** The ontogeny and cloning of B cells in the bursa of Fabricius, *Immunol. Today*, 6, 223, 1985.

51. **Malkovský, M. and Medawar, P. B.,** Is immunological tolerance (non-responsiveness) a consequence of interleukin 2 deficit during recognition of antigen?, *Immunol. Today*, 5, 340, 1984.

52. **Malkovský, M., Medawar, P., Hunt, R., Palmer, L., and Doré, C.,** A diet rich in vitamin A acetate or *in vivo* administration of interleukin-2 can counteract a tolerogenic stimulus, *Proc. R. Soc. London Ser. B*, 220, 439, 1984.

53. **Malkovský, M., Medawar, P. B., Thatcher, D. R., Toy, J., Hunt, R., Rayfield, L. S., and Doré, C.,** Acquired immunological tolerance of foreign cells is impaired by recombinant interleukin 2 or vitamin A acetate, *Proc. Natl. Acad. Sci. U.S.A.*, 82, 536, 1985.

54. **Feng, H. M., Glasebrook, A. L., Engers, H. D., and Louis, J. A.,** Clonal analysis of T cell unresponsiveness to alloantigens induced by neonatal injection of F_1 spleen cells into parental mice, *J. Immunol.*, 131, 2165, 1984.

55. **Wood, P. J., Strome, P. G., and Streilein, J. W.,** Clonal analysis of helper and effector T-cell function in neonatal transplantation tolerance: clonal deletion of helper cells determines lack of *in vitro* unresponsiveness, *Immunogenetics*, 20, 185, 1984.

56. **Jian, Y. and Qiuzhao, H.,** Role of IL-2 in the abrogation of neonatally induced transplantation tolerance in mice, *Acta Acad. Med. Shanghai*, 16, 259, 1989.

57. **Loveland, B., Hunt, R., and Malkovsky, M.,** Autologous lymphoid cells exposed to recombinant interleukin-2 *in vitro* in the absence of antigen can induce the rejection of long-term tolerated skin allografts, *Immunology*, 59, 159, 1986.

58. **Essery, G., Feldmann, M., and Lamb, J. R.,** Interleukin-2 can prevent and reverse antigen-induced unresponsiveness in cloned human T lymphocytes, *Immunology*, 64, 413, 1988.

59. **Tempelis, C. H., Hála, K., Krömer, G., Schauenstein, K., and Wick, G.,** Failure to alter neonatal transplantation tolerance by the injection of interleukin-2, *Tranplantation*, 45, 449, 1988.

60. **Carnaud, C., Ishizaka, S., and Stutman, O.,** Early loss of precursors of CTL and IL 2-producing cells in the development of neonatal tolerance to alloantigens, *J. Immunol.*, 133, 45, 1984.

61. **Mohler, K. M. and Streilein, J. W.,** Tolerance to class II major histocompatibility complex molecules is maintained in the presence of endogenous interleukin 2-producing, tolerogen-specific T lymphocytes, *J. Immunol.*, 139, 2211, 1987.

62. **Goldings, E. A.,** Regulation of B cell tolerance by macrophage-derived mediators: antagonistic effects of prostaglandin E_2 and interleukin 1, *J. Immunol.*, 136, 817, 1986.

63. **Weigle, W. O., Scheuer, W. V., Hobbs, M. V., Morgan, E. L., and Parks, D. E.,** Modulation of the induction and circumvention of immunological tolerance to human γ-globulin by interleukin 1, *J. Immunol.*, 138, 2069, 1987.

64. **Levich, J. D., Signorella, A. P., Wittenberg, G., and Weigle, W. O.,** Macrophage handling of a tolerogen and the role of IL 1 in tolerance induction in a helper T cell clone *in vitro*, *J. Immunol.*, 138, 3675, 1987.

65. **Bendtzen, K.,** Induction of antigen-specific immunological unresponsiveness by inhibitors of human lymphocyte-activating factors, *Scand. J. Immunol.*, 14, 427, 1981.

66. **Weigle, W. O., Gahring, L. C., Romball, C. G., and Goodman, M. G.,** The effect of lipopolysaccaride desensitization on the regulation of *in vivo* induction of immunologic tolerance and antibody production and *in vitro* release of IL-1, *J. Immunol.*, 142, 1107, 1989.

67. **Lorenz, R. G. and Allen, P. M.,** Processing and presentation of self antigens, *Immunol. Rev.*, 106, 115, 1988.

68. **Crispe, N.,** Mechanisms of self-tolerance, *Immunol. Today*, 9, 329, 1988.

69. **Fowlkes, B. J., Schwartz, R. H., and Pardoll, D. M.,** Deletion of self-reactive thymocytes occurs at a $CD4^+8^+$ precursor stage, *Nature (London)*, 334, 620, 1988.

70. **MacDonald, H. R., Hengartner, H., and Pedrazzini, T.,** Intrathymic deletion of self-reactive cells prevented by neonatal anti-CD4 antibody treatment, *Nature (London)*, 335, 174, 1988.

71. **von Boehmer, H., Teh, H. S., and Kisielow, P.,** The thymus selects the useful, neglects the useless and destroys the harmful, *Immunol. Today*, 10, 57, 1989.

72. **Kisielow, P., Blüthmann, H., Staerz, U. D., Steinmetz, M., and von Boehmer, H.,** Tolerance in T-cell-receptor transgenic mice involves deletion of immature $CD4^+8^+$ thymocytes, *Nature (London)*, 333, 742, 1988.

73. **Kappler, J. W., Staerz, U., White, J., and Marrick, P. C.,** Self-tolerance eliminates T cells specific for Mls-modified products of the major histocompatibility complex, *Nature (London)*, 332, 35, 1988.

74. **Kappler, J. W., Roehn, N., and Marrack, P.,** T cell tolerance by clonal elimination in the thymus, *Cell*, 49, 273, 1987.

75. **Hausman, P. B. and Stobo, J. D.,** Specificity and function of a human autologous reactive cell, *J. Exp. Med.*, 149, 1537, 1979.

76. **Glimcher, L. H., Longo, D. L., Green, I., and Schwartz, R. H.,** Murine syngeneic mixed lymphocyte response. I. Target antigens are self Ia molecules, *J. Exp. Med.*, 154, 1652, 1981.

77. **Kotani, H., Mitsuya, H., Benson, E., James, S. P., and Stober, W.,** Activation and function of an autoreactive T cell clone with dual immunoregulatory activity, *J. Immunol.*, 140, 4167, 1988.

78. **Bandeira, A., Coutinho, A., Carnaud, C., Jacquemart, F., and Forni, L.,** Transplantation tolerance correlates with high levels of T- and B-lymphocyte activity, *Proc. Natl. Acad. Sci. U.S.A.*, 86, 272, 1989.

79. **Miller, J. F. A. P., Morohan, G., Allison, J., Bhathal, P. S., and Cox, K. O.,** T-cell tolerance in transgenic mice expressing major histocompatibility class I molecules in defined tissues, *Immunol. Rev.*, 107, 109, 1989.

80. **Zamoyska, R., Waldmann, H., and Matzinger, P.,** Peripheral tolerance mechanisms prevent the development of autoreactive T cells in chimiras grafted with two minor incompatible thymuses, *Eur. J. Immunol.*, 19, 111, 1989.

Chapter 8

FEATURES OF CELLULAR IMMUNE SYSTEMS IN AVIAN SPECIES OTHER THAN CHICKENS

Haruo Matsuda and Takeshi Mikami

TABLE OF CONTENTS

I. INTRODUCTION

In recent years, a considerable amount of new knowledge has accumulated on cell-mediated immunity (CMI) in the chicken. However, research on CMI of other avian species, including turkeys, Japanese quails, and ducks, has been limited. There are several reasons for the lack of interest in understanding immune mechanisms of birds other than chickens: (1) the economic importance of these birds differs from one country to the next (due to the differences in eating habits of people), and (2) the prevailing assumption that the cellular immune mechanisms of these birds are very similar to those of chickens. This assumption has discouraged research laboratories from getting involved in immune studies involving birds of species other than chickens and has thus restricted our knowledge on the comparative aspects of avian immunology. Most studies conducted on CMI in birds other than the chicken have involved delayed hypersensitivity and lymphocyte transformation. In this review, the current state of knowledge on cellular immunity in three species of birds including turkeys, quails, and ducks will be discussed. Some interesting and unique features of the immune system of these birds will be noted.

II. CELLULAR IMMUNITY IN THE TURKEY

There are many reports[1-9] on studies of CMI in turkeys because of the economic importance of this bird in some countries.

A. DELAYED HYPERSENSITIVITY

The CMI response to tuberculin and phytohemagglutinin (PHA) in chickens has been demonstrated to be a T-dependent reaction.[10-14] McCorkel et al.[7] have investigated CMI to PHA, *Mycobacterium avium* (MA), and *M. tuberculosis* (MT) in turkey poults. They found that the kinetics of the responses were similar to those of rodents and other birds including chickens and Japanese quails. The cutaneous basophil hypersensitivity (CBH) response of turkeys to PHA occurred 18 to 36 h following a single injection and was similar to that in chickens.[13,15-17] However, the delayed hypersensitivity response to MA and MT required a period of 2 to 3 weeks following initial sensitization.[13,18]

As in the chicken, the wattle test with mycobacterium has also been used in the turkey.[11,12] Turkeys possess a dewlap that resembles the wattle of a chicken. The dewlap may be a suitable site for antigen injection. Rose and Bradley[18] recommended the use of skin around the ear, frontal process, and body as the sites for antigen injection.

The histological examination of the site of PHA injection revealed that granulocytic cells invaded the dermis within 2 h of injection, and the number of invading cells increased with time. By 6 h postinjection, large numbers of lymphocytes were also observed in the dermis.[6] On the other hand, skin reactions of turkeys to MA or hapten 2,4-dinitrophenyl conjugated to bovine γ-globulin (DNP-BGG)[18] were observed 48 h following inoculation. Edema usually accompanied the cellualr infiltration at the site of antigen injection. The infiltrating cells included mononuclear cells and granulocytes. As in the chicken, cellular immune reactions may be demonstrated in turkeys at hatching,[16,17] although maximum responsiveness is attained after 2 to 4 weeks of age.[7] Interestingly, the delayed hypersensitivity response of 8-week-old turkeys was lower in magnitude than that of young poults. This unusual finding suggested a unique pattern of maturation of the immune functions in turkeys.[7] Further studies are required to understand the maturation of CMI in turkeys.

Delayed-type hypersensitivity response has been used in turkey and chicken to examine immunosuppressive effects of ochratoxin A (OA), a nephrotoxic mycotoxin produced by *Penicillium virdicatum* and *Aspergillus ochraceus*.[19-22] OA caused lymphoid-cell depletion in the thymus of turkeys[19,20] accompanied by reduced delayed hypersensitivity reaction to a variety of antigens.[20,22]

B. LYMPHOCYTE TRANSFORMATION

Blastogenic response of lymphocytes to mitogens or antigens is often used as a measure of CMI. As in mammals, PHA and concanavalin A (Con A) act as T-cell mitogens in chickens.[20-27] Although turkey lymphocytes also respond to these mitogens,[1-5,7-9,18,28] there is little information regarding the specificity of lymphocyte transformation in this animal. Exposure of turkeys to infectious agents may compromise lymphocyte blastogenic response.[1,3-5,8,9]

Lymphocytes recovered from turkeys immunized with chlamydia bacteria underwent blastogenic response upon *in vitro* exposure to purified chlamydia organisms.[2]

III. CELLULAR IMMUNITY IN THE QUAIL

Japanese quail is widely used as an experimental animal in avian research. Compared to chickens, turkeys, and ducks, quails have the advantage of being small in size and thus requiring much less experimental space. Further, the quail is easy to handle and has a large accessible wing vein resembling the cephalic vein of the chicken. The well-developed wing vein of quails permits ease of intravenous injection as well as ease of obtaining blood samples.[29] Because of these advantages, immune responses in the quail have been reported in several studies.[30-37]

A. DELAYED HYPERSENSITITIVY

The CMI reactions to tuberculin[18,29] and PHA[38] in quails are similar to those seen in chickens and turkeys. The wattle test originally developed in chickens cannot be used in the quail because the quail lacks an anatomic site equivalent to the wattle of the chicken. For the delayed hypersensitivity test in the quail, several sites were compared for antigen inoculation. The sites included wing-web,[18,29,38] body skin,[18,29] and the anal area.[18,29] Grossly detectable delayed hypersensitivity reaction was apparent only if the antigen was inoculated in the anal area. Histologically, delayed hypersensitivity reaction in the quail was similar to that seen in the turkey and the chicken.

B. CELL-MEDIATED IMMUNITY INDUCED BY ROUS SARCOMA VIRUS

The quail is highly sensitive to Schmidt-Ruppin strain of Rous sarcoma virus (SR-RSV) belonging to subgroup A of avian retroviruses.[30] The tumors induced by SR-RSV in the quail show a high rate of spontaneous regression. Following tumor repression, the animals remain resistant to subsequent challenge with large doses of SR-RSV.[30] Several immunologic parameters of tumor regression have been examined.[31-33] Surgical thymectomy, but not bursectomy, prevented tumor regression. Thus, CMI played an important role in the inhibition of tumor growth. The cytotoxic activity of spleen cells from bursectomized quails, whose sarcomas had regressed, was much higher than that of the spleen cells from non-bursectomized quails. On the other hand, spleen cells from thymectomized birds which had progressively growing tumors were not cytotoxic. Studies on the SR-RSV system in quail has led to several significant findings such as the recognition of a humoral arming factor which confers cytotoxic activity on the normal spleen cells in the sera of the tumor-regressor quails,[34,35] a role of alternative complement pathway in host responses to SR-RSV-induced tumors,[39] and the isolation and ontogenic features of the third component of complement.[36,37]

C. NATURAL KILLER CELLS

The natural killer (NK) cell system in the quail,[40-42] as well as the chicken,[43-45] is well studied. Further, it is known that the NK cell acitivity in quails is suppressed by α-fetoprotein (AFP) which is present in the chicken amniotic fluid and that the suppression of the activity is caused by AFP-induced suppressor cells.[42]

IV. CELLULAR IMMUNITY IN THE DUCK

It is well established that ducks, especially wild ducks, play an important role as a natural reservoir for certain infectious agents such as influenza virus[46] and Newcastle disease virus.[47] The immune mechanisms in the duck are not well understood. Published studies have revealed some interesting observations.

Higgins and Chung[48] used common immunological techniques for the purification, identification, cultivation, and functional assessment of duck lymphocyte subpopulations. The immunological characteristics of duck lymphocytes recovered from blood or lymphoid organs such as thymus, bursa of Fabricius, spleen, and cervical lymph node were different from those of lymphocytes of chickens or mammals. The proportions and organ distribution of lymphocytes with surface immunoglobulin (SmIg) or receptors for peanut agglutinin (PNA) did not follow a pattern consistent with an expected distribution of T and B cells. In two fractions (mean densities 1.026 and 1.068 g/cm^3) of duck blood spearated by Percoll® gradients, cells in the upper fraction, but not in the lower fraction, responded to the mitogenic effect of PHA, Con A, pokeweed mitogen, and rabbit anti-duck Ig serum. However, the expressions of SmIg and receptors for PNA did not differ in the lymphocytes of the two fractions. In addition, although chicken T lymphocytes are easily recovered from nylon wool column as nonadherent cells,[49,50] the duck T cells apparently remained adherent to the nylon wool fibers. The mitogenic response to PHA and Con A was associated with the nylon wool adherent cell fraction. Because ducks seem to be phylogenetically close to amphibians and reptiles,[48] the immunological techniques established for chickens and mammals may not apply to ducks.

Chang[51] reported that vaccination of ducks with a virulent live *Pasteurella multocida* (PM) induced high levels of systemic humoral and cell-mediated immune responses which were measured by a passive hemagglutination test and lymphocyte transformation test to the PM antigens, respectively. The level of immune responsiveness was correlated with protection against disease. The identity of the immune cells involved in protection needs to be established.

V. CONCLUSIONS

The lymphoreticular tissues of birds have broad patterns of organization similar to mammals. Cellular immune mechanisms in the avian species other than the chicken have not been well examined. Functionally, lymphoid cells of turkeys and quails are similar to those of chickens. Duck lymphocytes, however, appear quite unique and may reflect the phylogenetic proximity of this animal to amphibians and reptiles.

REFERENCES

1. **Maheswaran, S. K., Thies, E. S., and Due, S. K.,** Studies on *Pasteurella multocida.* III. *In vitro* assay for cell-mediated immunity, *Avian Dis.,* 20, 332, 1976.
2. **Page, L. A.,** Stimulation of cell-mediated immunity to chlamidiosis in turkeys by inoculation of chlamydial bacterin, *Am. J. Vet. Res.,* 39, 473, 1978.
3. **Maheswaran, S. K. and Thies, E. S.,** *Pasteurella multocida* atigen induce *in vitro* lymphocyte immunostimulation, using whole blood from cattle and turkeys, *Res. Vet. Sci.,* 26, 25, 1979.
4. **Maheswaran, S. K., Due, S. K., and Thies, E. S.,** Studies on *Pasteurella multocida.* IX. Levamisole-induced augmentaiton of immune response to a live fowl cholera vaccine, *Avian Dis.,* 24, 71, 1980.
5. **Nagaraja, K. V. and Pomeroy, B. S.,** Cell-mediated immunity against turkey coronaviral enteritis (Bluecomb), *Am. J. Vet. Res.,* 41, 915, 1980.

6. **McCorkle, F. M., Simmons, D. G., and Luginbuhl, G. H.,** Delayed hypersensitivity reponse in *Alcaligenes faecalis* infected turkey poults, *Avian Dis.,* 26, 782, 1982.

7. **McCorkle, F. M., Luginbuhl, G. H., Simmons, D. G., Morgan, G. W., and Thaxton, J. P.,** Ontogeny of delayed hypersensitivity in young turkeys, *Dev. Comp. Immunol.,* 7, 517, 1983.

8. **Giambrone, J. J., Diener, U. L., Davis, N. D., Panangala, V. S., and Hoerr, F. J.,** Effects of aflatoxin on young turkeys and broiler chickens, *Poult. Sci.,* 64, 1678, 1985.

9. **Giambrone, J. J., Diener, U. L., Davis, N. D., Panangala, V. S., and Hoerr, F. J.,** Effects of purified aflatoxin on turkeys, *Poult. Sci.,* 64, 859, 1985.

10. **Warner, N. L., Ovary, Z., and Kantor, F. S.,** Delayed hypersensitivity reactions in normal and bursectomized chickens, *Int. Arch. Allergy Appl. Immunol.,* 40, 719, 1971.

11. **Klesius, P. H., Kramer, T., Burger, D., and Malley, A.,** Passive transfer of coccidian oocyst antigen and diphtheria toxoid hypersensitivity in calves across species barriers, *Transplant. Proc.,* 7, 499, 1985.

12. **Subba Rao, D. S. V. and Glick, B.,** The production of a lymphocyte inhibitory factor (LyIF) by bursal and thymic lymphocytes, in *Avian Immunology,* Benedict, A. A., Ed., Plenum Press, New York, 1977, 87.

13. **Goto, N., Kodama, H., Okada, K., and Fujimoto, Y.,** Suppression of phytohemagglutinin skin response in thymectomized chickens, *Poult. Sci.,* 57, 246, 1978.

14. **McCorkle, F. M., Stinson, R., and Glick, B.,** A biphasic graft vs. host response in aging chickens, *Cell. Immunol.,* 46, 208, 1979.

15. **Stadecker, M. J., Lukic, M., Dvorak, A. M., and Leskowitz, S.,** The cutaneous basophil response to phytohemagglutinin in chickens, *J. Immunol.,* 118, 1564, 1977.

16. **Palladino, A. A., Brebenall, M. D., and Thorbecke, G. J.,** Requirements for induction of delayed hypersensitivity in the chicken, *Dev. Comp. Immunol.,* 2, 121, 1978.

17. **McCorkle, F. M., Olah, I., and Glick, B.,** The morphology of the phytohemagglutinin-induced cell response in the chicken wattle, *Poult. Sci.,* 59, 616, 1980.

18. **Rose, M. E. and Bradley, J. W. A.,** Delayed hypersensitivity in the fowl, turkey and quail, *Avian Pathol.,* 6, 313, 1977.

19. **Chang, C.-F., Doerr, J. A., and Hamilton, P. B.,** Experimental ochratoxicosis in turkey poults, *Poult. Sci.,* 60, 114, 1981.

20. **Dwivedi, P. and Burns, R. B.,** Ochratoxicosis A in broilers and turkeys: a comparative immunopathological study, in Proc. Abstr. XVII World Poultry Congress and Exhibition, Helsinki, Finland, August 1984, Section 4B10, 559.

21. **Burns, R. B. and Dwivedi, P.,** The natural occurrence of ochratoxin A and its effects in poultry. A review. II. Pathology and immunology, *World Poutl. Sci. J.,* 42, 48, 1986.

22. **Dwivedi, P. and Burns, R. B.,** Immunosuppressive effects of ochratoxin A in young turkeys, *Avian Pathol.,* 14, 213, 1985.

23. **Greaves, M. F., Roitt, I. M., and Rose, M. E.,** Effect of bursectomy on the responses of chicken peripheral blood lymphocytes to phytohemagglutinin, *Nature (London),* 17, 43, 1968.

24. **Alm, G. V.,** *In vitro* studies of chicken lymphoid cells. I. Phytohemagglutinin induced DNA, RNA and protein synthesis in spleen cells from control-irradiated and bursectomized-irradiated chickens, *Acta Pathol. Microbiol. Scand.,* 78B, 632, 1979.

25. **Toivanen, P. and Toivanen, A.,** Bursal and postbursal stem cells in chickens: functional characteristics, *Eur. J. Immunol.,* 3, 585, 1973.

26. **Lee, L. F.,** *In vitro* assay of mitogen stimulation of avian peripheral lymphocytes, *Avian Dis.,* 18, 602, 1974.

27. **Weber, W. T.,** Avian B lymphocyte subpopulations: origins and functional capacities, *Transplant. Rev.,* 24, 113, 1975.

28. **Maheswaran, S. K., Thies, E. S., and Greimann, C.,** A micromethod for evaluating turkey lymphocyte responses to phytomitogens, *Am. J. Vet. Res.,* 36, 1397, 1975.

29. **Karlson, A. G., Thoen, C. O., and Harrington, R.,** Japanese quail: susceptibility to avian tuberculosis, *Avian Dis.,* 14, 39, 1970.

30. **Yamanouchi, K., Haymai, M., Fukuda, A., and Kobune, F.,** Tumor development and induction of resistance by Rous sarcoma virus in Japanese quail, *Jpn. J. Med. Sci. Biol.,* 21, 393, 1968.

31. **Yamanouchi, K. and Hayami, M.,** Cellular immunity induced by Rous sarcomas in Japanese quail. I. Effect of anti-lymphocyte serum on oncogenesis of Rous sarcoma virus, *Jpn. J. Med. Sci. Biol.,* 23, 395, 1970.

32. **Yamanouchi, K., Hayami, M., Miyakura, S., Fukuda, A., and Kobune, F.,** Cellular immunity induced by Rous sarcoma virus in Japanese quail. II. Effect of thymectomy and bursectomy on oncogenesis of Rous sarcoma virus, *Jpn. J. Med. Sci. Biol.,* 24, 1, 1971.

33. **Hayami, M., Hellström, I., Hellström, K. E., and Yamanouchi, K.,** Cell-mediated destruction of Rous sarcomas in Japanese quails, *Int. J. Cancer,* 10, 507, 1972.

34. **Hayami, M., Hellström, I., Hellström, K. E., and Lannin, D. R.,** Further studies on the ability of regressor sera to block cell-mediated destruction of Rous sarcomas, *Int. J. Cancer,* 13, 43, 1974.
35. **Hayami, M., Ito, M., Yoshikawa, Y., and Yamanouchi, K.,** Temporal analysis of cellular cytotoxicity and humroal factors during progression of Rous sarcomas in Japanese quails, *Jpn. J. Med. Sci. Biol.,* 29, 11, 1976.
36. **Kai, C., Yoshikawa, Y., Yamanouchi, K., and Okada, H.,** Isolation and identification of the third component of complement of Japanese quails, *J. Immunol.,* 130, 1814, 1983.
37. **Kai, C., Yoshikawa, Y., Yamanouchi, K., Okada, H., and Morikawa, S.,** Ontogeny of the third component of complement of Japanese quails, *Immunology,* 43, 463, 1985.
38. **Galvin, M. J., Thaxton, J. P., McRee, D. I., and Hall, C. A.,** Immunity in late juvenile and young adult Japanese quail as related to microwave radiation during embryogeny, *Int. J. Radiat. Biol.,* 42, 673, 1982.
39. **Yoshikawa, Y., Yamanouchi, K., Hishiyama, M., and Kobune, K.,** Lysis of RSV-transformed Japanese quail cells by a factor from normal quail serum, *Int. J. Cancer,* 21, 658, 1978.
40. **Yamada, A., Haymai, M., Yamanouchi, K., and Fujiwara, K.,** Detection of natural killer cells in Japanese quail, *Int. J. Cancer,* 26, 381, 1980.
41. **Yamada, A. and Hayami, M.,** The role of natural killer cells in tumor growth assessed by induction of their suppressor cells in Japanese quails, *Jpn. J. Med. Sci. Biol.,* 34, 161, 1981.
42. **Yamada, A. and Hayami, M.,** Suppression of natural killer cell activity by chicken α-fetoprotein in Japanese quail, *J. Natl. Cancer Inst.,* 70, 735, 1983.
43. **Sharma, J. M. and Coulson, B. D.,** Presence of natural killer cells in specific pathogen-free chickens, *J. Natl. Cancer Inst.,* 63, 527, 1979.
44. **Lam, K. M. and Linna, T. J.,** Transfer of natural resistance to Marek's disease (JMV) with non-immune spleen cells. I. Studies of cell population transferring resistance, *Int. J. Cancer,* 24, 662, 1979.
45. **Lam, K. M. and Linna, T. J.,** Transfer of natural resistance to Marek's disease (JMV) with non-immune spleen cells. II. Further characterization of the protecting cell population, *J. Immunol.,* 125, 715, 1980.
46. **Kida, H., Yanagawa, R., and Matsuoka, Y.,** Duck influenza lacking evidence of disease signs and immune response, *Infect. Immun.,* 30, 547, 1980.
47. **Kawamura, M., Mikami, T., Kodama, H., and Izawa, H.,** Pathogenicity and immunogenicity in chickens of Newcastle disease virus isolated from wild ducks, *Arch. Virol.,* 95, 149, 1987.
48. **Higgins, D. A. and Chung, S.-H.,** Duck lymphocytes. I. Purification and preliminary observations on surface markers, *J. Immunol. Methods,* 86, 231, 1986.
49. **Stinson, R. E., McCorkle, F., and Glick, B.,** Nylon wool column separation of chicken thymic-derived (T) and bursal-derived (B) lymphocytes, *Poult. Sci.,* 57, 518, 1978.
50. **Lamont, S. J. and Van Alten, P. J.,** Characteristics of nylon fiber adherence-separated chicken splenocytes, *J. Immunol. Methods,* 40, 181, 1981.
51. **Chang, C.-F.,** *In vitro* assay for humoral and cell-mediated immunity of pasteurellosis in ducks, *J. Chin. Soc. Vet. Sci.,* 13, 67, 1987.

Chapter 9

ROLE OF CELLULAR IMMUNITY IN NEOPLASTIC AND NONNEOPLASTIC VIRAL DISEASES

J. M. Sharma, S. J. Prowse, and J. J. York

TABLE OF CONTENTS

I. INTRODUCTION

Birds raised under natural conditions are vulnerable to environmental exposure to a number of pathogenic viruses that may cause neoplastic or nonneoplastic disease. Because of potential economic loss due to viral infections, commercial chicken and turkey flocks are routinely vaccinated with antiviral vaccines. The vaccines are not always effective, and epornitics of viral disease may occur in vaccinated poultry flocks. Thus, there has been much interest in studies on antiviral resistance mechanisms and the role of viral immunity in protection against disease.

The purpose of this presentation is to review cell-mediated immune responses in some of the common neoplastic and nonneoplastic viral infections of poultry. Among the neoplastic viruses, Marek's disease virus (MDV) of chickens has been studied most extensively and will be emphasized here. Viruses that cause avian leukosis and reticuloendotheliosis (RE) will also be considered. For each neoplastic virus infection, we will briefly describe the characteristics of the disease caused by the virus followed by a description of the cell-mediated immune response of the host and the role of this immunity in pathogenesis of the disease.

Cell-mediated immune responses to nonneoplastic avian viruses have not been well examined and thus will not be emphasized here. The role of cellular immunity in some of the common avian viruses will be reviewed briefly. These will include infectious bronchitis virus (IBV), Fowlpox virus, Newcastle disease virus (NDV), and infectious laryngotracheitis virus. The role of cellular immunity in other common viral infections such as reovirus, encephalomyelitis virus, infectious bursal disease virus, fowl adenovirus, and avian influenza is not well documented.

II. CELLULAR IMMUNITY IN NEOPLASTIC VIRAL DISEASES

A. MAREK'S DISEASE
1. Characteristics of the Disease

Marek's disease (MD) is the most common naturally occurring neoplastic disease of commercial chickens. This disease is caused by a cell-associated herpesvirus that tends to infect most commercial chickens during the first few days of life. In unprotected flocks, MD is liable to cause a high rate of mortality. At the present time, the disease is under control because of the widespread use of highly effective vaccines.

Natural disease occurs primarily in the chicken, although birds of certain other avian species may either be infected experimentally or may contain natural antibodies to the virus.[1] Inoculation of high doses of virulent MDV in turkeys often results in tumor formation.[2,3]

In susceptible chickens lacking antibodies to MDV, exposure to virulent MDV initiates a series of rapidly progressing events. Initially, within 3 to 7 d of exposure, the virus causes extensive necrotic changes in the lymphoid organs. This early phase is characterized by cytolytic infection of B cells[4] and appearance of abundant viral internal antigens detectable by immune fluorescent assays using anti-MDV antibody. Lytically infected cells do not produce significant quantities of enveloped infectious virions. Infectious cell-free virus is produced only by the feather follicle epithelium later in the infectious cycle.[5]

Accompanying the early cytolytic infection is a severe but transient depression in the ability of T cells to respond to mitogens *in vitro*.[6-9] This immunodepressive effect appears to be mediated by activated suppressor macrophages.[10] The early cytolytic phase rarely lasts more than 3 to 4 d, and most birds recover from this phase. Subsequently, the virus establishes a permanent latent infection in T lymphocytes. The mechanism of the dramatic switch from lytic to latent phase is not known. Of interest is a recent finding that the lymphocytes obtained from chickens undergoing the cytolytic phase secrete interferon (IFN) *in vitro*.[11]

Lymphocytes obtained prior to the initiation of the lytic phase or after the end of the lytic phase did not produce detectable IFN *in vitro*. If lymphocyte-derived IFN is also produced *in vivo*, the IFN may have a role in restricting the early cytolytic phase of MDV infection.

The latent infection occurs primarily in T lymphocytes although some B cells may also become latently infected.[4] Early lytic infection of B lymphocytes may activate T cells that acquire immune associated antigen (Ia) antigens and become susceptible to virus infection.[12] The latent infection persists through the life of the host.

The onset of latent infection is accompanied by lymphoid-cell proliferation, and some latently infected lymphocytes become neoplastically transformed and produce tumors. The virus transforms T lymphocytes in the chicken and T or B lymphocytes in the turkey.[3,13] Neoplastically transformed cells exhibit a new surface antigen designated Marek's disease tumor-associated surface antigen (MATSA).[14] This is likely a cell differentiation antigen because a certain proportion of mitogen-stimulated T lymphoblasts may express MATSA.[15]

The lymphoproliferation may be detected in a number of tissues, although peripheral nerves are specially prone to lymphoid cell accumulation. The affected chickens develop varying degrees of neurological disorders, most commonly leg paralysis. Chickens bearing progressive MD tumors also become immunodepressed in both humoral and cellular immune systems. T cells from tumor-bearing chickens become persistently deficient in mitogenic responsiveness.[9] Several mechanisms may be responsible for mitogenic hyporesponsiveness.[9,10,16,17] Although MDV causes immunodepression, the infected chickens develop vigorous humoral and cellular immune responses against the virus.[18]

The outcome of infection with MDV is determined by a number of factors. Chickens exposed to nonpathogenic isolates of MDV may develop persistent viremia but no disease. Virulent isolates may also fail to cause progressive disease under the following circumstances:

1. Chickens may be genetically resistant to tumor formation. The major histocompatibility complex (MHC)-related resistance has been well documented in MD and appears to be associated with the B^{21} allele[19] although other alleles and loci outside of MHC may also control resistance.[20,21]
2. If the virus exposure is delayed, the chickens may develop age-resistance to MD. Newly hatched chickens are most susceptible to clinical MD, but chickens become resistant as they get older.[22,23]
3. Prior vaccination may protect highly susceptible chickens against pathogenic effects of MDV. Vaccines may consist of turkey herpesvirus (HVT), nonpathogenic serotype 2 MDV, or attenuated isolates of virulent serotype 1 MDV.[24]

Natural and vaccine-induced resistance is immunologically mediated. Studies involving experimentally induced immunodepression revealed that chickens deficient in humoral immunity remained resistant to MD, although deficiency in the cellular immune competence compromised resistance.[25-28] Several laboratories have examined the role of cell-mediated immunity in resistance to MD.

2. Role of T Cells

The first evidence that MDV elicits a cell-mediated immune response in chickens was obtained in an *in vivo* study. When chickens affected with MD were injected intradermally with preparations of MD viral antigens, a local delayed-type hypersensitivity (DTH) reaction was observed.[29] This observation was followed by a number of reports that described *in vitro* assays that measured cellular immunity. The assays included the migration-inhibition assay,[30] plaque-reduction assay,[31-34] and cytotoxicity assays that utilized radioisotope release.[35-36] The latter two tests have been examined in some detail and will be described further.

The plaque-reduction assay reported by Ross,[31,32] and later by others,[33,34] measured antiviral T-cell response in chickens. Lymphocytes isolated from chickens vaccinated with MD vaccines were cytotoxic *in vitro* to virus-infected lymphoid or nonlymphoid target cells and reduced the ability of the target cells to induce plaques in permissive monolayer cell cultures. The effector cells of this cytotoxic activity were identified as T lymphocytes, and the cytotoxic activity was not restricted by MHC. Plaque inhibition occurred whether the virus-infected target cells were syngeneic or allogeneic to the effector lymphocytes.[32,37]

In the 4- or 8-h ^{51}Cr-release assays, lymphocytes obtained from spleen or circulation of virus-exposed birds, or from virus-induced solid tumors, are reacted *in vitro* with ^{51}Cr-labeled target cells.[35,36,38-41] The target cells consist of cells of *in vitro* propagating lines derived from MD tumors. The target cells may also be labeled with ^{3}H-proline[42] or ^{35}S-methionine.[43] The cytotoxic reactivity of the effector cell population is quantitated by the amount of radioactive label released from the target cells. The cytotoxic effector cells detactable in spleen or peripheral blood leukocytes (PBL) of MDV-exposed birds appear shortly after infection and remain detectable for varying intervals. In most studies, the cytotoxic activity was transient and peaked about 1 week after virus infection. The time of peak cytotoxic activity coincided with the time when lymphocytic infection was prominent and detectable MATSA-bearing cells first appeared in infected chickens.[44] The cytotoxic effector cells were identified as T lymphocytes because the cytotoxic activity of spleen cells was abrogated by treatment with polyclonal anti-T-cell serum.[45] This cytotoxic activity was best expressed if the cytotoxic cells were allogeneic to the tumor target cells. The reactivity was poorly expressed in syngeneic effector-target combinations.[46,47]

The antigen(s) against which the cytotoxic activity is directed are not known. Because the cytotoxic cells reacted against tumor targets and the activity coincided with the appearance of MATSA-bearing cells,[44] some of the activity may be directed against MATSA present on tumor target cells. However, other antigens must also be involved because tumor target cells on which MATSA was either blocked with anti-MATSA antibody or removed enzymatically remained susceptible to T-cell lysis.[48]

The role of cytotoxic T cells in resistance to MD is not clear because the level of detectable cytotoxicity in individual chickens could not always be correlated with the outcome of infection.[40,49] The cytotoxic cells were best expressed in highly susceptible chickens destined to develop progressive tumors,[36,42] and MDV-induced solid tumors lacked detectable cytotoxic T cells.[50] On the other hand, vaccines that protected chickens against oncogenesis by MDV also induced cytotoxic T cells,[39,41] overall cytotoxic activity was higher in groups of chickens resistant to tumor formation than in those with high incidence of mortality and tumors.[40,49] The appearance of T-cell cytotoxicity against tumor targets is a prominent feature of the pathogenesis of MDV in chickens, and additional studies are warranted to examine the role of these cells in disease.

3. Role of Macrophages

Infection with MDV results in activation of macrophages, and suppressor functions associated with normal macrophages become enhanced.[51] Macrophages from virus-infected chickens are highly phagocytic for the virus[52] and may restrict MDV replication *in vitro*.[53-55] Macrophages in collaboration with B lymphocytes may inactivate cell-free MDV.[56] Inhibition of mitogenic response of T cells from chickens undergoing early cytolytic phase of virus infection also appears to be mediated by suppressor macrophages.[57] Macrophages also inhibit *in vitro* DNA synthesis by line cells derived from MD tumors.[58]

Macrophage proliferation, induced by injecting silica in chickens, delayed the appearance of clinical MD and reduced the number of viral-antigen positive cells in the thymus and bursa.[59] Furthermore, inhibition of macrophage functions by injecting chickens with anti-macrophage serum or trypan blue resulted in elevated levels of circulating virus and enhanced tumor incidence.[52] Cell suspensions made from MD tumors had a macrophage-like population of cells that were cytotoxic *in vitro* for MDV-transformed lymphoid cells.[50] These adherent effector cells were inactivated by pretreatment with carbonyl iron and carrageenan. Because the tumors with macrophage-mediated cytotoxicity progressed and killed the host, the role of intratumoral cytotoxic macrophages was not clear.[50]

4. Role of Natural Immune Cells

Natural killer (NK) cells and effector cells of antibody-dependent cellular cytotoxicity (ADCC) have been reported in chickens,[60] and both activities may be important in the pathogenesis of MD.[32,33,61-63]

There was a difference in the NK cell activity between susceptible and resistant chickens exposed to pathogenic MDV.[63] In chickens of line P, a highly susceptible line, MDV caused a progressive debilitating disease characterized by high incidence of gross tumors and death. The NK reactivity in the spleen cells of these chickens was significantly lower than in age-matched virus-free hatchmates. On the other hand, in line N chickens that were resistant to MD, exposure to MDV resulted in no clinical disease and elevated NK levels. MD vaccines that protected chickens against oncogenic effects of MDV also induced elevated NK levels.[63,64] In another study, resistance to the JMV transplant, a virus-free MD tumor-cell transplant, was also associated with NK cell reactivity. Spleen cells from 8-week-old chickens resistant to JMV due to age transferred resistance to younger, highly susceptible chickens.[61,62] The spleen cells that transferred resistance to JMV did not have characteristics of macrophages, T cells, or B cells and were thus considered to be NK cells.

One of us compared progressive and regressive MD tumors of chickens for the presence of NK cells.[50] The incidence and levels of NK activity were greater in the regressive tumors than in progressive tumors, thus suggesting a possible role of NK cells in tumor regression. In the tumor-bearing chickens, the NK cell activity was greater in the tumors than in the spleen.

The effector cells of ADCC have been described in birds infected with MDV or vaccinated with MD vaccines,[32,33,65] although the role of this effector mechanism in MD is not clear and needs to be examined.

B. AVIAN LEUKOSIS AND SARCOMA TUMORS

1. Characteristics of the Disease

Viruses of avian leukosis and sarcoma (ALS) group are C-type retroviruses. The replication of these RNA viruses is characterized by the formation of DNA provirus with the help of the enzyme reverse transcriptase. The DNA provirus becomes linearly integrated into the host genome and is subsequently transcribed into viral RNA which is then translated to produce the precursors and structural proteins of the virion.[66]

The ALS group is composed of two types of viruses: (1) avian leukosis viruses (ALV) that cause lymphoid tumors after a long latent period and (2) avian sarcoma virus (ASV) and acute defective leukemia viruses (DLV) that cause acute neoplasms after a short latent period. The genome of the acutely transforming viruses contains an oncogene, v-onc, that is responsible for initiating neoplastic transformation in cells. ASVs that cause transformation of connective tissue cells contain the *src* gene, which is similar to the *src* gene present in normal cells. Rous sarcoma virus (RSV) is the best-studied prototype of the ASVs. ALVs and DLVs usually do not transform fibroblasts. The slow-transforming viruses lack the oncogene. The oncogene-lacking ALVs induce neoplastic transformation by inserting themselves in the host genome in such a way that the insertion activates oncogenes present in the host cell genome.[67,68]

The ALS viruses have been classified into several subgroups designated by letter alphabets. The subgroups important for chickens include subgroups A, B, C, D, and E.

Viruses isolated from pheasants have been identified as subgroups F and G. The subgroup distribtion is based on differences in the viral coat glycoproteins.[69] Subgroups A, B, C, and D are exogenous viruses because they may be transmitted horizontally or vertically among chickens. Subgroup E viruses are endogenous viruses and are transmitted genetically in a Mendelian fashion. Cellular DNA of almost all normal chickens carry DNA proviral sequences of subgroup E virus.

The pathogenic manifestations of the various viruses in the ALS group is highly variable and depends on many factors. In general, the ALVs cause B-cell lymphomas, the DLVs cause leukemias, and the ASVs cause sarcomas.

Three types of pathologic responses may be observed in birds following infection with ALS viruses:

1. Infection may result in tumor development. Depending upon the virus, the tumors may appear after a long latent period, such as with ALVs, or may be acute, such as with DLVs.
2. ALS viruses may induce nonneoplatic lesions. Birds may develop wasting disease manifested by anemia, hepatitis, and immunodepression. This syndrome associated with certain leukosis viruses has been reported to occur under experimental conditions.[70-72]
3. Infection may not cause overt disease but may reduce flock performance by reducing production and compromising egg quality.[73]

Among the ALVs, viruses of subgroup A are of most importance because these viruses are widely distributed in commercial chicken flocks and may occasionally cause a high incidence of tumors in chickens. The chickens generally acquire infection with the virus either congenitally or as neonates. Congenital infection often results in immunological tolerance to the virus and a high incidence of tumors.[74,75] Chickens infected after hatching may not become tolerant to the virus, but may remain vulnerable to tumor development. The virus initiates neoplastic transformation of cells in the bursa of Fabricius. Microscopic loci of neoplastically transformed cells may be detected in the bursa at about 4 weeks of age although grossly detectable metastatic tumors generally do not appear until after 14 weeks of age. The tumors are bursa-dependent and are comprised of transformed B lymphocytes.[76] Gross tumors may be present in a variety of organs including bursa, liver, kidneys, spleen, ovaries, etc.

2. Role of Cellular Immunity in Avian Leukosis

As noted above, congenital transmission of ALV may result in immunological tolerance to the virus. Tolerant chickens develop persistant viremia but no detectable immune responses to the virus. Nontolerant infection results in the development of antibody against viral antigens. The antibody may control the level of circulating infectious virus.

Specific cell-mediated immune responses following natural infection with ALV have not been reported. Bauer et al.[77] used an *in vitro,* microcytotoxicity assay to demonstrate that lymphocytes of chickens given repeated intramuscular injections of ALV were cytotoxic for virus-infected and virus-transformed target cells. Neither the nature of the effector cells nor the identity of the target antigens were reported. It is not known if a similar cytotoxic immune response plays a role in the pathogenesis of natural ALV-induced disease. In some birds, foci of neoplastically transformed cells in the bursal follicles may regress, and this regression may be immunologically mediated.[78] The nature of protective immunity and the involvement of cellular immunity in protection need to be examined. Thymectomy did not affect the disease response.[79]

3. Role of Cellular Immunity in Avian Sarcoma Viruses

Although ASVs are not a common field problem, they have been used extensively as experimental models to study the role of cell-mediated immunity in tumorigensis. These viruses cause tumors in chickens after a short latent period, and some of the tumors frequently undergo spontaneous regression,[80,81] thus allowing the opportunity to compare progressing and regressing tumors. Experimental tumors induced by RSV have been examined extensively.

Studies with RSV have shown that tumor regression is immunologically mediated, and cellular immunity plays the principal protective role. Several laboratories have demonstrated that neonatal thymectomy consistently enhanced tumor progression in chickens and quails.[82-84] Perry et al.[85] compared histologic appearance of progressing and regressing RSV tumors. They noted that regressing tumors contained a higher proportion of lymphocytes than the progressing tumors, and there was an interesting difference in the spatial arrangement of lymphocytes and tumor cells between regressing and progressing tumors. Lymphocytes infiltrating regressive tumors had a polar accumulation of organelles at the point of contact between the lymphocytes and the tumor cells. Such an organelle arrangement was not seen in progressing tumors.

Several *in vitro* assays have been used to demonstrate cellular immune responses to RSV in chickens and quails. Israel and Wainberg[86] showed that PBL of chickens bearing RSV tumors proliferated *in vitro* if exposed to antigens derived from supernatant or extracts of cultures of virus-transformed cells. The development of this lymphoblastic response closely parallelled tumor development. The response appeared within 2 weeks following RSV inoculation and disappeared after tumor regression was complete. The antigens to which immune cells in the PBL responded *in vitro* were recognized as internal viral proteins P15 and P27 coded by the *gag* gene.[87]

Inoculation with ASVs also induced cytotoxic lymphocytes in chickens and quails.[77,84,88-92] The cytotoxic activity in the spleens of virus-infected birds appeared within 2 weeks of inoculation and remained detectable for several weeks after the tumor had regressed. The cytotoxic reactivity of effector cells was directed against virus-induced glycoproteins, embryonic antigens, and a transformation-specific antigen unrelated to structural constituents of the virus.[92] Wainberg et al.[91] examined the susceptibility of RSV-induced tumor cells to lysis by immune effector cells. Cells from progressive tumors that were actively producing infectious virus were much more susceptible to lysis than were the cells from regressive tumors that did not produce virus. Furthermore, autologous virus particles inhibited target-cell destruction by the effector cells.[91] This study demonstrated that viral antigens served as the target antigens for immune effector cells. The cytotoxic effector cells were presumed to be T lymphocytes, although their identity was not firmly established. There is also some confusion on the role of the MHC in the expression of immune cytotoxic reactivity. Some of the antigens recognized by the effector cells on the surface of susceptible target cells may be similar to the alloantigens coded by the MHC.[93]

Presence of specific immune effector cells in RSV-infected chickens was also demonstrated by the migration-inhibition test. Soluble tumor extract inhibited *in vitro* migration of PBL from chickens undergoing tumor regression.[94] Specific migration inhibition was significantly more pronounced in PBL from tumor regressors than in PBL from tumor progressors.

There is evidence that NK cells may play a role in regression of ASV-induced tumors.[91] Normal NK cell activity of spleen cells of chickens was not affected by the presence of regressing RSV tumors. Presence of progressing tumors inhibited normal NK cell activity. Of further interest was the observation that cells comprising regressing RSV tumors were susceptible to the cytotoxic effect of NK effector cells, whereas cells of progressing tumors were resistant.[91] This result indicated that regression of RSV tumors may be immunologically mediated by an active participation by NK cell activity. The target antigens recognized by NK cells were different from those recognized by immune cytotoxic effector cells. Presence of autologous virus in the *in vitro* reaction inhibited the cytotoxicity of immune effector cells but not of NK cells.[91] Studies in Japanese quails have shown that treatment with α-fetoprotein present in the chicken amniotic fluid induced suppressor cells that inhibited normal NK cell activity in the quail.[95] The inhibition of normal NK reactivity by α-fetoprotein resulted in a higher incidence of progressive RSV tumors than in controls that had normal NK cell levels.[96]

Participation of macrophages in regression of ASV-induced tumors is not well understood. Activation of macrophages by injecting BCG at the site of the tumor enhanced tumor progression apparently because macrophages served as targets for active virus replication.[97] Increased virus levels facilitated tumor progression by enhancing cell transformation. Possible protective role of macrophages in virus-free regressive tumors needs to be examined.

C. RETICULOENDOTHELIOSIS
1. Characteristics of the Disease

RE is a natural disease of turkeys, although chickens, ducks, geese, pheasants, quail, and guinea fowl may contain antibodies to the RE virus (REV) or may become infected by experimental exposure to the virus. Although the chicken is not the most common natural host of REV, the disease is important for chickens because on several occasions large populations of commercial chickens have been inoculated with cell-culture-propagated vaccines inadvertently contaminated with REV.[98-100] The REV infection resulted in immunodepression and poor flock performance.

RE is caused by a group of retroviruses that are antigenically distinct from the ALS group of avian retroviruses.[101-105] The strains of REV may be differentiated into nondefective and replication-defective strains. The replication-defective viruses have deletions in the *gag-pol* region of the genome and contain the transforming gene *rel* in the *env* region.[103-105] The counterpart sequences of the viral oncogenes have been identified in the genome of normal avian cells, particularly in turkey cells.[103,106] The nondefective strains of REV cause a runting-disease syndrome characterized by nonneoplastic lesions that may involve a number of organs. For instance, chickens inoculated with nondefective REV become pale and stunted and may develop thymic and bursal atrophy as well as necrosis of liver and spleen.[107,108] The runting disease syndrome has been studied most extensively in the chicken, although similar syndromes may also occur in ducks and turkeys.[109,110] Nondefective REV may also induce bursa-dependent lymphomas after a long latent period.[111] These lymphomas appear identical to the B-cell lymphoma induced by ALVs. The similarity of the relationship of the proviral genome of REV and avian leukosis virus to c-*myc* indicates that both types of lymphomas may be initiated by a common mechanism.[112]

Replication-defective REV causes acute, rapidly progressing tumors in a variety of organs particularly in liver and spleen.[113] These tumors are usually fatal within 3 weeks of virus inoculation. The target cells of viral transformation have not been identified and appear to be undifferentiated mononuclear cells.

Chickens infected with REV may develop tolerance to the virus if the virus exposure occurs shortly after hatching;[114,115] exposure at subsequent age results in antibody development and cellular immunity. Antibodies may be detected by several serologic assays.[116] Immune responses may have a protective role in RE.[117,118]

2. Role of Cellular Immunity

REV induces profound immunodepression in birds. Both the nondefective and the replication defective viruses induce a rapid and dramatic inhibition of the mitogenetic response of T cells.[119-121] The mitogenetic inhibition is mediated by a suppressor cell population induced by the virus.[122] The suppressor cells inhibit the proliferative but not the cytotoxic functions of lymphoid cells.[123,124] REV infection delayed allograft rejection.[124]

Two specific cytotoxic reactions have been described in REV-infected chickens. Maccubbin and Schierman[125,126] noted that spleen cells obtained from chickens 7 d following REV exposure were cytotoxic for REV-transformed line cells. Cyclophosphamide treatment enhanced the cytotoxic activity, and the enhancement was attributed to the removal of bursa-dependent suppressor T cells. Most importantly, cytotoxicity was detectable only if the effector cells and target cells shared the same MHC. The cytotoxic activity of the effector cells was directed against viral membrane antigens on target cells. Walker et al.[124] reported the presence of cytotoxic cells in spleen and PBL of chickens infected 7 d previously with REV tumor cells. The antigens against which this cytotoxic activity was directed were not identified, although infector cells lysed both virus producing and nonproducing REV-transformed tumor cells. The cytotoxicity was measured in an 18-h ^{51}Cr-release assay, but the identity of the effector cells was not determined.

Cell-mediated immune responses in RE may be involved in resistance to the disease, since Linna et al.[118] showed that surgical thymectomy in chickens enhanced tumor incidence and mortality. Surgical and chemical bursectomy had a similar enhancing effect.

II. CELLULAR IMMUNITY IN NONNEOPLASTIC VIRAL DISEASES

A. INFECTIOUS BRONCHITIS VIRUS

Cellular immunity has been implicated in resistance to IBV by virtue of the lack of correlation between protection and antibody responses. Lymphocyte transformation in response to IBV antigens was described by Timms et al.[127] PBL from infected chickens proliferated following cultivation with IBV antigens. The response peaked at 12 d after infection with an average stimulation index of 5.5 and declined to be essentially absent by 30 d postinfection despite the continued presence of high levels of antibody.

Secondary proliferative responses were examined in chickens immunized with a live vaccine and challenged with a virulent virus.[128] The secondary responses in vaccinated challenged birds were not consistently higher than the primary responses of birds which received only the challenge infection. Furthermore, no cellular immune responses could be detected in vaccinated chickens at the time of challenge.

Chubb et al.[129] measured DTH responses to IBV infection. A low DTH reaction was detected, and it declined 2 to 3 weeks after vaccination. DTH reaction was not detected in birds immunized with a high dose of virus, although the birds were protected against virus challenge. The lack of responsiveness may be due to the possible blocking of the DTH reaction by antibody.[130]

Cytotoxic lymphocytes in the spleen and blood of IBV-infected birds were demonstrated by Chubb et al.[131] The kinetics of the response were similar to those seen for lymphocyte transformation and DTH; all responses lasted about 3 weeks after infection. The cytotoxic response was only seen when autologous cells were used as both targets and effector cells, suggesting that the response was restricted by the MHC. However, the use of IBV-infected autologous macrophages from immunized birds as targets makes these data difficult to interpret because of possible antiviral activity of the immune macrophages.

In summary, the cell-mediated immune responses to IBV appeared to be short lived, arising soon after infection and lasting for 2 to 3 weeks. Surprisingly, birds that resisted challenge infection did not necessarily have detectable specific cellular immunity prior to challenge. Thus, the role of cellular immunity in protection against IBV is not clear.

B. FOWLPOX VIRUS

It is well established that fowlpox vaccines induce immunity against virulent strains of fowlpox virus. However, the immune mechanisms are unclear. Dharsana and Spradbrow[132] showed that a DTH reaction could be detected 5 d after the administration of a fowlpox vaccine. The response lasted longer than 33 d and correlated with results of a leukocyte migration inhibition assay conducted with cells from the same birds.

It was demonstrated by Morita[133] that bursectomized birds were able to survive infection with fowlpox virus in the absence of detectable antibody, indirectly suggesting the importance of cellular immunity in recovery from fowlpox infection. Furthermore, healing of lesions correlated with cellular immunity as determined by leukocyte migration-inhibition assays. There was no correlation between healing and antibody levels. Thus, immunity to fowlpox virus appears to have a cell-mediated component, although the immune responses have not been well characterized.

C. NEWCASTLE DISEASE VIRUS

Because antibody-mediated mechanisms (particularly local antibody responses) are thought to be important in immunity to Newcastle disease,[134] the role of cell-mediated immunity has not been extensively studies. Marino and Hanson[135] used bursectomized chickens to study the role of antibody and cellular immunity in vaccinated and challenged chickens. They showed that bursectomized chickens were able to respond to vaccination and resist a challenge infection, although the virus persisted longer in the bursectomized chickens than in the unbursectomized controls. While this suggested a protective role for cellular immunity, antibody may also be involved because the bursectomized chickens had developed antibody, albeit 10 to 100 times less than the unbursectomized chickens. Low secondary cytotoxic response was detected after *in vitro* stimulation of cells primed *in vivo* with Newcastle disease virus.[136]

D. INFECTIOUS LARYNGOTRACHEITIS VIRUS

There is little evidence of a direct correlation between levels of neutralizing antibody and protection against infection with infectious laryngotracheitis virus;[137] therefore, cellular immunity is implicated in protection. Indirect evidence for the role of cellular immunity is provided by experiments performed in bursectomized chickens. The absence of specific serum antibody in vaccinated chickens that were surgically bursectomized at 1 d of age and treated with cyclophosphamide did not affect their ability to resist subsequent challenge infection.[138,139] Similarly, hormonal bursectomy and treatment with cyclophosphamide abrogated local antibody response in the trachea following vaccination although the vaccinated chicken remained resistant to clinical symptoms and replication of the challenge virus in tracheal cells. These observations suggested that cell-mediated mechanisms, rather than antibody, are involved in vaccinal protection.[140] The protective role of cell-mediated immunity in infectious layngotracheitis was further implicated in a study in which spleen cells from immune donors successfully transferred protection.[141]

Strong DTH response was detected until at least 5 weeks following vaccination with a live infectious laryngotracheitis virus vaccine, although the DTH response in chickens vaccinated with subunit glycoprotein vaccines did not correlate with protection.[142]

IV. SUMMARY AND CONCLUSIONS

Cell-mediated immunity plays an important role in resistance against a number of avian neoplastic viruses. Immune responses in chickens infected with MDV have been examined extensively. This virus causes rapidly growing T-cell tumors in chickens. Although MDV causes generalized immunodepression in chickens, infected chickens develop well-pronounced cellular and humoral immune responses against the virus. Natural and vaccine-induced resistance is compromised in thymectomized but not in bursectomized chickens. T-cell-mediated immunity plays a role in disease resistance, and several *in vitro* assays may be used to quantitate the activity of T-effector cells. The antigen(s) against which T-cell immunity is directed have not been clearly defined. There is strong evidence that non-T immune cells, particularly NK cells, may also be important in resistance to MD. Elevated levels of NK cells were detected in spleens of resistant chickens and in regressing MD tumors.

Among retrovirus-induced tumors, the role of cellular immunity has been best examined in experimentally induced RSV tumors. Several laboratories have shown that thymectomy consistently enhanced RSV tumor progression in chickens. Immune cells recovered from tumor bearers had cytotoxic activity and proliferated *in vitro* upon exposure to viral protein antigens. Presence of specific immune effector cells in RSV-infected chickens was also demonstrated by the migration-inhibition assays. There is evidence that immunologic regression of RSV tumors may be mediated by participation of NK cells. A role of cell-mediated immunity is also implicated in RE. Thymectomy-enhanced REV tumors in chickens and spleen cells obtained from REV-infected chickens were cytotoxic *in vitro* to REV-transformed syngeneic target cells. Thymectomy did not enhance tumors induced by ALVs, and convincing evidence suggesting a role for cellular immunity in the pathogenesis of ALV-induced disease is lacking.

Cellular immune responses induced by nonneoplastic avian viruses have not been well examined. Because experimental immunodepression in the humoral immune system did not abrogate resistance against several common nononcogenic viruses, the role of cellular immunity in disease resistance may be implicated. The nature of cellular immunity and the effector cells involved are not well known.

REFERENCES

1. **Calnek, B. W. and Witter, R. L.**, Marek's disease, in *Diseases of Poultry*, 8th ed., Hofstad, M. S., Barnes, H. J., Calnek, B. W., Reid, W. M., and Yoder, H. W., Jr., Eds., Iowa State University Press, Ames, 1984, 325.
2. **Paul. P. S., Sautter, J. H., and Pomeroy, B. S.**, Susceptibility of turkeys to Georgia strain of Marek's disease virus of chicken origin, *Am. J. Vet. Res.*, 38, 1653, 1977.
3. **Elmubarak, A. K., Sharma, J. M., Witter, R. L., Nazerian, K., and Sanger, V. L.**, Induction of lymphomas and tumor antigen by Marek's disease virus in turkeys, *Avian Dis.*, 25, 911, 1981.
4. **Calnek, B. W., Schat, K. A., Ross, L. J. N., Shek, W. R., and Chen, C. L. H.**, Further characterization of Marek's disease virus-infected lymphocytes. I. *In vivo* infection, *Int. J. Cancer*, 33, 389, 1984.
5. **Calnek, B. W., Adldinger, H. K., and Kahn, D. E.**, Feather follicle epithelium: a source of enveloped and infectious cell-free herpes virus from Marek's disease, *Avian Dis.*, 14, 219, 1970.
6. **Lu, Y. S. and Lapen, R. F.**, Splenic cell mitogenic response in Marek's disease: comparison between non-infected tumor-bearing infected chickens, *Am. J. Vet. Res.*, 35, 977, 1974.
7. **Lee, L. F., Sharma, J. M., Nazerian, K., and Witter, R. L.**, Suppression and enhancement of mitogen response in chickens infected with Marek's disease virus and the herpesvirus of turkeys, *Infect. Immun.*, 21, 474, 1978.
8. **Schat, K. A., Schultz, R. D., and Calnek, B. W.**, Marek's disease: effect of virus pathogenicity and genetic susceptibility on responses of peripheral blood lymphocytes to concanavalin A, in *Advances in Comparative Leukemia Research*, Bentvelzen, P., Hilgers, J., and Yohn, D. S., Eds., Elsevier/North-Holland, Amsterdam, 1978, 183.
9. **Theis, G. A., McBride, R. A., and Schierman, L. S.**, Effects of lymphocytes from Marek's disease infected chickens on mitogenic responses of syngeneic normal chicken spleen cells, *J. Immunol.*, 118, 887, 1977.
10. **Lee, L. F., Sharma, J. M., Nazerian, K., and Witter, R. L.**, Suppression of mitogen-induced proliferation of normal spleen cells by macrophages from chickens inoculated with Marek's disease virus, *J. Immun.*, 20, 1554, 1978.

11. **Sharma, J. M.,** Interferon production *in vitro* by spleen cells of chickens undergoing early lympholytic phase of Marek's disease virus infection, in *Advances in Marek's Disease Research,* Proc. 3rd Int. Symp. Marek's Disease, Kato, S., Horiuchi, T., Mikami, T., and Hirai, K., Eds., Japanese Association on Marek's Disease, Osaka, Japan, 1988, 227.

12. **Calnek, B. W.,** Pathogenesis of Marek's disease — a review, in Proc. Int. Symp. Marek's Disease, Calnek, B. W. and Spencer, J. L., Eds., Japanese Association on Marek's Disease, Osaka, Japan, 1984, 374.

13. **Powell, P. C., Howes, K., Lawn, A. M., Mustill, B. M., Payne, L. N., Rennie, M., and Thomas, M. A.,** Marek's disease in turkeys: the induction of lesions and the establishment of lymphoid cell lines, *Avian Pathol.,* 13, 201, 1984.

14. **Witter, R. L., Stephens, E. A., Sharma, J. M., and Nazerian, K.,** Demonstration of a tumor associated surface antigen in Marek's disease, *J. Immunol.,* 115, 177, 1975.

15. **McColl, K., Calnek, B. W., Schat, K. A., Lee, L. F., and Harris, W. V.,** Expression of a putative tumor-associated surface antigen on normal versus Marek's disease virus transformed lymphocytes, *J. Natl. Cancer Inst.,* 79, 991, 1987.

16. **Theis, G. A.,** Subpopulations of suppressor cells in chickens infected with cells of a transplantable lymphoblastic leukemia, *Infect. Immun.,* 34, 526, 1981.

17. **Katsutoshi, K., Arai, T., and Oki, Y.,** Immunosuppression and its mechanisms in chickens affected with Marek's disease lymphoma, in Proc. 3rd Int. Symp. Marek's disease, Kato, S., Horiuchi, T., Mikami, T., and Hirai, K., Eds., Japanese Association on Marek's disease, 1988, 237.

18. **Sharma, J. M.,** Immunology of Marek's disease, in Proc. 3rd Int. Symp. Marek's Disease, Kato, S., Horiuchi, T., Mikami, T., and Hirai, K., Eds., Japanese Association on Marek's disease, 1988, 204.

19. **Pazderka, F., Longenecker, B. M., Law, G. R. J., Stone, H. A., and Ruth, R. F.,** Histocompatibility to chicken population selected for resistance to Marek's disease, *Immunogenetics,* 2, 93, 1981.

20. **Gilmour, D. G., Brand, A., Donnelly, N., and Stone, H. A.,** BU-1 and Th-1, two loci determining surface antigens of B or T lymphocytes in the chicken, *Immunogenetics,* 3, 549, 1976.

21. **Fredericksen, T. L., Longenecker, B. M., Pazderka, F., Gilmour, D. G., and Ruth, R. F.,** A T cell antigen system of chickens: LY-4 and Marek's disease, *Immunogenetics,* 5, 535, 1977.

22. **Witter, R. L., Sharma, J. M., Solomon, J. J., Champion, L. R.,** An age-related resistance of chickens to Marek's disease: some preliminary observations, *Avian Pathol.,* 2, 43, 1973.

23. **Calnek, B. W.,** Influence of age at exposure on the pathogenesis of Marek's disease, *J. Natl. Cancer Inst.,* 51, 929, 1973.

24. **Witter, R. L.,** Principles of vaccination, in *Marek's Disease,* Payne, L. N., Ed., Martinus Nijhoff, Boston, 1985, 203.

25. **Purchase, H. G. and Sharma, J. M.,** Amelioration of Marek's disease and absence of vaccine protection in immunologically deficient chicks, *Nature (London),* 248, 419, 1974.

26. **Sharma, J. M., Witter, R. L., and Purchase, H. G.,** Absence of age resistance in neonatally thymectomized chickens as evidence for cell-mediated immune surveillance in Marek's disease, *Nature (London),* 253, 477, 1975.

27. **Payne, L. N., Rennie, M. C., Powell, P. C., and Rowell, J. G.,** Transient effect of cyclophosphamide on vaccinal immunity to Marek's disease, *Avian Pathol.,* 7, 295, 1978.

28. **Gupta, S. K., Kharole, M. U., and Kalra, D. S.,** Role of thymus-dependent immune system in HVT protection against Marek's disease, *Avian Dis.,* 26, 134, 1982.

29. **Byerly, J. L. and Dawe, D. L.,** Delayed hypersensitivity reaction in Marek's disease virus infected chickens, *Am. J. Vet. Res.,* 33, 2267, 1972.

30. **Fauser, I. S., Purchase, H. G., Long, P. A., Velicer, L. F., Mallman, H., Fauser, H. T., and Winegar, G. O.,** Delayed hypersensitivity and leucocyte migration inhibition in chickens with BCG or Marek's disease infection, *Avian Pathol.,* 2, 55, 1973.

31. **Ross, L. J. N.,** Antiviral T cell-mediated immunity in Marek's disease, *Nature (London),* 268, 644, 1977.

32. **Ross, L. J. N.,** Mechanisms of protection conferred by HVT, in *Resistance and Immunity to Marek's Disease,* Biggs, P. M., Ed., EEC Publication, Luxembourg, 1980, 289.

33. **Kodama, H., Sugimoto, C., Inage, F., and Mikami, T.,** Antiviral immunity against Marek's disease virus infected chicken kidney cells, *Avian Pathol.,* 8, 33, 1979.

34. **Adldinger, H. K.,** Cell-mediated cytotoxicity of blood leukocytes from Marek's disease virus infected chickens directed against viral and tumor-associated antigens, in *Advances in Comparative Leukemia Research,* Yohn, D. S., Lapin, B. A., and Blakeslee, J. R., Eds., Elsevier/North-Holland, Amsterdam, 1980, 407.

35. **Powell, P. C.,** Studies on Marek's disease lymphoma-derived cell lines, *Bibl. Haematol,* 43, 348, 1976.

36. **Sharma, J. M. and Coulson, B. D.,** Cell-mediated cytotoxic response to cells bearing Marek's disease tumor-associated surface antigen in chickens infected with Marek's disease virus, *J. Natl. Cancer Inst.,* 58, 1647, 1977.

37. **Schat, K. A. and Heller, D. H.,** A chromium-release assay for the study of cell-mediated immune responses to Marek's disease antigens, in Proc. Int. Symp. on Marek's Disease, Calnek, B. W. and Spencer, J. L., Eds., American Association for Avian Pathology, Kennett Square, PA, 1985, 306.

38. **Sharma, J. M.,** Immunopathology of Marek's disease, in *Animal Models of Comparative and Developmental Aspects of Immunity and Disease,* Gershwin, M. E. and Cooper, E. L., Eds., Pergamon Press, Oxford, 1978, 132.

39. **Sharma, J. M., Witter, R. L., and Coulson, E. D.,** Development of cell-mediated immunity to Marek's disease tumor cells in chickens inoculated with Marek's disease vaccines, *J. Natl. Cancer Inst.,* 61, 1273, 1978.

40. **Confer, A. N. and Adldinger, H. K.,** Cell-mediated immunity in Marek's disease: cytotoxic responses in resistant and susceptible chickens and relation to disease, *Am. J. Vet. Res.,* 41, 307, 1980.

41. **Schat, K. A. and Calnek, B. W.,** *In vitro* cytotoxicity of spleen lymphocytes against Marek's disease tumor cells: induction by SB-1, and apparently nononcogenic Marke's disease virus, in *Resistance and Immunity to Marek's Disease,* Biggs, P. M., Eds., EEC Publication, Luxembourg, 1980, 301.

42. **Dambrine, G., Coudert, F., and Cauchy, L.,** Cell-mediated cytotoxicity in chickens infected with Marek's disease virus and the herpesvirus of turkeys, in *Resistance and Immunity to Marek's Disease,* Biggs, P. M., Ed., CEC Publ. EUR 6470 EN, EEC Brussels, Luxembourg, 1980, 320.

43. **Kitamoto, N., Ikuta, K., Kato, S., and Yamaguchi, S.,** Cell-mediated cytotoxicity of lymphocytes from chickens inoculated with herpesvirus of turkey against Marek's disease lymphoma cell line (MSB-1), *Biken J.,* 22, 11, 1979.

44. **Murthy, K. K. and Calnek, B. W.,** Pathogenesis of Marek's disease: early appearance of Marek's disease tumor-associated surface antigen in infected chickens, *J. Natl. Cancer Inst.,* 61, 849, 1978.

45. **Sharma, J. M.,** Cell-mediated immunity to tumor antigen in Marek's disease: susceptibility of effector cells to antithymocyte serum and enhancement of cytotoxic activity by *Vibrio cholerae* neuraminidase, *Infect Immun.,* 18, 46, 1977.

46. **Schat, K. A., Shek, W. R., Calnek, B. W., and Abplanalp, H.,** Syngeneic and allogeneic cell mediated cytotoxicity against Marek's disease lymphoblastoid tumor cell lines, *Int. J. Cancer,* 29, 187, 1982.

47. **Powell, P. C., Mustill, B. M., and Rennie, M.,** The role of histocompatibility antigens in cell-mediated cytotoxicity against Marek's disease tumor-derived lymphoblastoid cell lines, *Avian Pathol.,* 12, 461, 1983.

48. **Schat, K. A. and Murthy, K. K.,** *In vitro* cytotoxicity against Marek's disease lymphoblastoid cell lines after enzymatic removal of Marek's disease tumor-associated surface antigen, *J. Virol.,* 34, 130, 1980.

49. **Confer, A. W., Adldinger, H. K., and Buening, G. M.,** Cell-mediated immunity in Marek's disease: correlation of disease-related variables with immune responses in age-resistant chickens, *Am. J. Vet. Res.,* 41, 313, 1980.

50. **Sharma, J. M.,** Presence of adherent cytotoxic cells and nonadherent natural killer cells in progressive and regressive Marek's disease tumors, *Vet. Immunol. Immunopathol.,* 5, 125, 1983.

51. **Sharma, J. M.,** *In vitro* suppression of T-cell mitogenic response and tumor cell proliferation by spleen macrophages from normal chickens, *Infect. Immun.,* 28, 914, 1980.

52. **Haffer, K., Sevoian, M., and Wilder, M.,** The role of the macrophage in Marek's disease: *in vitro* and *in vivo* studies, *Int. J. Cancer.,* 23, 648, 1979.

53. **Lee, L. F.,** Macrophage restriction of Marek's disease virus replication and lymphoma cell proliferation, *J. Immunol.,* 123, 1088, 1979.

54. **Kodama, H., Mikami, T., Inoue, M., and Izawa, H.,** Inhibitory effects of macrophages against Marek's disease virus plaque formation in chicken kidney cultures, *J. Natl. Cancer Inst.,* 63, 1267, 1979.

55. **Powell, P. C., Hartley, K. J., Mustill, B. M., and Rennie, M.,** Studies on the role of macrophages in Marek's disease of the chicken, *J. Reticuloendothial Soc.,* 34, 289, 1983.

56. **Schat, K. A. and Clanek, B. W.,** *In vitro* inactivation of cell-free Marek's disease herpesvirus by immune peripheral blood lymphocytes, *Avian Dis.,* 22, 693, 1978.

57. **Lee, L. F., Sharma, J. M., Nazarian, K., and Witter, R. L.,** Suppression and enhancement of mitogen response in chickens infected with Marek's disease virus and the herpesvirus of turkeys, *Infect. Immun.,* 21, 474, 1978.

58. **Ozaki, K., Kodama, H., Onuma, M., Izawa, H., and Mikami, T.,** *In vitro* suppression of proliferation of Marek's disease lymphoma cell line (MDCC-MSB-1) by peritoneal exudate cells from chickens infected with MDV or HVT, *Zentralbl. Veterinaermed.,* 30, 223, 1983.

59. **Higgins, D. A. and Calnek, B. W.,** Some effects of silica treatment of Marek's disease, *Infect. Immun.,* 13, 1054, 1976.

60. **Sharma, J. M.,** Avian cellular immune effector mechanism — a review, *Avian Pathol.,* 13, 357, 1984.

61. **Lam, K. M. and Linna, T. J.,** Transfer of natural resistance to Marek's disease (JMV) with nonimmune spleen cells. I. Studies of cell population transferring resistance, *Int. J. Cancer,* 24, 662, 1979.

62. **Lam, K. M. and Linna, T. J.,** Transfer of natural resistance to Marek's disease (JMV) with non-immune spleen cells. II. Further characterization of the protecting cell population, *J. Immunol.,* 125, 715, 1980.

63. **Sharma, J. M.,** Natural killer cell activity in chickens exposed to Marek's disease virus: inhibition of activity in susceptible chickens and enhancement of activity in resistant and vaccinated chickens, *Avian Dis.,* 25, 882, 1981.

64. **Heller, E. D. and Schat, K. A.,** Enhancement of natural killer cell activity by Marek's disease vaccines, *Avian Pathol.,* 16, 51, 1987.

65. **Lee, L. F., Powell, P. C., Rennie, M., Ross, L. J. N., and Payne, L. N.,** Nature of genetic resistance to Marek's disease in chickens, *J. Natl. Cancer Inst.,* 66, 789, 1981.

66. **Cooper, C. S.,** New methods for detecting cellular transforming genes, in *RNA Tumor Virus,* Vol. 218, Weiss, R., Teich, N., Varmus, H., and Coffin, J., Eds., Cold Spring Harbor Laboratory, Cold Spring Harbor, NY, 1982, 1122.

67. **Cooper, G. M. and Neiman, P. E.,** Transforming genes of neoplasms induced by avian lymphoid leukosis viruses, *Nature (London),* 287, 656, 1980.

68. **Fung, Y. K. T., Lewis, W. G., Crittenden, L. B., and Kung, H.-J.,** Activation of the cellular oncogene c-erb B by LTR insertion. Molecular basis for induction of erythroblastosis by avian leukosis virus, *Cell,* 33, 357, 1983.

69. **Hanafusa, H.,** Etiology — viral carcinogenesis, in *Cancer: A Comprehensive Treatise,* Vol. 2, Becker, F. F., Ed., Plenum Press, New York, 1975, 49.

70. **Weiss, R. A. and Frisby, D. P.,** Are avian endogenous viruses pathogenic?, in *10th Int. Symp. Comp. Leukosis and Related Diseases,* Yohn, D. S., Eds., Elsevier/North Holland, New York, 1981.

71. **Crittenden, L. B., Fady, A. M., and Smith, E. J.,** Effect of endogenous leukosis virus genes on response to infection with avian leukosis and reticuloendotheliosis viruses, *Avian Dis.,* 26, 279, 1982.

72. **Smith, R. E. and Schmidt, E. V.,** Induction of anemia by avian leukosis viruses of five subgroups, *Virology,* 117, 516, 1982.

73. **Gavora, J. S., Spencer, J. L., Gowe, R. S., and Harris, D. L.,** Lymphoid leukosis virus infection: effects on production and mortality and consequences in selection for high egg production, *Poult. Sci.,* 59, 2165, 1980.

74. **Wainberg, M. A. and Phillips, E. R.,** Immunity against avian sarcomas — a review, *Isr. J. Med. Sci.,* 12, 388, 1976.

75. **Kurth, R. and Bauer, H.,** Cell-surface antigens induced by avian RNA tumor viruses detection bv a cytotoxic microassay, *Virology,* 47, 426, 1972.

76. **Purchese, H. G. and Gilmour, D. G.,** Lymphoid leukosis in chickens chemically bursectomized and subsequently inoculated with bursa cells, *J. Natl. Cancer Inst.,* 55, 851, 1975.

77. **Bauer, H., Kurth, R., Rohrschneider, L., and Gelderblom, H.,** Immune response to oncornaviruses and tumor-associated antigen in the chicken, *Cancer Res.,* 36, 598, 1976.

78. **Purchese, H. G.,** The pathogenesis and pathology of neoplasm caused by avian leukosis viruses, in *Developments in Veterinary Virology. Avian Leukosis,* DeBoer, G. F., Ed., Martinus Nijhoff, Boston, 1987, 171.

79. **Peterson, R. D. A., Purchase, H. G., Brumester, B. R., Cooper, M. D., and Good, R. A.,** Relationships among visceral lymphomatosis, bursa of bricius, bursa-dependent lymphoid tissue of the chicken, *J. Natl. Cancer Inst.,* 36, 585, 1966.

80. **Rubin, H.,** The immunologic basis for non-infective Rous sarcomas. Cold Spring Harbor Symposium, *Avian Biol.,* 27, 441, 1962.

81. **Freire, P. M. and Duran-Reynals, F.,** Growth and regression of the Rous sarcoma as a function of the age of the host, *Cancer Res.,* 13, 386, 1953.

82. **Yamanouchi, K., Hayami, M., Miyakura, S., Fukuda, A., and Kolbune, F.,** Cellular immunity induced by Rous sarcoma virus in Japanese quail. II. Effect of thymectomy and bursectomy on oncogenies of Rous sarcoma virus, *Jpn. J. Med. Sci. Biol.,* 24, 1, 1971.

83. **Cotter, P. F., Colliner, W. M., Dunlop, W. R., and Corbett, A. C.,** The influence of thymectomy on Rous sarcoma regression, *Avian Dis.,* 20, 75, 1976.

84. **Wainberg, M. A., Beiss, B., Wahi, R., and Israel, E.,** Thymic dependence of cell-mediated immunity to avian sarcomas in chickens, *Cell. Immunol.,* 45, 344, 1979.

85. **Perry, L. L., Wight, T. N., Collins, W. M., and Dunlop, W.,** Differentiation of progressive versus regressive Rous virus-induced avian sarcoma according to tumor and infiltrating lymphocyte fine structure, *Poult. Sci.,* 57, 80, 1978.

86. **Israel, E. and Wainberg, M. A.,** Immune stimulation of sensitized chicken lymphocytes by avian retrovirus proteins, *J. Immunol.,* 118, 2237, 1977.

87. **Wainberg, M. A. and Israel, E.,** Immune stimulation of sensitized chicken lymphocytes by avian retrovirus proteins, *J. Gen. Virol.,* 60, 391, 1982.

88. **Hayami, M., Hellstrom, I., Hellstrom, K. E., and Yamanouchi, K.,** Cell-mediated destruction of Rous sarcomas in Japanese quails, *Int. J. Cancer,* 10, 507, 1972.

89. **Bensasson, Z., Doljanski, F., and Weiss, D. W.,** Specific killing of RSV-transformed cells *in vitro* by lymphoid cells from RSV tumor-bearing chickens, *Isr. J. Med.,* 9, 258, 1973.

90. **Hayami, M., Ignjatovic, J., and Bauer, H.,** Avian retrovirus induced cell-mediated cytotoxicity which is directed against virus-transformed or chemically-transformed Japanese quail cells as well as against primary embyonic cells, *Int. J. Cancer,* 20, 729, 1977.

91. **Wainberg, M., Beaupre, S., Geiss, B., and Israel, E.,** Differential susceptibility of avian sarcoma cells derived from different periods of tumor growth to natural killer cell activity, *Cancer Res.,* 43, 4774, 1987.

92. **Ignjatovic, J., Rubsamen, H., Hayami, M., and Bauer, H.,** Rous sarcoma virus-transformed avian cells express four different cell surface antigens that are distinguishable by a cell mediated cytotoxicity blocking test, *J. Immunol.,* 120, 1663, 1978.

93. **Heinzelmann, E. W., Zsigray, R. M., and Collins, W. M.,** Cross-reactivity between RSV-induced tumor antigen and B5 MHC alloantigen in the chicken, *Immunogenetics,* 13, 29, 1981.

94. **Cotter, P. F., Collins, W. M., Dunlop, W. R., and Corbett, A. C.,** Detection of cellular immunity to Rous tumors of chickens by the leukocyte migration inhibition reaction, *Poult. Sci.,* 55, 1008, 1976.

95. **Yamada, A., Hayami, M., Yamanouchi, K., and Fujiwara, I.,** Detection of natural killer cells in Japanese quails, *Int. J. Cancer,* 26, 381, 1980.

96. **Yamada, A. and Hayami, M.,** Suppression of natural killer cell activity by chicken fetoprotein in Japanese quails, *J. Natl. Cancer Inst.,* 70, 753, 1983.

97. **Wainberg, M. A. and Israel, E.,** Enhancement of avian sarcoma virus-induced tumor growth after pretreatment with BCG, *Infect. Immun.,* 22, 328, 1978.

98. **Yuasa, N., Yoshida, I., and Taniguchi, T.,** Isolation of a reticuloendotheliosis virus from chickens inoculated with Marek's disease virus, *Natl. Inst. Anim. Health Q. (Tokyo),* 16, 141, 1976.

99. **Jackson, C. A. W., Dunn, S. E., Smith, D. I., Gilchrist, P. T., and MacQueen, P. A.,** Proventriculitis "nakanuke" and reticuloendotiosis in chickens following vaccination with herpesvirus of turkeys (HVT), *Aust. Vet. J.,* 53, 457, 1977.

100. **Motha, M. X. J.,** Effects of reticuloendotheliosis virus on the response to chickens to infectious laryngotracheitus virus, *Avian Pathol.,* 11, 475, 1982.

101. **Mizutani, S. and Temin, H. M.,** Lack of serological relationship among DNA polymerases of avian leukosis — sarcoma viruses, reticuloendotheliosis viruses, and chicken cells, *J. Virol.,* 12, 440, 1973.

102. **Moelling, K., Gelderblom, H., Pauli, G., Friis, R., and Bauer, H.,** A comparative study of the avian reticuloendotheliosis virus: relationship to murine leukemia virus and viruses of the avian sarcoma leukosis, *Virology,* 65, 546, 1975.

103. **Chen, I. S. Y., Mak, T. W., O'Rear, J. J., and Temin, H. M.,** Characterization of reticuloendotheliosis virus strain T DNA and isolation of novel varient of reticuloendotheliosis virus strain T by molecular cloning, *J. Virol.,* 40, 800, 1981.

104. **Cohen, R. S., Wong, T. C., and C. Lai, M. M.,** Characterization of transformation — and replication — specific sequences of reticuloendotheliosis virus, *Virology,* 113, 672, 1981.

105. **Rice, R. R., Hibsch, M. A., Gonda, H. R., Bose, H. R., and Gilden, R. V.,** Genome of reticuloendotheliosis virus: characterization by use of cloned proviral DNA, *J. Virol.,* 42, 237, 1982.

106. **Wong, T. C. and Lai, M. M. C.,** Avian reticuloendotheliosis virus contains a new class of oncogene of turkey origin, *Virology,* 111, 289, 1981.

107. **Witter, R. L., Purchase, H. G., and Burgoyne, G. H.,** Peripheral nerve lesions similar to those of Marek's disease by infection with reticuloendotheliosis virus, *J. Natl. Cancer Inst.,* 45, 567, 1970.

108. **Purchase, H. G. and Witter, R. L.,** The reticuloendotheliosis viruses, *Curr. Top. Microbiol. Immunol.,* 71, 103, 1975.

109. **Paul, P. S., Pomeroy, K. A., Sarma, P. S., Johnson, K. H., Barnes, D. M., Kumar, M. C., and Pomeroy, B. S.,** Naturally occurring reticuloendotheliosis in turkeys: transmission, *J. Natl. Cancer Inst.,* 56, 419, 1976.

110. **McDougall, J. S., Biggs, P. M., and Shilleto, R. W.,** A leukosis in turkeys associated with infection with reticuloendotheliosis virus, *Avian Pathol.,* 7, 557, 1978.

111. **Witter, R. L. and Crittenden, L. B.,** Lymphoma resembling lymphoid leukosis in chickens inoculated with reticuloendotheliosis virus, *Int. J. Cancer,* 23, 673, 1979.

112. **Noori-Daloii, M. R., Swift, R. A., Kung, H. J., Crittenden, L. B., and Witter, R. L.,** Specific integration of REV proviruses in avian bursal lymphomas, *Nature (London),* 294, 574, 1981.

113. **Robinson, F. R. and Twiehaus, M. J.,** Isolation of the avian reticuloendotheliosis virus (strain T), *Avian Dis.,* 18, 278, 1974.

114. **Ianconescu, M. and Aharonovici, A.,** Persistent viremia in chickens subsequent to *in vivo* inoculation of reticuloendotheliosis virus, *Avian Pathol.,* 7, 237, 1978.

115. **Witter, R. L., Smith, E. J., and Crittenden, L. B.,** Tolerance, viral shedding, and neoplasia in chickens infected with nondefective reticuloendotheliosis viruses, *Avian Dis.,* 25, 374, 1981.

116. **Smith, E. J. and Witter, R. L.,** Detection of antibodies against reticuloendotheliosis viruses by an enzyme linked immunosorbent assay, *Avian Dis.,* 27, 225, 1983.

117. **Hu, C. -P. and Linna, T. J.,** Serotherapy of avian reticuloendotheliosis virus-induced tumors, *Ann. N. Y. Acad. Sci.,* 277, 634, 1976.
118. **Linna, T. J., Hu, C., and Thompson, K. D.,** Development of systemic and local tumors induced by avian reticuloendotheliosis virus after thymectomy or bursectomy, *J. Natl. Cancer Inst.,* 53, 847, 1974.
119. **Carpenter, C. R., Bose, H. R., and Rubin, A. S.,** Contact-mediated suppression of mitogen-induced responsiveness by spleen cells in reticuloendotheliosis virus-induced tumorigenesis, *Cell. Immunol.,* 33, 392, 1977.
120. **Rup, B. J., Hoelzer, J. D., and Bose, H. R.,** Helper viruses associated with avian acute leukemia viruses inhibit the cellular immune response, *Virology,* 116, 61, 1982.
121. **Scofield, V. L. and Bose, H. R.,** Depression on mitogen response in spleen cells from reticuloendotheliosis virus-infected chickens and their suppressive effect on normal lymphocyte response, *J. Immunol.,* 120, 1321, 1978.
122. **Carpenter, C. R., Rubin, A. S., and Bose, H. R.,** Suppression of the mitogen-stimulated blastogenic response during reticuloendotheliosis virus-induced tumorigenesis: investigations into the mechanism of action of the suppressor, *J. Immunol.,* 120, 313, 1978.
123. **Carpenter, C. C., Kempf, K. E., Bose, H. R., and Rubin, A. S.,** Characterization of the interaction of reticuloendotheliosis virus with the avian lymphoid system, *Cell. Immunol.,* 39, 307, 1978.
124. **Walker, M. H., Rup, B. J., Rubin, A. S., and Bose, H. R.,** Specificity in the immunosuppression induced by avian reticuloendotheliosis virus, *Infect. Immun.,* 40, 225, 1983.
125. **Maccubin, D. and Schierman, L.,** Evidence for association of viral and MHC antigens on reticuloendotheliosis virus-transformed cells of chickens, *Fed. Proc.,* 41, 698, 1982.
126. **Maccubin, D. and Schierman, L.,** Cytotoxic reactivity to reticuloendotheliosis virus-transformed cells is MHC-restricted in the chicken, *Fed. Proc.,* 42, 439, 1983.
127. **Timms, L. M., Bracewell, C. D., and Alexander, D. J.,** Cell mediated and humoral immune response in chickens infected with avian infectious bronchitis, *Br. Vet. J.,* 136, 349, 1980.
128. **Timms, L. M. and Bracewell, C. D.,** Cell mediated and humoral immune response of chickens to live infectious bronchitis vaccines, *Res. Vet. Sci.,* 31, 182, 1981.
129. **Chubb, R. C., Huynh, V., and Bradley, R.,** The induction and control of delayed type hypersensitivity reactions induced in chickens by infectious bronchitis virus, *Avian Pathol.,* 17, 371, 1988.
130. **Crowle, A. J.,** Delayed hypersensitivity in the mouse, *Adv. Immunol.,* 20, 197, 1975.
131. **Chubb, R. C., Huynh, V., and Law, R.,** The detection of cytotoxic lymphocyte activity in chickens infected with infectious bronchitis virus or fowlpox virus, *Avian Pathol.,* 16, 395, 1987.
132. **Dharsana, R. and Spradbrow, P. B.,** The demonstration of cell-mediated immunity in chickens vaccinated with fowlpox virus, *Zentralbl. Veterinaermed. Reihe B,* 32, 628, 1985.
133. **Morita, C.,** Role of humoral and cell-mediated immunity on the recovery of chickens from fowlpox virus infection, *J. Immunol.,* 111, 1495, 1973.
134. **Powell, P. C.,** Immune mechanisms in infections of poultry, *Vet. Immunol. Immunopathol.,* 15, 87, 1987.
135. **Marino, O. C. and Hanson, R. P.,** Cellular and humoral response of *in ovo*-bursectomized chickens to experimental challenge with velogenic Newcastle disease virus, *Avian Dis.,* 31, 293, 1987.
136. **Cannon, M. J. and Russell, P. H.,** Secondary *in vitro* stimulation of specific cytotoxic cells to Newcastle disease virus in chickens, *Avian Pathol.,* 15, 731, 1986.
137. **Jordan, F. T. W.,** Immunity to infectious laryngotracheitis, in *Avian Immunology,* Rose, M. E., Payne, L. N., and Freeman, B. M., Eds., British Poultry Science, Edinburgh, U.K., 1981, 245.
138. **Robertson, G. M.,** The role of bursa-dependent responses in immunity to infectious laryngotracheitis, *Res. Vet. Sci.,* 22, 281, 1977.
139. **Fahey, K. J., Bagust, T. J., and York, J. J.,** Laryngotracheitis herpesvirus infection in the chicken: the role of humoral antibody in immunity to a graded challenge infection, *Avian Pathol.,* 12, 505, 1983.
140. **Fahey, K. J. and York, J. J.,** unpublished results, 1989.
141. **Fahey, K. J., York, J. J., and Bagust, T. J.,** Laryngotracheitis herpesvirus infection in the chicken. II. The adoptive transfer of resistance with immune spleen cells, *Avian Pathol.,* 13, 265, 1984.
142. **York, J. J.,** Immunogens of Infectious Laryngotracheitis Virus, Ph.D. thesis, University of Melbourne, Melbourne, Australia, 1989.

Chapter 10

CELL-MEDIATED IMMUNITY IN PARASITIC AND BACTERIAL DISEASES

Hyun S. Lillehoj

TABLE OF CONTENTS

I. INTRODUCTION

Recent studies in viral, bacterial, and parasitic diseases suggest that host responses to microbial infections are complex and involve both humoral as well as cellular immune mechanisms. Although detailed immune mechanisms involved in host resistance against most poultry diseases are not yet understood, some studies suggest that cell-mediated immune mechanisms play a major role in disease resistance. The main topic of this chapter will focus on the intestinal infections, such as coccidiosis, cryptosporidiosis, and salmonellosis, since they represent economically important poultry diseases. Leucocytozoonosis is also included in this chapter since there have been increased problems with this disease in Southeast Asia, including Japan and Korea. Since it is crucial to understand the intestinal immune system to develop any immunological control strategy against intestinal diseases, the first part of this chapter will review current understanding of the avian intestinal immune system and mucosal immune response; the assessment will provide a conceptual overview of the complex cellular and molecular events involved in the intestinal immune response to enteric pathogens.

In mammals, it is well established that major histocompatibility complex (MHC) genes and non-MHC genes influence both the host immune response to infectious agents and disease resistance against microbial infections. Although immunogenetic studies of avian MHC lag behind, recent availability of molecular probes and genetically defined chicken strains now enables study of the role of host genetic factors influencing immunity to intestinal diseases in this species. A brief summary of current knowledge on the biochemical and functional aspects of the chicken MHC will be included in this review. In addition, specific examples will be used to illustrate how new biotechnical developments have enhanced our understanding of the immunobiology of host-parasite interactions. Since there is only limited information concerning the immune mechanisms in most poultry diseases, studies carried out in other animal species will be used wherever relevant.

II. HOST FACTORS INFLUENCING ANTIMICROBIAL RESPONSES

A. GASTROINTESTINAL IMMUNE SYSTEMS

Host responses to intestinal microbial infections leading to the elimination of microbes involve the complex interplay of soluble factors, leukocytes, and epithelial, endothelial, and other physiological components of gut-associated lymphoid tissues (GALT). GALT represent only one component of the mucosa-associated lymphoid tissues (MALT), which also include the bronchial, salivary, nasopharyngeal, and genitourinary lymphoid tissues. GALT have evolved with specialized features that reflect their role as the first line of defense on mucosal surfaces; these include antigen-presenting cells, immunoregulatory cells, and effector cell types distinct from their counterparts in the systemic immune system. Due to the uniqueness of location of GALT and their constant exposure to environmental antigenic challenge, investigation of the immune system is crucial in understanding food allergies, tolerance, and immune responses to intestinal infections. Recent technical advances in molecular and cellular immunology have facilitated understanding of the ontogeny, structure, and function of GALT. Isolation and flow cytometric analysis of intestinal lymphoid cells now enable researchers to dissect various components of GALT and to investigate the role of subpopulations of intestinal lymphocytes in disease processes. Following infection, macrophage-dependent antigenic activation of T and B cells initiates a series of antigen-specific and nonspecific responses involving secretory immunoglobulins, local cells, and locally produced cytokines. One of the salient features of the secretory immune system is the intraepithelial transport of immunoglobulins into the lumen of the gut. External transport of secretory immunoglobulins from blood or tissue fluids into external mucosae of the alimentary, respiratory, genitourinary, and nasolacrimal tracts contributes a major source of immunoglobulins to the intestine. In contrast to mammals, limited information is available concerning the intestinal immune system of chickens. However, research of the avian intestinal immune system assumes a high priority because the development of vaccines against intestinal infections such as coccidiosis, colibacillosis, salmonellosis, and intestinal viral infections has become an industrial priority. The advent of new molecular technqiues to manipulate the genomes of various pathogens and enhanced understanding of interaction of GALT with peripheral lymphoid organs will soon enable new approaches to vaccination against enteric pathogens.

1. Gut-Associated Lymphoid Tissues

GALT in chickens include the bursa of Fabricius, cecal tonsils (CTs), Peyer's patches (PPs), and lymphocyte aggregates in the intraepithelium and in the lamina propria (LP) of the intestinal wall of the gastrointestinal tract. PP are lymphoid aggregates in the intestine which possess a morphologically distinct lymphoepithelium with microfold (M) cells, follicles, a B-cell-dependent subepithelium zone, and a T-cell-dependent central zone.[1,2] GALT contain unique phagocytic cells such as M cells that possess numerous vacuoles reflecting active pinocytosis.[3] Within the gastrointestinal mucosa, lymphocytes in the epithelium (intraepithelial lymphocytes, IEL) are morphologically separated by a basement membrane from the underlying lamine propria lymphocytes (LPL). GALT, largely represented by PP, are important sites of immunoglobulin A (IgA) synthesis in mammals and contain a large subpopulation of B lymphocytes committed to IgA secretion.[4] Recent studies showed that administration of oral antigen leads to the appearance of clonal precursor cells that mature into cells secreting mostly IgA.[5] Moreover, such precursors were found to be more numerous in mucosal tissues than in the spleen and in greater abundance in conventional animals vs. germ-free animals.[6] The polymeric IgA antibody is produced by plasma cells in GALT and is selectively transported through epithelial cells into external secretions. Following immunization with gut luminal antigens, antigen-sensitized, IgA-committed B cells and T cells leave PP via efferent lymphatics, pass through mesenteric lymph nodes, and enter the bloodstream through the thoracic duct. From the blood, IgA-committed B cells migrate to and selectively localize in distant mucosal tissues (e.g., mammary, salivary, and lacrimal glands) and in the LP regions of the gastrointestinal and upper respiratory tract, where they differentiate into plasma cells.

Intestinal IEL are mainly T cells and, to a lesser extent, non-T, non-B cells, whereas LPL are relatively enriched with immunoglobulin-producing B cells.[7-10] IEL from chickens contain 80% lymphocytes, 10 to 15% monocytes, approximately 5% mononuclear cells, and <1% polymorphonuclear leukocytes and plasma cells.[1] Cells isolated from mechanical scraping of the muscularis mucosa showed that small intestinal LPL contain 80% lymphocytes, 20% monocytes, and <1% polymorphonuclear leukocytes. Mononuclear cells isolated from epithelium and LP were reported to contain immunoglobulin positive cells, but the percentage was higher in LPL (29.5%) than in IEL (7.9%) or spleen cells (19.4%).

PP represent the major inductive stie for IgA responses to ingested antigens and pathogenic microorganisms in the gastrointestinal tract. In mammals, PP contain approximately 40% B lymphocytes, a high percentage (12 to 16%) of which bear surface IgA and are committed to IgA synthesis.[5] Of the PP cells, 40% are regulatory T cells, which include 40 to 50% inducer and helper cells, and 15 to 20% cytotoxic and suppressor T cells. A significant percentage of PP T cells bear Fc receptors for IgA and are important in regulation of IgA isotype responses.[5] PP also contain accessory cells such as macrophages (5 to 9%) and functional dendritic cells. In contrast, CT lymphocytes are mainly IgG- and IgM-staining B cells, a relatively small quantity are IgA-expressing cells.[1]

Molecular complexes similar to human and murine CD3, CD4, and CD8 antigens have been identified in chickens.[11-13] The predominant subset of IEL T lymphocytes expresses CD3 polypeptides (γ, δ, ϵ, and ξ) that are noncovalently associated with the $\gamma\delta$-chain receptor heterodimer of the antigen-specific T-cell receptor (TCR) referred to as TCR1.[14] Another subset of T lymphocytes expresses CD3 polypeptide chains in association with the $\alpha\beta$-chain receptor heterodimer called TCR2.[12] the ontogeny of T cells bearing different TCRs has been studied recently.[12,15] Early in fetal development, precursor thymocytes pass through the thymus and acquire distinct functions. TCR1 is expressed on a small percentage of thymocytes by embryonic day 11, increases to 30% of thymocytes by day 15, and then declines to about 5% of the cells by hatching. Thymocytes bearing TCR2 and CD3 appear after 15 d of fetal development and then quickly increase in number to exceed the level of TCR1$^+$ lymphocytes. Among the 85% of blood T cells that are CD3$^+$, 16% are TCR1$^+$.[16] TCR1$^+$ cells in the blood and the thymus lack both CD4 and CD8 molecules, and approximatley 75% of splenic TCR1$^+$ cells express the avian CD8.[14] Most TCR1$^+$ cells localized in the splenic sinusoids and the intestinal epithelium express the CD8 antigen.[14] In contrast, TCR2$^+$ cells, a majority of which express the CD4 homologue, are found primarily in the splenic periarteriolar sheath (PAL) and the LP of the intestine. In contrast to this finding, a recent study suggested that both TCR1$^+$ and TCR2$^+$ cells are present in the IEL and LP of the chicken gut.[17] Thus, although it is clear that TCR1$^+$ and TCR2$^+$ cells represent separate lineages of T cells, the differential tissue homing patterns of the TCR1$^+$ and TCR2$^+$ cells observed in some mammalian systems may not be present in chickens. Germinal centers detected in the CT contain scattered TCR2$^+$ CD4$^+$ cells, but no TCR1$^+$ cells. Neither subset is present in the intestinal mucosa at hatching, and only occasional TCR1$^+$ or TCR2$^+$ cells are found in the intestine of 3-d-old chicks.[14] By 6-d posthatching, both subsets are present, and the number of these cells reaches adult levels by 1 month of age. The percentages of TCR1$^+$ and TCR2$^+$ T cells in newborn and adult SC and TK chicken strains showed that the level of cells in IELs did not reach adult levels until 4 to 5 weeks after hatching.[17] TK chickens in general contained a substantially higher number of TCR1$^+$ cells compared to SC chickens; the results suggested a genetic influence on local T-cell development. In adult SC chickens, IELs and LPLs of the duodenum and jejunum contained similar numbers of TCR1$^+$ and TCR2$^+$ cells, whereas those of the ceca contained a higher number of TCR1$^+$ cells.[17]

In chickens, as in mammals, T cells can be separated into CD4 and CD8 antigen-expressing subpopulations on the basis of their function.[11,13] Chicken T cells expressing a homologue of the mammalian CD4 antigen represent 20% of spleen cells, 40 to 45% of blood leukocytes, and 79 to 80% of thymocytes. During ontogeny, CD4 antigen appears on thymocytes at embryonic day 13, and the frequency of CD4 antigen-bearing cells increases rapidly to approximately 90% by the end of the embryonic period. In the periphery, CD4 cells can be observed in substantial numbers only after hatching; by the end of the first month, adult levels have been reached. CD4 cells seem to occupy certain characteristic histological locations; they are mainly localized in the PAL tissue of the spleen and the LP in the intestine. The appearance of CD8$^+$ T cells during embryonic development of chickens is very similar to that of CD4$^+$ T cells; by the end of embryogenesis, most thymocytes express both of these molecules. In the periphery, up to 50% of spleen cells are CD8$^+$, whereas only 15% of blood leukocytes carry this antigen. Thymic and peripheral blood T cells expressing TCR1 are negative for CD4 and CD8 antigens, whereas 70% of splenic and IEL TCR1 cells in the intestine bear CD8 antigen. A recent study[17] showed that in 2-month-old SC chickens reared in a clean (but not germ-free) environment, the composition of T and B cells in intraepithelium and LP depended upon the region from which these cells were isolated. Intestinal cells bearing the CD8 antigen were present in both the intraepithelium and the LP of the gut, although IEL and LPL of the duodenum contained substantially higher numbers of CD8[+] cells compared to those of jejunum and ceca.

A third type of cell mediating intestinal immunity is the natural killer (NK) cell. NK cells constitute a population of non-T, and non-B, nonmacrophage mononuclear cells with characteristic morphology and which are capable of spontaneous cytotoxicity against a wide variety of syngeneic, allogeneic, and xenogeneic target cells. NK cells lack immunological memory and MHC restriction, thus, their cellular lineage is debatable.[18,19] There is much confusion concerning the phenotypic characterization of human leukocytes mediating natural cytotoxicity. Although specific antigenic markers for NK cells have been described in some mammalian species, monoclonal antibodies specific for chicken NK cells have not been reported. Rabbit anti-asialo GM1 antibody, known to be relatively specific for NK cells in many mammalian species,[20,21] stains avian IEL cells.[22] NK-cell activity has been reported to be present in the intestinal IEL populations of mice,[23,24] rats,[25] and guinea pigs.[26] In chickens, NK cell activity has been demonstrated in the spleen[27,28] and peripheral blood,[29,30] thymus,[31] bursa,[31] and intestine.[31,32] Great variability in cytotoxic potential has been observed among NK cells of different lymphoid organs; strain variation in NK cell activity was also demonstrated.[32] NK cell activity and cytotoxic potential increased with age and were not fully developed until 6 weeks after hatching.[31]

Postnatal development of other parameters of the intestinal immune system in chickens has also been studied.[1] The proventriculus, Meckel's diverticulum, and PP generally contained germinal centers beginning at 12 weeks of age. At 5 d posthatching, CT were macroscopically visible and contained B cells with membrane-bound IgM, IgG, or IgA, as well as some IgG and IgM plasma cells. In older chickens, the size of CT and the number of plasma cells gradually increased. The number of PP also varies depending upon age. The PP and CT of chickens were easily identified at 10 d post-hatching. As birds aged, the intestinal lymphoid aggregates underwent involution; by 20 weeks the lymphoid follicles became less distinct and fewer in number, and there appeared to be a relative depopulation of the subepithelial zone in both the CT and PP. Not only did the morphologic characteristics of the PP vary with age, but their abundance and distribution also changed. PP were not evident at hatching, but could be identified in the intestine by day 1 or 2 and increased to a maximum of five at 16 weeks of age; their number then decreased in association with morphological involution, and at 52 to 58 weeks of age only a single PP was evident. The number of IEL cells was also sparse in the newborn animal, subsequently rising in number.[33] In germ-free animals few IEL were found, but they attained normal levels upon antigen exposure, suggesting that the presence of IEL cells in the small intestine is a function of intraluminal antigenic stimulation.

2. Effector Functions Associated with Gut-Associated Lymphoid Tissues

The roles of various components of the immune response of GALT in host defense against microbial infections have been studied extensively.[34] Tremendous architectural changes in the intestine occur during infection and inflammation following exposure to microbes, including increases in permeability, infiltration of cells, mucin elaboration, enzyme synthesis, and immunoglobulin production. Specific and nonspecific factors can restrict the colonization of microbes, e.g., secretory immunoglobulins and mucin. Complex interactions between lymphocytes, epithelial cells, dendritic cells, and local macrophages are involved in both secretory immunoglobulin and mucin production during the host defense process. Three general functions of the GALT immune system include: (1) antigen presentation, (2) production of antibodies, and (3) activation of cell-mediated immunity.

a. Antigen Presentation

Two basic types of lymphocytes are involved in antigen-specific responses: (1) B lymphocytes that express surface immunoglobulin (SIg) molecules with exquisite specificities for antigen and (2) T lymphocytes that recognize processed antigens on antigen-presenting cells (APC). After binding of antigen to B cells that express SIg, cell division and clonal expansion occur, and immunoglobulins with antigen specificity identical to that of SIg are secreted from the differentiated B cells. In contrast, T cells recognize antigens that have been enzymatically degraded into smaller fragments by the APC, and binding occurs only in conjunction with gene products encoded by MHC genes expressed by the APC. Recent studies have provided direct molecular evidence that antigenic peptides derived from protein antigens bind to MHC class I[35] and class II molecules.[36] Interaction of the TCR-CD3 complex with self-MHC class I and II molecules and bound peptide antigen induces a cascade of events that results in T-cell activation.

Immunization with viable or nonviable antigens through the gut induces the production of local antibody and cellular responses. The initial steps involve antigen uptake, processing, and presentation. The mode of antigen uptake by the gut cells depends upon the nature and type of antigen. APC in the gut have been suggested to be dendritic cells, macrophages, and epithelial cells. The dome region of the PP is covered by an epithelium which contains a unique cell type, the M cell; these cells are follicular-associated epithelial (FAE) cells.[3] M cells are actively pinocytic and phagocytic for both soluble and particulate antigens (e.g., viruses and bacteria) in the lumen of the gut. M cells can present antigen to underlying lymphoreticular cells, leading to the sensitization of lymphoid cells present in distinct T- and B-cell zones in the PP.

b. Antibody-Mediated Immune Mechanisms

In chickens, IgA and IgM are the predominant immunoglobulins in the external intestinal secretions. Although IgG is found in the gut, it is believed to be derived from the circulation or leaked from the lymphatics following permeability changes occurring during infection. Secretory IgM, which is pentameric, is effective in elimination of microbes. However, secretory IgA (sIgA) has been characterized the best. Several distinctive features are important for the IgA to function as a secretory antibody, including the ability of the IgA monomer to polymerize. In addition, sIgA is able to associated with a 15-kDa joining (J)-chain peptide and a 70-kDa protein, the secretory component (SC) produced by epithelial cells. The IgA-SC complex is internalized in endocytic vesicles, transported across the cytoplasm, and exocytosed onto the external surface of the epithelium. A minor source of IgA in secretions is derived from blood via the hepatobiliary IgA transport system. In contrast to the transepithelial IgA pathway, hepatocytes express a specific receptor for blood IgA.[37] Polymeric IgA injected into the blood is cleared into the bile in less than 3 h.[38]

The major functions of sIgA include prevention of environmental antigen influx into internal body compartments, neutralization of viruses and microbial toxins, and prevention of adherence and colonization of mucosal surfaces by microbial pathogens. Secretory antibodies may attach to the surface of the pathogen and prevent binding to the epithelium by direct blockage, steric hindrance, induction of a conformational changes, or reduction of motility. In this manner, microorganisms would be susceptible to the natural cleaning functions of the mucosae. The role of secretory immunoglobulins has been documented in agammaglobulinemic humans. However, the role of secretory immunoglobulins is less clear in some poultry infections. Despite the absence of immunologbulins, agammaglobulinemic chickens are resistant to reinfection with coccidiosis[39] and to leucocytozoonosis.[40] Therefore, although the primary role of sIgA is to prevent invasion of microbes in the intestine, it is less certain whether sIgA limits the course of major infections once established.

c. Cell-Mediated Immune Mechanisms

Cell-mediated immune responses include antigen-specific as well as antigen-nonspecific activation of various cell populations, including T lymphocytes, NK cells, and macrophages. T lymphocytes are comprised of two functionally distinct subpopulations distinguishable by their surface phenotypes. Cytotoxic T lymphocytes (CTL) recognize foreign antigens in the context of MHC class I molecules, whereas T helper cells recognize antigens in association with MHC class II molecules. Although CTL activity has been demonstrated in the intestine of mammals, MHC-restricted IEL CTL activity has yet to be shown in chickens. Recently, there has been increased interest in the selective homing of TCR1[+] cells to the intestinal epithelium in mice.[41] Studies in humans[34] and a recent study in chickens[17] showed that TCR2[+] T cells are present in intestinal IEL. Thus, species differences as well as other host-related factors can influence location of different T-cell populations in the gut, and great caution should be exercised in generalizing from findings obtained under controlled conditions.

A considerable interest in gut mucosal lymphoid populations, particularly IEL NK cells, has developed in recent years.[43] NK cells have been postulated to play an important role as a primary host-defense mechanism against tumors, bacteria, and viruses, as well as in the homeostasis of normal tissues.[42] It has been suggested that IEL NK cells are active in the first line of host defense because of their close proximity to the gut, where a variety of antigenic substances are introduced.[43] The observation that chicken intestinal IEL contain NK cells that can mediate spontaneous cytotoxicity[31,32] suggests that NK cells may play an important role in local defense. Kinetic studies showed that cytotoxicity was detectable from 2 h after incubation, with progressive increase to 16 to 18 h. Furthermore, NK cell activity was higher in the jejunum or ileum than in the duodenum or cecum. Following the infection of chickens with *Eimeria*, the agent causing coccidiosis, there is an increase in asialo GM1-bearing cells and cells with NK markers, suggesting that IEL NK cells may be involved in defense against invasion of the gut mucosa by coccidia.[22]

B. MAJOR HISTOCOMPATIBILITY COMPLEX GENES AND NON-MAJOR HISTOCOMPATIBILITY COMPLEX GENES

1. Structure and Function of Major Histocompatibility Complex Genes and Proteins

The immune response is a genetically controlled process; many of the pertinent genes are located in the MHC. The MHC was originally defined by its influence on tumor rejection in mice.[44] The chicken MHC, or *B* complex, was first described by Briles and co-workers[45] in 1950. As in mammals, the *B* complex has been shown to control the same wide range of immunological reactions such as resistance to autoimmune, viral, bacterial, and parasitic diseases.[46] Furthermore, non-immunity-related traits such as reproduction, hatchability, growth rate, feed use efficiency, and body weight are also influenced.[46] The *B* complex is located on the 16th chromosome and is closely linked to the nucleolar organizer region (NOR) containing DNA encoding ribosomal RNA.[47] *B*-complex genes and proteins are divided into three classes (I, II, and IV). Unlike the mammalian MHC, class III genes encoding components of the complement system are not found in the *B* complex. Class I, II, and IV genes are also designated *B-F*, *B-L*, and *B-G*, respectively. Molecular cloning of *B*-complex class I, II, and IV genes has been accomplished.[48-51] Five independent class II genes and six independent class I genes have been identified. The chicken *B* complex appears very different from mammalian MHCs in that the distances between class I and class II regions, as well as between genes within a region, are shorter. The close proximity of class I and class II genes is probably responsible for the very low frequency of observed recombination between them. Another distinctive feature of the avian MHC is the tight association of *B*-complex genes with unique genes such as that encoding the guanine nucleotide-binding protein (C12.3) which influences lymphocyte proliferation.[49]

The class I antigens (HLA-A, B, and C in man; H-2K, D, and L in mice; and *B-F* in chickens) are the classical transplantation antigens expressed by virtually all nucleated cells that function as restricting elements for CTL. Molecular analysis of *B-F* antigens showed an α chain of 40 to 45 kDa bound to a 12-kDa β$_2$-microglobulin.[52] The class II or Ia gene products (HLA-DR, DP, DQ in man; I-E and I-A in mice; *B-L* in chickens) restrict antigen presentation to T-helper lymphocytes; these gene products are composed of two noncovalently glycosylated polypeptide chains, an α chian (33 to 34 kDa) and a β chain (28 to 29 kDa) that are expressed on the surface of B lymphocytes, cells of the myeloid lineage, and activated T cells.[53] The *B-G* (class IV) subregion is tightly linked to the *B-F* and *B-L* subregion and encodes a family of highly polymorphic 40- to 46-kDa proteins associated with red blood cells[54] but not involved in skin-graft rejection, graft vs. host reaction, or mixed lymphocyte reaction.[55,56]

2. Influences on Immune Response and Disease Resistance

MHC genes have a profound effect on the ability of animals to respond to specific antigens. Immune-response (Ir) genes, located in the subregion containing class II genes, were first discovered in guinea pigs by Benacerraf and co-workers;[57] these genes directly influence T-cell-mediated immunity and indirectly, through helper T cells, affect humoral immune responses. Control of the immune system by Ir genes can now be better explained as a consequence of characterization of the cell surface glycoproteins encoded by them. These proteins bind to peptide fragments produced by intracellular degradation of protein antigens in a manner suitable for recognition by T cells. Failure to bind and subsequently present a peptide results in selective unresponsiveness due to an apparent defect in antigen presentation. On the other hand, not all peptides that bind to MHC molecules elicit a T-cell response for the simple reason for size limitation in the TCR repertoire. In chickens, the MHC has been shown to influence humoral immune response to simple, chemically defined antigens and to complex antigens.[58,59] Furthermore, interaction between T cells and B cells in the antibody response to T-dependent antigens, macrophage presentation of antigens to T cells, and splenic germinal center formation are also controlled by class II gene products of the *B* complex.[60] Recent studies indicated that class I antigens are important determinants of CTL recognition of virus-infected chicken cells.[61,62]

It is well established that certain disease conditions are more (or less) likely to occur in hosts carrying a particular MHC marker. Both MHC and non-MHC genes have been associated with disease susceptibility and disease resistance. Examples of MHC control of resistance to disease in chickens include virally induced diseases such as Marek's disease (MD), lymphoid leukosis, and Rous sarcomas. The best observed correlation between disease resistance to MD virus and MHC type has been seen in *B*-21 chickens.[46] However, the role of non-MHC-linked genes in the pathogenesis of MD needs to be investigated further, since a recent study suggests that susceptibility to MD may also be controlled by a non-MHC gene.[49] In Rous sarcoma, certain *B* haplotypes are linked with regression as a dominantly inherited trait while others permit progressive growth and metastasis.[63,64] However, until the molecular structure of the chicken MHC is better defined, caution should be exercised in interpreting the reported disease associations with *B*-complex genes.

The advent of molecular biological techniques and the availability of genetically defined, *B*-congenic, and recombinant chicken lines now enable continued analysis of *B*-complex genes and the role of *B*-gene products in host immunity. Avian genome manipulation to improve economically important traits, as well as traits associated with immunity and disease resistance, will soon be feasible.

III. IMMUNITY TO PARASITIC DISEASES

The protozoa include a number of parasites that cause serious problems in poultry. Three major protozoan diseases, coccidiosis, cryptosporidiosis, and leucocytozoonosis, will be considered in this review. Coccidiosis is caused by *Eimeria* species, intestinal protozoan parasites that seriously impair the growth and feed utilization of both livestock and poultry. Infection with *Eimeria* is self-limiting; the protozoan extensively destroys the intestinal epithelium. Recently, interest has been increasing in another coccidium species, *Cryptosporidium*, which parasitizes man and domestic animals. *Cryptosporidium* causes enteritis and diarrhea in domestic animals. In man, the protozoan is self-limiting in immunocompetent humans, but causes persistent, often life-threatening diarrhea in immunodeficient patients. *Leucocytozoon* species represents another group of intracellular parasites that cause severe economic loss in Southeast Asia. Leucocytozoonosis, unlike coccidiosis and cryptosporidiosis, is transmitted by biting midges.

The desire to develop vaccines against these parasites has promoted immunological studies. Protozoa differ greatly from viruses and bacteria in their methods of transmission and in the nature of disease manifestations, the significance of which should be considered in the development of control strategy. Host responses to intracellular parasites involve many facets of the immune response, including nonspecific as well as antigen-specific components. In general, antibodies and cell-mediated immune responses are two major hallmarks of infection. Specific antibodies have been shown to play a major role in some bacterial and viral infections; however, in most parasitic infections in mammals and chickens, cell-mediated immunity (CMI) has been shown to provide major protection. Current understanding of the molecular and cellular aspects of CMI suggests that an intricate and complex interplay of different cell populations and cytokines is involved not only in the pathogenesis of the infections but also in the development of protective immunity against intracellular parasitic infections. Elucidation of the events leading to protection following protozoal infection and identification of protective immunity is the focus of several current clinical and veterinary immunology studies. Since knowledge of the life history of parasites within the host is essential for understanding immunological aspects of the host-parasite relationships, the life cycles of relevant parasites, will be summarized briefly in the current review.

A. COCCIDIOSIS

1. Biology of *Eimeria*

Avian coccidiosis is caused by intracellular protozoan parasites belonging to several different species of *Eimeria;* in many respects these *Eimeria* species resemble *Plasmodium,* the agent responsible for human malaria. There are at least seven known species of coccidia that infect poultry. *Eimeria* parasites exhibit a marked specificity for both the species they infect and the tissue they parasitize within the host, although a few exceptions have been reported.[65] *Eimeria* are obligate intracellular parasites with a complicated life cycle involving both asexual (schizony) and sexual (gametogony) phases of development. Chickens are infected through ingesting oocyst-contaminated food and water. Once in the gut, sporozoites excyst from the oocysts and parasitize epithelial cells. Here they pass through the basement membrane into the LP, are engulfed by macrophages[66] or IEL,[67] and are carried to the glands of Lieberkuhn in the cecum. In the cecum, the sporozoites leave the macrophages or IEL and enter the epithelial cells of the gland, where subsequent development occurs. The sporozoites differentiate into spherical trophozoites and undergo asexual multiplication via nuclear fission (merogony or schizogony). The number of asexual generations is usually limited and is thought to be genetically determined. The last generation of merozoites undergo sexual multiplication (gamogony) to form a zygote. The prepatent period (the interval between infection and oocyst shedding) is slightly over 5 d. The patent period (duration of shedding) lasts from 6 to 9 d.

2. Humoral Response to Parasites

Chickens infected with *Eimeria* parasites show a variety of immune responses. Circulating antibodies specific for various stages of coccidial parasites are usually detectable within 1 week of the inoculation of oocytes, reach a peak level 1 to 2 months later, and then decline, but persist in the circulation.[68-70] The level and duration of antibody responses are influenced by the host age, genetics, dose of inoculum, and species of *Eimeria*.[69] Locally produced antibodies have been detected in bile and intestinal secretions.[69,71-73] Secretory antibodies are usually detectable 7 d postinoculation (DPI) and peak 10 to 14 DPI.[72,74] In general, secondary infection does not increase the titers of serum or secretory antibodies.[68,75] Using an *in vitro* lymphoproliferation assay, detectable T-cell response to sporozoite antigens is detected 7 to 10 DPI.[76] The peak T-cell proliferative response is usually observed 14 DPI and quickly wanes after 21 DPI unless secondary inoculation is given. Sporozoites, merozoites, and soluble protein secreted from cultured parasites stimulate T-cell proliferation. In addition, significant changes in the number of large mononuclear cells other than T and B cells in peripheral blood and intestine were reported;[77] phagocytic activity of macrophages was enhanced following treatment with serum antibodies or with normal serum.[78]

The roles of various components of the immune system after *Eimeria* infection in the development of protective immunity have been investigated. Antibodies, both circulating in the blood and locally present in the gut, may play some role during the early phase of infection, but there is no convincing evidence for any significant role of antibodies in anticoccidial immunity.[39,70,79,80] In most instances, infection of bursectomized chickens, showed no effect on the development of protective immunity following secondary inoculation, although bursectomized chickens were more susceptible following primary infection. In general, patency is not appreciably prolonged in T- and B-cell-deficient hosts; an exception was chickens treated with corticosteroids, where it was shown that the patency of *E. mivati* infection persisted.[81] The levels of serum or secretory antibodies do not correlate with protection,[82,83] and attempts to transfer protection using *Eimeria*-immune antibodies have yielded inconsistent results.[84,70] The results show that antibodies are not involved in host resistance to coccidial challenge infection despite numerous effects of antibodies on penetration and development of coccidial parasites.[85,86] However, the results suggest that antibodies could have a deleterious effect on sporozoites and merozoites if they come into close contact with the parasites.

3. Cell-Mediated Immunity to Parasites

The scope of cellular immune responses evoked by coccidial infection encompasses both nonspecific and specific components and includes soluble factors, NK cells, macrophages, helper T cells, and CTL. Two aspects of immunity to *Eimeria* will be considered: (1) innate resistance, which refers to a nonspecific immune response following primary infection; and (2) acquired immunity, which refers to an antigen-specific immune response that occurs following secondary infection. Innate immunity is responsible for elimination of parasites during the early phase of primary infection, whereas acquired immunity to *Eimeria* is usually considered in the context of respect to its effect on secondary and subsequent infections. Immunity to challenge infection usually results in the reduction in oocyst number and amelioration of clinical signs and is influenced by many factors associated with host and parasties.[69,70] The great majority of *Eimeria* species are relatively immunogenic; a single infection of an immunocompetent host will induce some degree of protective immune response to reinfection. Antigens associated with developing asexual stages have been shown to be more immunogenic than those of sexual stages.[79,87,88] In immune hosts, sporozoites enter the gut early after infection, but they are prevented from developing;[70,87] these sporozoites, when taken 24 to 48 h following infection, resume normal development upon transfer to a nonimmune host.[89] Thus, acquired immunity to coccidiosis may involve immune mechanisms that either reduce the number of intracellular sporozoites or inhibit the natural progression of parasite development.

a. Role of Natural Killer Cells

Innate immunity responsible for parasite elimination involves nonspecific components of immunity such as NK cells or macrophages.[22,89-92] In mammals, the effector cells responsible for natural, non-MHC-restricted cytotoxicity are complex and heterogeneous. Besides classical NK cells, lymphokine-activated killer (LAK) cells,[93] macrophages, and granulocytes express natural cytotoxicity.[94] Among lymphocyte subpopulations, non-MHC-restricted cytotoxic lymphocytes[95] and lymphocytes of B-cell phenotype[96] can lyse NK-sensitive tumor targets or virally infected murine cells. Chicken splenic effector cells responsible for natural resistance to MD were non-T, non-B, and nonphagocytic in nature.[27] Chicken phagocytic and adherent cells,[30] as well as granulocytes,[97] were also reported to be effector populations capable of killing tumor cells of allogeneic or xenogeneic origin.

Several positive correlations between NK cell activity and genetically determined disease resistance to murine malaria[90,91] and coccidia[22] were noted. Augmentation of NK cell activity has been induced following infection with a number of intracellular parasites, including *Leishmania, Trypanosoma,* and *Toxoplasma.*[42] Increase in NK cell activity occurred in the early stages of infection; the observation suggests direct or indirect roles that NK cells may have in the control of parasite proliferation and the outcome of infection.

IEL of chickens contain effector cells that can mediate NK cell activity against chicken tumor cells.[31,32] Recent studies on the nature of IEL mediating NK activity centered around their role in the local immune defense against viruses, bacteria, and parasites. In coccidiosis, ultrastructural studies indicate that eimerian sporozoites are transported to the crypts via the LP by cells resembling macrophages[67] or by cells described as granulated IELs.[66] The levels of NK cell activity in splenic and IEL are increased above normal coinciding with parasite elimination.[22] Furthermore, strain differences in NK cell responses were noted which correlated with genetically controlled disease susceptibility seen following primary infection.[32] Thus, these cells may be involved in immunosurveillance against eimerian parasites.

The enhancement of IEL NK cell activity observed during the post-patent period following *Eimeria* infection is accompanied by an increase in the number of IEL expressing the asialo GM1 antigen, which is expressed on cells mediating nonspecific cytotoxicity in mammals.[20] Further phenotypic characterization of chicken NK cells will be helpful in understanding their ontogeny, phylogeny, and roles in mucosal and systemic immunosurveillance against infectious agents. In particular, the relationship between IEL NK cells and TCR1[+] CD8[+] IEL cells needs to be investigated in view of the controversy involving these cells.[41]

b. Role of Macrophages

Macrophages are known to exert an active defense against many viral, bacterial, and intracellular parasites in mammals and chickens. The role of macrophages in coccidiosis has been suggested.[78,92,98-100] Macrophages exhibit enhanced phagocytosis of sporozoites and sporocysts in the presence of immune serum.[99] Macrophages showed enhanced cytotoxicity against *Eimeria* when activated by lymphokines secreted by T-cell lymphomas, immune T cells stimulated by sporozoites or merozoites, or normal spleen cells stimulated with concanavalin A (Con A) or phytohemagglutinin (PHA).[92] Furthermore, macrophages from immune chickens were capable of enhanced phagocytosis and intracellular killing of ingested sporozoites. The peak phagocytic activity was found after 3 to 5 weeks postinoculation in *E. tenella* and *E. maxima* infections with continuation of phagocytic activity through a subsequent 1- to 9-week period.[78]

c. Role of T Cells and Cytokines

After the initial infection with coccidia, a long-lasting species-specific immunity develops that is characterized by strong antigen-specific lymphocytic responsiveness *in vitro.*[76] Delayed-type hypersensitivity (DTH) is detectable within 1 week of infection and continues for several weeks postinfection.[101] Chickens with immunosuppressed CMI are highly susceptible to challenge infection with *Eimeria* even though they have high levels of antibodies.[39] T cells obtained from chickens immune to coccidiosis proliferate and secrete cytokines that activate cytotoxic effector cells and macrophages.[92] Although the final proof that lymphokines are involved in protection awaits the availability of recombinant avian lymphokines, these results suggest that CMI plays a predominant role in the host protective response.

In immune chickens, considerable numbers of sporozoites are capable of invading intestinal enterocytes but are unable to develop into mature, first-generated schizonts.[70] T-lymphocyte-derived soluble factors, or lymphokines, are involved in the immune defense against coccidia as in other host-parasite interactions.[102-111] Indeed, earlier studies demonstrated release of leukocyte migration inhibition factor (LIF) or macrophage migration inhibition factor (MIF) during coccidiosis.[108] MIF and LIF activities were not observed at 4 DPI, but they were detectable at 1 to 3 weeks postinfection with *E. tenella*.

A role of γ-interferon (γ-IFN) in anticoccidial immunity has been suggested. γ-IFN was detected during infection with *E. tenella*.[107] γ-IFN release from spleen cells of infected chickens was not detectable until 35 DPI, whereas serum antibodies were detected by 10 d and peaked by 20 DPI. No γ-IFN release was detected from intestinal IEL in the study; this may have been due to a lack of T helper cells, which are primarily responsible for γ-IFN release. Chickens treated with γ-IFN inducer showed enhanced resistance to *Eimeria* infection.[102] However, until avian recombinant γ-IFN becomes available, the role of γ-IFN in coccidiosis cannot be definitively established from these results.

Interspecies transfer of anticoccidial immunity or CMI using transfer factor (TF) has been reported.[109,110] Nonresponsive chickens were induced to respond to antigens as tested by an *in vitro* assay using TF. Transfer of delayed wattle response with TF could not be demonstrated unless the recipient chickens had been previously primed with a homologous antigen used to induce TF. Bovine TF also initiated antigen-specific CMI *de novo* in nonimmune SPF and SC chickens. Bovine TF action was rapid; it occurred in less than 1 d and lasted at least 35 d.

Various chicken lymphokine preparations contained inhibitory factors that suppressed the development of eimerian parasites *in vitro*, including cell-free supernatant from the JMV T-cell lymphoma, normal spleen cells activated with Con A, or immune spleen cells stimulated with sporozoites.[92] Cell-free supernatants from the cultures also conferred significant protection against *Eimeria* infections when given *in vivo* to normal chickens that were subsequently challenged with live eimerian parasites. Normal macrophages or a macrophage cell line pretreated with the supernatant preparations showed *in vitro* inhibitory activity against *Eimeria*. The inhibitory activity had no direct cytotoxic effect on sporozoites and did not inhibit cell invasion. Cell-free, noninfectious supernatants produced by the JMV lymphoblastoid cell line, a Marek's disease virus (MDV)-transformed T-cell line, also inhibited MDV infection and showed broad antimicrobial activity both *in vivo* and *in vitro*.[112,113] Similar mechanisms involving lymphokine-activated macrophages have been described in bovine *Eimeria* infections,[114,115] as well as other intracellular parasitic infections such as toxoplasmosis[105,116-118] and leishmaniasis.[119,129]

4. Genetic Factors Influencing Immunity

The genetic constitution plays a significant role in determining susceptibility or resistance to *Eimeria* infections.[68,82,83,121-124] In mammals, both MHC and non-MHC genes have been found to influence the protective immune responses against most parasitic helminths.[125-127] Genetic variation in the host response to coccidiosis following primary and secondary infections has been reported either by directly comparing different chicken strains[68,82,122,123] or by selection of the resistance traits.[121,124] The results from these studies showed that genes associated with various blood group alloantigens segregated with disease resistance. However, they did not provide clear evidence for involvement of *B*-complex genes, since the nature of genetic differences in the chicken strains is not clearly understood.

The relative importance of MHC and background genes in the genetic control of primary and secondary infections to *E. tenella* and *E. acervulina* was recently examined using genetically well-defined strains of chickens congenic for *B*-complex genes.[82,83] Eight $15I_5$-*B*-congenic chickens, developed by more than ten backcrossings of the donor strain to the parental $15I_5$ chickens with genetic difference at the *B*-complex,[128] were used to investigate the effect of *B*-complex gene differences on host immunity to coccidiosis. In addition, several inbred stains of chickens that shared the same *B* haplotypes with some of the $15I_5$-*B*-congenic chickens, but expressed different background, were also studied to elucidate the role of non-MHC-linked genes in controlling susceptibility. Wide variations in host response to *E. tenella*[83] and *E. acervulina*[82] were noted following initial and challenge infections among the chicken strains.[82,83] When screened for oocyst production, the different strains segregated into three distinct nonoverlapping groups, suggesting that the susceptibility to coccidiosis among inbred chickens may be controlled by multiple genes. The differences seen in resistance to challenge infection and cellular immunity between relatively resistant *B*-congenic lines and susceptible lines was attributable to differences at the *B* complex. However, disease susceptibility was quite different in two chicken strains that shared the same *B* haplotype, but expressed different genetic background. Similar results were obtained by other investigators.[129] The observations strongly suggest that both MHC and non-MHC genes control the phenotypically expressed levels of disease susceptibility. Examination of disease resistance patterns following secondary infection suggested that there are distinct processes controlling two different phases of immunity; (1) an innate mechanism during primary infection and (2) an immune mechanism controlling acquired immunity following secondary inoculation. Some strains were highly susceptible to primary infection and resisted secondary challenge, whereas other strains resisted primary infection and were susceptible to secondary infection.

Two recombinant antigens were used to study the immune response of chickens infected with *E. acervulina*:[82] the p130 recombinant antigen (encoded by the cSZ-1 cDNA clone representing the p240/p160 immunodominant *E. acervulina* sporozoite surface antigen) and the p150 recombinant antigen (encoded by the cMZ-8 cDNA clone representing the P250 immunodominant *E. acervulina* merozoite surface antigen).[130] Immune sera obtained from *E. acervulina*-inoculated chickens contained circulating antibodies that showed strong immunoreactivity in immunoblots to the p150 but not to the p130 antigen. T-cell responses were observed against both antigens. In general, the cellular response, but not the antibody response, to the p150 recombinant antigen correlated with the degree of protection following challenge infection.

Underlying genetic factors that influence innate immunity in avian coccidiosis were investigated. When two different chicken strains with different levels of disease susceptibility to coccidiosis were compared, the efficiency of IEL NK cell activity was influenced by the host genetic background.[22,32] Relatively rapid induction of killing of tumor targets was observed in SC chickens, while delayed and less efficient killing by FP-strain IEL occurred. However, the cytotoxic potentials of SC and FP spleen cells were not significantly different. In SC chickens the cytotoxicity of IEL was similar to that of their spleen cells, whereas in FP chickens the cytotoxicity of IEL was lower than that of their spleen cells. This difference in NK cell activity is intriguing for the gut immunity implicated in avian coccidiosis in view of the life cycle of *Eimeria*. Whether or not sporozoites can enter NK cells among the IEL population is uncertain. However, the potential invasion of coccidia into IELs is of considerable importance to the study of mucosal immunity against the infection. Genetic susceptibility of different strains of chickens to coccidiosis may be determined at this level.

5. Parasite Antigens and Vaccine Development

The increasing incidence of drug-resistant eimerian parasites as well as the high economic costs involved in the production of existing anticoccidial drugs have limited the effectiveness of prophylactic medication. Therefore, there is increased interest in the development of immunologically based controls of coccidiosis. Although active infection results in complete protection against reinfection, eimerian parasites have evolved with complex life cycles involving both intra- and extracellular stages in the gut. Due to the localized nature of infection, effective methods of stimulating immunity must include activation of local effector mechanisms. Currently, two different immunization methods[131] are being exploited: (1) induction of protection using live parasites through the "trickle method"[132] with a graded, low dose of parasites; and (2) oral inoculation of attenuated parasites developed either through embryo adaptation or selection of precociousness.[133] However, commercialization of either method will depend upon the development of safe, reproducible, and efficient delivery methods. The ideal vaccine using live parasites may rely on oral immunization with attenuated parasites using the "trickle method", delivered in vectors that are stable, safe, and economical.

Because of potential limitations with live immunizations, several laboratories have focused on the development of recombinant coccidial vaccines.[82,130,134,135,138,139] Recent success in the induction of protective anticoccidial immunity using vaccines prepared from genetically engineered recombinant antigens indicates that this holds promise as an alternative strategy for the control of this disease.[135] Coccidial antigens that induce parasite-specific immunity have been identified and include surface, internal, and secretory antigens[136,138,139] of asexual as well as sexual stages.[70,138] Recombinant proteins derived from these antigens have been shown to elicit either humoral responses,[139] cellular responses,[82] or both[82,134] and confer a significant protection against live challenge.[82,134,135,139]

Immunization of chickens with the p150 recombinant antigen elicited anamnestic T- and B-cell responses following live parasite challenge.[134] This antigen contains an immunodominant epitope of the p230-250 merozoite protein which is recognized by immune serum and T cells obtained from chickens infected with *E. acervulina*.[82] Chickens infected with *E. acervulina* showed *in vitro* T-cell responses to the recombinant p150 antigen correlating with the level of disease protection. These findings suggested that the native p250 merozoite protein may be an immunodominant antigen eliciting a functionally important cellular response. Identification of other antigenic motifs eliciting protective T-cell responses will allow construction of second-generation recombinant proteins that contain relevant epitopes which may be even more efficient in the induction of a protective response.

The effect of antigen delivery and the genetic background of the host on vaccination with the p150 recombinant merozoite protein was studied.[134,135] One group of chickens was immunized intramuscularly with the recombinant protein in complete Freund's adjuvant (CFA), while another was inoculated orally with live *Escherichia coli* transformed with the recombinant plasmid carrying the cMZ8 cDNA encoding the p150 antigen (*E. coli* pCO_5cMZ8).[134] Among the group given intramuscular immunization, strain .6-2 (B^2B^2) showed significantly enhanced protection against *Eimeria acervulina* compared to other strains. In contrast, strains .C-12 ($B^{12}B^{12}$) and .P-13 ($B^{13}B^{13}$) showed increased protection among the groups given the live recombinant antigen. Subsequent challenge with the purified, native p250 protein showed that some strains immunized intramuscularly did not respond, but did respond when immunized orally with the live recombinant. Thus, Ir gene action may be epitope specific, as previously suggested by others.[140] In malaria, only T cells from congenic mouse strains bearing the I-A^b haplotype recognized the T-cell epitope contained within the tandemly repeated tetramer of the circumsporozoite protein of *Plasmodium falciparum*.[141] The finding that only certain chicken strains respond to the p150 merozoite recombinant antigen suggests that the presence of multiple T-cell epitopes in vaccines could improve their efficacy. Furthermore, since at least seven different species of *Eimeria* infect chickens, the development and implementation of such subunit faccines will depend upon either the cloning and expression of protective antigens from a combination of *Eimeria* species or the identification of a single cross-reactive antigen. A recent study showed a possibility of inducing cross protection against nonhomologous strains of parasites using a sporozoite recombinant antigen.[142]

Another approach to induce protective immunity uses immunization with anti-idiotype antibody.[143] Polyclonal or monoclonal anti-idiotype antibodies prepared against the idiotype of sporozoite-specific antibody were able to prime chicken T and B cells against *Eimeria tenella* sporozoites. Although the immunological mechanism involved in anti-idiotype antibody-induced protection against coccidiosis is not known, the method of immunization may offer an alternative approach to vaccination with parasite antigens.

In view of the complexity of the parasite life cycle and involvement of the local immune response, development of complete protection will probably require more than one mechanism. Therefore, it will be crucial to develop vaccines or alternative control strategies that elicit a wide spectrum of immune responses both locally and systemically. Effective administration of recombinant vaccines will depend on identification of protective antigens of many life stages as well as identification of optimal delivery systems. Delivery systems that produce persistent stimulation of the local immune system need to be explored.

B. CRYPTOSPORIDIOSIS

Cryptosporidiosis is considered an important enteric disease in animals and humans.[144-146] *Cryptosporidium* species are coccidian parasites that inhabit the microvillous border of epithelial surfaces. *Cryptosporidium* infection of chickens was first reported in 1929[147] and identified in 1955 as *C. meleagridis*.[148] Among the 20 different *Cryptosporidium* species known, *C. meleagridis* and *C. baileyi* specifically infect birds. Avian cryptosporidiosis manifests itself as a respiratory, alimentary, or renal disease.[149] Cryptosporidia will develop in many anatomical sites, but only if infectious oocysts or other developmental stages gain access to the pertinent sites. *C. meleagridis* infects mostly the lower one third of the ileum in quail and turkeys, causing severe enteritis with high morbidity and mortality.[148-150] *C. baileyi* infects bursa of Fabricius and cloaca without enteric disease.[151] When inoculated intratracheally or intra-abdominally, clinical disease results and parasites are found in the respiratory tract. Experimental intratracheal inoculation of *C. baileyi* oocysts results in severe and sometimes fatal respiratory disease in broiler chickens.[152] Cryptosporidia have also been reported from many anatomical sites in naturally infected avian hosts. Oocysts from the bursa of Fabricius were found to infect the cloaca, bursa, terminal colon, cecum, trachea, bronchi, air sacs, salivary gland ducts, and nasal turbinates of experimentally inoculated chickens. Bursa pathology includes disturbed growth and diffuse, chronic, superficial, purulent, protozoal bursitis with mucosal epithelial hyperplasia.[153] Histopathological changes include hypertrophy and hyperplasia of infected epithelial surfaces. Infiltrates of macrophages, heterophils, lymphocytes, and plasma cells are usually present. Microscopic lesions in enteric infections consisted of villous atrophy, villous fusion, crypt hyperplasia, and infiltration of the LP with large mononuclear cells, lymphocytes, and plasma cells.

1. Biology of *Cryptosporidium*

The genus *Cryptosporidium* belongs to the phylum Apicomplexa and is a member of Eimeriorida, of which *Eimeria* is also a member. The life cycle of the parasite is similar to that of other true coccidia (Eimeriorina) in that it can be subdivided into the following major developmental events:

1.   Excystation, release of infective sporozoites
2.   Merogony, asexual multiplication within the host cells
3.   Gametogony, formation of micro- and macrogametes

4.   Fertilization
5.   Oocyst wall formation
6.   Sporogony and sporozoite formation

The life cycle of mammalian isolates of *C. parvum* differs somewhat from that of other monoxenous coccidia (e.g., *Eimeria*) in that each intracellular stage of *C. parvum* is within a parasitophorous vacuole confined to the microvillous region of the host cell, whereas comparable stages of *Eimeria* species occupy parasitophorous vacuoles usually deep (perinuclear) within the host cells. Oocysts of *Cryptosporidium* sporulate while they are within the host cells and are infective when released in the feces, whereas *Eimeria* oocysts do not sporulate until they are passed outside of the host. *Cryptosporidium* has been transmitted to chickens by placing them in a battery brooder artificially contaminated with feces containing oocysts. Oocysts, once ingested, excyst in the gastrointestinal or respiratory tract and enter the microvillus of an epithelial cell, where they differentiate into trophozoites. In the case of intestinal development, the sporozoites invade the brush border of the enterocytes without entering the cytoplasm close to the nucleus; they appear to be intracellular but extracytoplasmic, although they have been found occasionally in the cytoplasm of M cells above the PP. Sporozoites also have been observed in macrophages in PP.[154] Trophozoites undergo nuclear division to form mature type I meronts with six or eight merozoites which recycle to produce additional type I merozoites. Three distinct types of meronts have been described in *C. baileyi*, whereas *C. parvum* has two distinct types.[149] Type I meronts, with four merozoites, do not recycle and develop into the sexual stage with a microgamont fertilizing a macrogamont to form a zygote. A type II meront leaves the meront to form microgametes or a macrogamont. The microgametes fertilizes the macrogamont, which then develops into an oocyst which, unlike *Eimeria*, sporulates *in situ*. Most of the zygotes (80%) form thick-walled oocysts that sporulate within the parasitophorus vacuole of the host cell before being passed in the feces as the environmentally resistant form that transmits the infection to another host. Some of the zygotes (20%) do not form an oocyst wall; rather, their sporozoites are surrounded only by a unit membrane. These thin-walled, autoinfective oocysts rupture and release sporozoites that reinitiate the endogenous cycle. Since oocysts sporulate when they are released from hosts, reinfection is hard to prevent. *C. baileyi* has both autoinfective, thin-walled oocysts and merozoites (type I) that can recycle, and heavy infections can result following exposure to small numbers of oocysts.[144] Oocysts are passed in the feces 4 to 5 d after oral inoculation and are usually passed for an additional 17 d. The prepatent period lasts from 3 to 6 d and the patent period from 4 to 24 d in immunocompetent hosts.

2. Host Immune Response and Immunity to Parasites

Immunocompetent hosts usually develop self-limited, short-term intestinal illnesses following oral exposure to *Cryptosporidium*, whereas most immunocompromised hosts develop prolonged, life-threatening illnesses.[144,145] Parasites have been found within the microvillous region of M cells covering the PP,[154] suggesting that M cells may initially bring cryptosporidia into close contact with the local immune system. The immune mechanisms responsible for disease resistance to reinfection to cryptosporidiosis is also not well understood. In humans, recovery from intestinal *C. parvum* infection is usually accompanied by parasite-specific antibodies directed against all life cycle stages of the parasites.[155] However, efforts to adoptively transfer protective immunity with hyperimmune serum failed.[156] These results suggest that although immune serum may have an effect on sporozoites if close contact is established, antibodies may not play a role in protection against disease.

Since the parasite appears to be confined to the microvillous region of the intestinal or respiratory mucosa, it is probable that local antibodies in concert with T cells may play a role in immunity. In the acquired immunodeficiency syndrome (AIDS) associated with a T helper cell defect, patients readily develop a prolonged, life-threatening cholera-like infection following *C. parvum* infection, whereas healthy humans clear the infection within 2 weeks.[144,145] The importance of T lymphocytes in the clearance of *C. parvum* has also been demonstrated in T-cell-deficient nude (Nu/Nu) mice.[157] Compared with their heterozygous (Nu/+) immunocompetent littermates, the T-cell-deficient nude mice fail to clear infection and progressively develop severe diarrhea.

Limited immunological studies of cryptosporidiosis have been carried out in chickens.[158] The autoinfective nature of cryptosporidia, unlike *Eimeria,* makes the development of resistance to this parasite difficult. The ability to develop immunity and clear infection was shown to depend upon the host age and immune maturity.[159] Chickens inoculated at 2 or 14 d of age excreted oocysts sooner and for longer periods of time with greater number of developing intracellular parasites than did chickens inoculated at 28 or 42 d of age.[160] Chickens routinely developed an immune response to primary intestinal or respiratory infections and developed resistance to reinfection.[159] Clearance of parasites from the intestine was accompanied by high titers of serum antibodies that recognized more than 20 distinct *C. baileyi* antigens and the appearance of DTH to tuberculin, to oocysts, and to sporozoite antigens. A single infection with *C. baileyi* elicited protective immunity in broiler chickens.[159] Antigen-specific serum antibodies reconizing several heterogeneous-molecular-weight bands in immunoblots were detected at 14 DPI when parasites were being cleared from the bursa of Fabricius and cloaca. The effects of experimental inoculation of chickens with *C. baileyi* on antibody and DTH responses to Newcastle disease virus (NDV) and infectious bursal disease virus (IBDV) were investigated.[161] Intramuscular immunization with an inactivated commercial vaccine containing NDV and IBDV in CFA 7 d after intratracheal *C. baileyi* inoculation produced a significant increase in NDV hemagglutination-inhibition titers and a decrease in DTH. In contrast, IBDV antibody titers were unchanged. Chickens receiving oral inoculation showed lower anti-NDV antibody titers only at higher parasite doses and lower anti-IBDV antibody titers at all doses, but no differences in DTH response. Although the immune mechanisms responsible for innate and acquired immunity to cryptospordiosis are not understood, it is likely that locally produced factors as well as effector cells in the gut may be important. Furthermore, it is apparent that induction of host immunity is driven by a T-lymphocyte-dependent process, but the role of nonlymphocytic mediators of immunity such as macrophages, NK cells, and polymorphonuclear leukocytes needs to be carefully characterized. Since this parasite develops in the mucosal surface, studies on immunity should focus on the intestinal immunity.

C. LEUCOCYTOZOONOSIS

1. Biology of Leucocytozoon

Leucocytozoonosis is caused by *Leucocytozoon caulleryi,* an intracellular parasite that affects blood and tissue cells of birds. *L. caulleryi* was initially described by Mathis and Leger[162] in 1909 and by Akiba et al.[163] in Japan in 1958. *L. caulleryi* affects the productivity of chickens through reduction in egg production, weight loss, and sometimes death.[164] The life cycle includes reproduction by schizogony (merogeny) in tissue cells, gametogony in erythrocytes or leukocytes, and sporogony in insects; the life cycles and ultrastructures of some life stages are similar to *Plasmodium.* Unlike *Eimeria* and *Cryptosporidium, L. caulleryi* is transmitted via an insect vector, the biting midges of the Culicoides species.[164] Leucocytozoonosis is prevalent in areas with a suitable ecology and ethology for dipterous invertebrate hosts, simulid flies, and culicoid midges. The mature gamonts are round and occupy host erythrotcytes and leukocytes about 20 μm in diameter. Schizogony occurs in many organs, but more often in lungs, liver, and kidneys. *L. caulleryi* parasites undergo the first and second generations of schizony in various tissues and organs of chickens. Sporozoites invade the endothelial cells of organs such as the liver, spleen, and lung and develop into first-generation schizonts which mature and release first-generation merozoites between 5 and 7 DPI. The first-generation merozoites penetrate the endothelial cells of blood vessels and form second-generation schizonts. After day 9, these are released from host cells, maturing as extracellular schizonts which release second-generation merozoites at 14 DPI.[164] The second-generation merozoites invade erythrocytes and become gametocytes at 19 DPI.

2. Immune Response to Parasites

Chickens that had recovered from a primary infection with *L. caulleryi* usually exhibited complete resistance to reinfection.[165,166] First-generation merozoites are present in the peripheral blood[167] 5 and 6 d after sporozoite challenge, but second-generation merozoites and gametocytes are not seen in most chickens recovering from a primary infection. The results indicate that protective immunity against *L. caulleryi* involves an immune response to the second-generation schizont stage.[166,167] Immunization of chickens with schizonts, but not soluble antigens obtained from chickens infected with *L. caulleryi,* resulted in substantial reduction in the severity of clincial symptoms following reinfection with sporozoites.[168] In chickens experimentally inoculated with sporozoites, the IgM response to *L. caulleryi* appeared at 10 DPI and peaked at 21 DPI. IgG antibodies against schizonts were detected 14 DPI and peaked at 8 to 10 weeks postinoculation.[169] In one study, a single inoculation with a small number of sporozoites produced parasitemia from 14 to 24 d after inoculation, but high levels of antiparasite antibodies continued for nearly 1 year.[169]

3. Cell-Mediated Immunity to Parasites

The role of B cells in the development of resistance to reinfection was examined in bursectomized and sham-bursectomized contol chickens.[170] Hormonal bursectomy produced higher susceptibility to primary infection with slightly prolonged patency compared to control chickens, but both bursectomized and sham-control chickens that survived primary infection demonstrated resistance to reinfection. Furthermore, pretreatment of chickens with cyclosporin A, and regimen shown to increase disease susceptibility to coccidiosis,[39] greatly enhanced susceptibility to challenge infection with *L. caulleryi.*[170] The results indicate that CMI, rather than humoral immunity, plays a major role in protection against luekocytozoonosis.

IV. IMMUNITY TO BACTERIAL INFECTIONS

A. SALMONELLOSIS

Bacterial infections causing intestinal diseases produce significant economic loss in poultry; these bacterial diseases include colibacillosis and salmonellosis. Although both diseases have been known for many years, information concerning host immunity is scarce. The current review will focus on salmonellosis because there is significant public concern about food safety dealing with this organism. Salmonellosis is an important foodborne disease and accounts for the majority of such outbreaks whenever the causative agent is identified.[171] The widespread occurrence of this disease in livestock challenges the most stringent measures of food harvesting, processing, monitoring, and control; there is no other zoonosis as complex in epidemiology and control as salmonellosis. Salmonellosis in animals can be divided into three categories. First are infections with clinical manifestations that are pathognostic, e.g., abortion in cattle, horses, and sheep and pullorum disease in poultry. Second are infections with clinical symptoms that are only indicative of a salmonellosis; these are often septicemic and are characterized by weakness, recumbency, and increased temperature. Diarrhea is usually one of the accompanying symptoms, and blindness may appear in poultry. Outbreaks of salmonellosis are most common in young animals, and the mortality rates are higher than in adults. Third are asymptomatic carrier infections that may occur in both man and animals.

Domestic poultry constitutes the largest single reservoir of *Salmonella* in animal populations. The two relatively host-specific and nonmotile members of the genus are *S. pullorum* and *S. gallinarum*, which cause pullorum disease and fowl typhoid, respectively. They are grouped separately from the motile salmonellae, which are designated "paratyphoid organisms". Pullorum disease and fowl typhoid frequently infect reproductive organs of adult chickens; they establish a chronic infection with direct passage of the organisms into the egg. It usually occurs as an acute systemic form in young chickens and poults, but in adults it is most often localized and chronic.[172]

A prominent epidemiological factor of zoonotic salmonellosis is the common carrier status of animals. A great number of mammals, birds, and reptiles are responsible for maintenance of the chain of infections. Among the non-host-adapted *Salmonella* serotypes, *S. typhimurium* occurs most often and is the most widely distributed type; this organism causes severe outbreaks of salmonellosis in many kinds of animal species, and it is frequently the cause of sporadic outbreaks of gastroenteritis in humans. Newly hatched and young chicks are more susceptible to the disease; they may be infected by a single bacterium.

1. Biology of *Salmonella*

The genus *Salmonella* belongs to the family *Enterobacteriaceae*. The bacterium is Gram-negative, nonsporogenic, facultatively anaerobic, and, with few exceptions, motile. Approximately 2200 serotypes are known to exist based on O antigen and numerous H-antigen groups recognized by the World Health Organization. Seven subspecies of *Salmonella* may be differentiated using DNA-DNA hybridization or biochemical properties. Epidemiologically, salmonellae can be classified into three main groups. The first group comprises *S. typhi* and *S. paratyphi* A and C, which infect only man and are spread either directly or indirectely (via food and water) from person to person.[172] The second group includes serovariants (serovars) that are host adapted for a particular species of vertebrates, e.g., *S. gallinarum* in poultry, *S. dublin* in cattle, *S. abortus equi* in horses, *S. abortus ovis* in sheep, and *S. choleraesuis* and *S. typhisuis* in swine; some of these are also pathogenic in humans (especially *S. dublin* and *S. choleraesuis*). The third group contains the majority of other *Salmonella* serovars with no particular host preference that infect both man and animals. Among the third reservoir of serovars are the principal agents of salmonellosis in poultry.

2. Immune Response to Bacteria

Immunity to *Salmonella* infection has been studied extensively in mice as an experimental model for human *S. typhi* and *S. paratyphi*. The widely used model for "enteric fever" is produced by parenteral infection of mice with virulent strains, such as *S. typhimurium* or *S. enteritidis*. *S. enteritidis* is a naturally occurring pathogen of mice that causes systemic symptoms pathologically similar to typhoid fever. Several experiments in mice showed that the cellular, rather than humoral, response is involved in protection;[173] they included (1) lack of correlation of anti-*Salmonella* antibody levels and protection against disese, (2) live *Salmonella*-induced DTH in close temporal association with the onset of antibacterial immunity in the liver and spleen, and (3) normal protection to infection with live virulent *Salmonella* in agammaglobulinemic mice.[174] In chickens, the uptake of *S. enteritidis* and *S. thompson* by wandering macrophages across the cecal mucosa has been visualized ultrastructurally.[175] *S. typhimurium* were recovered mostly from the CT and persisted until 33 DPI.[176] Infected chickens usually produce agglutinating-type antibodies within 3 to 10 DPI.[171] As in mice, there is a lack of correlation between resistance to infection and the level of serum and biliary antibodies; resistance correlates with the development of CMI.[176,177] Compared to chickens receiving a killed *S. gallinarum* vaccine, immunization with a live vaccine produced significantly higher MIF at 10 and 21 DPI after challenge with live bacteria.[177]

3. Genetic Factors Influencing Immunity

Although there is a paucity of information on the genetic control of disease susceptibility to salmonellosis in chickens, extensive analysis of murine thphoid caused by *S. typhimurium* serves as a model for the genetic control of resistance to this organism and as a probe to evaluate mechanisms of immunity to typhoid fever.[178] In mice orally infected with *S. typhimurium,* the bacteria either multiply in the small bowel or penetrate the intestinal mucosa and enter in the PPs of the small intestine. The bacteria gain access to the circulation via the lymphatic system, enter the reticuloendothelial system (RES), and multiply within splenic and hepatic tissues. A secondary bacteremia ensues followed by systemic dissemination of the organism. When mice of different inbred strains are inoculated via the same route, they exhibit dose-dependent variable susceptibility to *S. typhimurium.*[178] Recent studies indicate that several distinct or closely linked genes act at different phases of infection to control specific and nonspecific immunity involved in disease resistance to salmonellosis. The host gene that controls the early replication of *S. typhimurium* in splenic and hepatic tissues after intravenous (i.v.) or subcutaneous (s.c.) challenge was designated *Ity* (for immunity to *typhimurium*); it is located on chromosome 1 and is not linked to the MHC.[178] The *Ity* gene is closely linked or identical to the gene designated *Lsh* that controls the extent to which *Leishmania donovani* replicates in the RES of mice during the first few weeks of parasitic disease.[179] Recently, Skamene et al.[180] found that the distribution of the *Bcg* gene, which regulates the early phase of resistance to *Mycobacterium bovis* bacille Calmette-Guerin (BCG), is identical to the pattern of *S. typhimurium* and *L. donovani* responses. The result suggests that resistance to all three microorganisms may be regulated by a single gene.

The mode of genetic control of innate immunity to salmonellosis appears to involve resident murine macrophages.[181,182] Mice genetically resistant (*Ity*^{r}) behaved as if they were highly susceptible to *Salmonella* if they were also homozygous for the defective allele of the endotoxin response gene located on chromosome 4. These two traits have been linked in C3H/HeJ mice (endotoxin hyporesponsive). C3H/HeJ mice were unable to restrict the net multiplication of *S. typhimurium* in their spleen, and their macrophages were not activated by lipopolysaccharide (LPS). The gene which controls the late phase of the anti-*Salmonella* response is designated *xid* (for X-linked immunodeficiency); mice carrying this gene tend to die later in the course of murine typhoid. Most macrophage and T-cell functions of *xid* mice appear to be normal,[183] but the initiation of an immunoglobulin G (IgG) anti-*Salmonella* antibody response in *xid* mice is delayed. The data indicate that enhanced disease susceptibility to *S. typhimurium* seen in *xid* mice is due to their inability to make an adequate protective antibody response that is apparently required for survival of infected mice later in the course of murine typhoid. In *Ity*^{r} nu/nu mice, no significant differences were observed in the growth patterns of *Salmonella* in the RES organs of T-cell deficient animals and their nu/+ littermates for up to 13 d after i.v. challenge. Thereafter, net *Salmonella* multiplication was greater in nu/nu than in nu/+ mice; the results suggested that T cells are necessary for the late phase of the protective anti-*Salmonella* antibody response and/or development of acquired cellular immunity.[177,178]

Genetically controlled variations in the host response to salmonellosis have been noted among different breeds of chickens.[184,185] Analysis of the antibody response to *S. pullorum* in segregating B^1B^1 populations suggested polygenic control.[184] The 9R strain of *S. gallinarum* produces hepatic and splenic lesions without mortality in meat-type and brown-egg-producing strains of chickens, but not in leghorns.[185] White leghorns had fewer *Salmonella* bacteria in the spleen, lower fecal excretion, and a shorter period of systemic infection than did the brown-egg-producing strain when the birds were inoculated subcutaneously at 1 d of age. There was no significant difference in the serological responses between white leghorn and meat-type birds.[185]

4. Vaccine Development

Information on protective *Salmonella* antigens is limited. The antigenic differences between two *Salmonella* species and existence of variants of *S. pullorum*, but no *S. gallinarum*, were reported.[171] *S. pullorum* contains a thermostable toxin to which several rodents are susceptible, but to which chickens are resistant; thus, the toxin may not be important. Endotoxin secreted by *S. gallinarum* results in clinical illness within a few hours after i.v. injection in chickens with significant reduction in body temperature and bursa weight.[186] A smooth (9S) or rough (9R) attenuated vaccine, but not a killed vaccine, produced good protection against oral challenge with *S. gallinarum*.[187] Immunity induced by the 9R strain vaccine lasted for 12 weeks, whereas immunity induced by 9S lasted at least 32 weeks. The 9R strain did not elicit antibodies, was nonlethal to 1-d-old chicks, and did not cause a drop in egg production in laying hens. The 9S strain vaccine produced agglutinins, killed 1-d-old chicks, and caused a marked drop in egg production. In chickens given cyclophosphamide during the first 3 to 5 d of life, there was a marked depression in the humoral antibody response but no effect on their ability to develop tuberculin sensitivity or on their immune response to a live *S. gallinarum* vaccine.[172] Humoral antibody titers frequently do not correlate with protection. In general, live vaccines stimulated greater CMI responses than did killed vaccines. Future studies on the identification of protective bacterial antigens of outer membrane proteins of *Salmonella* will provide necessary information for the development of subunit vaccine, since induction of protection has been shown to be possible using crude membrane proteins obtained from *Salmonella*.[188]

V. FUTURE AVENUES

It is clear that much remains to be studied concerning the role of MHC genes and immunological factors controlling intestinal immune responses to poultry pathogens. GALT operate in an extremely complex milieu compared to lymphoid tissues at other sites, and a variety of nonspecific environmental factors are likely to affect the response to enteric pathogens. Furthermore, innate and acquired immunity to microbes depends on host factors such as age, immune status, and genetic background of the host; the denoted factors can significantly influence the effective operation of the immune system. Thus, understanding the immunological responses involved in the development of protective immunity against poultry diseases should precede the development of a vaccine. With increasing public health concerns of salmonellosis and other infections via contamination of poultry products, it is important that better control strategies be developed. Vaccination against many different microbes using live *E. coli*,[135] *Salmonella*,[189] or a fowl pox vector[190] should be explored further. A novel approach involving the insertion of the MHC genes conferring disease resistance into the germlines of chickens will improve the genetic stock of poultry.

REFERENCES

1. **Befus, A. D., Johnston, N., Leslie, G. A., and Bienenstock, J.,** Gut-associated lymphoid tissue in the chicken. I. Morphology, ontogeny and some functional characteristics of Peyer's patches, *J. Immunol.*, 125, 2626, 1980.
2. **Owen, R. L. and Jones, A. L.,** Epithelial cell specialization within human Peyer's patches: an ultrastructural study of intestinal lymphoid follicles, *Gastroenterology*, 66, 189, 1974.
3. **Bockman, D. E. and Cooper, M. D.,** Pinocytosis by epithelium associated with lymphoid follicles in the bursa of Fabricius, appendix and Peyer's patches. An electron microscopic study, *Am. J. Anat.*, 136, 455, 1973.
4. **Kiyono, H., Kurita, T., Suzuki, I., Eldridge, J. H., Morrison, J. F., and McGhee, J. R.,** IgA-specific regulatory T cells in the mucosal system, in *Mucosal Immunity and Infections at Mucosal Surfaces*, Strober,

W., Lamm, M. E., McGhee, J. R., and James, S. P., Eds., Oxford University Press, New York, 1988, 63.

5. **Kiyono, H., Mosteller-Barnum, L., Pitts, A., Williamson, S., Michalek, S., and McGhee, J.,** Isotype specific immunoregulation, *J. Exp. Med.,* 161, 731, 1985.

6. **McGhee, J. R., Kiyono, H., and Alley, C. D.,** Gut bacterial endotoxin: influence on gut-associated lymphoreticular tissue and host immune function, *Surf. Immunol. Res.,* 3, 241, 1984.

7. **Ferguson, A.,** Intraepithelial lymphocytes of the small intestine, *Gut,* 18, 921, 1980.

8. **Guy-Grand, D., Griscelli, C., and Vassalli, P.,** The mouse gut T lymphocyte, a novel type of T cell. Nature, origin and traffic in mice in normal and graft-versus-host conditions, *J. Exp. Med.,* 148, 1661, 1978.

9. **Arnaud-Battandier, F., Lawrence, E. C., and Blaese, R. M.,** Lymphoid populations of gut mucosa in chickens, *Dig. Dis. Sci.,* 25, 252, 1980.

10. **Chiba, M., Bartnik, W., ReMine, S. G., Thayer, W. R., and Shorter, R. G.,** Human colonic intrae-pithelial and lamina proprial lymphocyte: cytotoxicity *in vitro* and the potential effects of the isolation method on their functional properties, *Gut,* 22, 177, 1981.

11. **Chan, M. M., Chen, C.-L. H., Ager, L. L., and Cooper, M. D.,** Identification of the avian homologue of mammalian CD4 and CD8 antigens, *J. Immunol.,* 140, 2133, 1988.

12. **Chen, C. H., Cihak, J., Losch, U., and Cooper, M. D.,** Differential expression of two T cell receptors, TCR1 and TCR2, on chicken lymphocytes, *Eur. J. Immunol.,* 18, 539, 1988.

13. **Lillehoj, H. S., Lillihoj, E. P., Weinstock, D., and Schat, K.,** Functional and biochemical characterization of chicken T lymphocyte antigens, *Eur. J. Immunol.,* 18, 2059, 1988.

14. **Bucy, R. P., Chen, C.-L. H., Cihak, J., Losch, U., and Cooper, M. D.,** Avian T cells expresses gamma delta receptors localize in the splenic sinusoids and the intestinal epithelium, *J. Immunol.,* 141, 2200, 1988.

15. **Vainio, O. and Lassila, O.,** Chicken T cells: differentiation antigens and cell-cell interactions, *Crit. Rev. Poult. Biol.,* 2, 97, 1989.

16. **Sowder, J. T., Chen, C.-L. H., Ager, L. L., Chan, M. M., and Cooper, M. D.,** A large subpopulation of avian T cells express a homologue of the mammalian T gamma/delta receptor, *J. Exp. Med.,* 167, 315, 1988.

17. **Lillehoj, H. S. and Chung, K. S.,** Intestinal immunity and genetic factors influencing colonization of microbes in the gut, in *Proc. Colonization Control of Human Bacterial Enteropathogens in Poultry,* Atlanta, Georgia, September 27 to 29, 1989.

18. **Reynolds, C. W. and Ortaldo, J. R.,** Natural killer activity: the definition of a function rather than a cell type, *Immunol. Today,* 8, 172, 1989.

19. **Herberman, R. B. and Holden, H. T.,** Natural cell-mediated immunity, *Adv. Can. Res.,* 27, 305, 1978.

20. **Kasai, M., Iwamori, M., Nagai, Y., Okumura, K., and Tada, T.,** A glycolipid on the surface of mouse natural killer cells, *Eur. J. Immunol.,* 10, 175, 1980.

21. **Keller, R., Bachi, T., and Okumura, K.,** Discrimination between macrophages and NK-type tumoricidal activities via anti-asialo GM1 antibody, *Exp. Cell. Biol.,* 51, 158, 1983.

22. **Lillihoj, H. S.,** Intestinal intraepithelia and splenic natural killer cell responses to eimerian infections in inbred chickens, *Infect. Immun.,* 57, 1879, 1989.

23. **Dillon, S. B. and MacDonald, T. T.,** Functional properties of lymphocytes isolated from murine small intestinal epithelium, *Immunology,* 52, 501, 1984.

24. **Tagliabue, A., Befus, D., Clark, D. A., and Bienenstock, J.,** Characteristics of natural killer cells in the murine intestinal epithelium and lamina propria, *J. Exp. Med.,* 155, 1785, 1982.

25. **Flexman, J. P., Shellam, G. R., and Mayrhofer, G.,** Natural cytotoxicity, responsiveness to interferon and morphology of intraepithelial lymphocytes from the small intestine of the rat, *Immunology,* 48, 733, 1983.

26. **Arnaud-Battandier, F., Bundy, B. M., O'Neill, M., Bienenstock, J., and Nelson, D. L.,** Cytotoxic activities of gut mucosal lymphoid cells in guinea pigs, *J. Immunol.,* 121, 1059, 1978.

27. **Lam, K. M. and Linna, T. J.,** Transfer of natural resistance to Marek's disease (JMV) with nonimmune spleen cells. II. Further characterization of protecting cell population, *J. Immunol.,* 125, 715, 1980.

28. **Sharma, J. M. and Okazaki, M.,** Natural killer cell activity in specific pathogen-free chickens, *J. Natl. Cancer Inst.,* 63, 527, 1981.

29. **Leibold, W., Janotte, G., and Peter, H. H.,** Spontaneous cell mediated cytotoxicity (SCMC) in various mammalian species and chickens: selective reaction pattern and different mechanisms, *Scand. J. Immunol.,* 11, 203, 1980.

30. **Fleischer, B.,** Effector cells in avian spontaneous and antibody-dependent cell-mediated cytotoxicity, *J. Immunol.,* 125, 1161, 1980.

31. **Lillihoj, H. S. and Chai, J. Y.,** Comparative natural killer cell activities of thymic, bursal, splenic and intestinal intraepithelial lymphocytes, *Dev. Comp. Immunol.,* 12, 629, 1988.

32. **Chai, J. Y. and Lillehoj, H. S.**, Isolation and functional characterization of chicken intestinal intra-epithelial lymphocytes showing natural killer cell activity against tumour target cells, *Immunology,* 3, 111, 1988.

33. **Jeurissen, S. H. M., Janse, E. M., Koch, G., and DeBoer, G. F.**, Postnatal development of mucosa-associated lymphoid tissue in chickens, *Cell Tiss. Res.,* in press.

34. **Brandtzaeg, P., Baklien, K., Bjerke, K., Rognum, T. O., Scott, H., and Valnes, K.**, Nature and properties of the human gastrointestinal immune system, in *Immunology of the Gastrointestinal Tract,* Miller, K. and Nicklin, S., Eds., CRC Press, Boca Raton, FL, 1987, 1.

35. **Bjorkman, P. J., Saper, M. A., Samraoui, B., and Bennett, W. S., Strominger, J. L., and Wiley, D. C.**, Structure of the human class I histocompatibility antigen, HLA-A2, *Nature (London),* 329, 506, 1987.

36. **Allen, P. M., Matsueda, G. R., Evans, R. J., Dunbar, J. B., Jr., Marshall, G., and Unanue, E. R.**, Identification of the T-cell and Ia contact residues of a T-cell antigenic peptide, *Nature (London),* 327, 713, 1987.

37. **Sanders, B. G. and Case, W. L.**, Chicken secretory immunoglobulin: chemical and immunological characterization of chicken IgA, *Comp. Biochem. Physiol.,* 56B, 273, 1977.

38. **Peppard, J. V., Rose, M. E., and Hesketh, P.**, A functional homologue of mammalian SC exists in chickens, *Eur. J. Immunol.,* 13, 566, 1983.

39. **Lillihoj, H. S.**, Effects of immunosuppression on avian coccidiosis. Cyclosporin A but not hormonal bursectomy abrogates host protective immunity, *Infect. Immun.,* 55, 1616, 1987.

40. **Isobe, T., Kohno, M., Suzuki, K., and Yoshihara, S.**, *Leucocytozoon caulleryi* infection in bursectomized chickens, in *Coccidia and Intestinal Coccidiomorphs,* INRA, Tours, France, 1989, 79.

41. **Janeway, C. A., Jones, B., and Hayday, A.**, Specificity and function of T cells bearing gamma delta receptors, *Immunol. Today,* 9, 73, 1988.

42. **Britten, V. and Hughes, H. P. A.**, American trypanosomiasis, toxoplasmosis and leishmaniasis: intracellular infections with different immunological consequences, *Clin. Immunol. Allergy,* 6, 189, 1986.

43. **Ernst, P., Befus, A. D., and Bienenstock, J.**, Leukocytes in the intestinal epithelium: a unique and heterogeneous compartment, *Immunol. Today,* 6, 50, 1985.

44. **Snell, G. D.**, The genetics of transplantation, *J. Natl. Cancer Inst.,* 14, 691, 1953.

45. **Briles, W. E., McGibbon, W. H., and Irwin, M. R.**, On multiple alleles affecting cellular antigens in chickens, *Genetics,* 35, 633, 1953.

46. **Bacon, L. D.**, Influence of the MHC on disease resistance and productivity, *Poult. Sci.,* 66, 802, 1987.

47. **Bloom, S. E. and Bacon, L. D.**, Linkage of the major histocompatibility (*B*) complex and the nucleolar organizer in the chicken, *J. Hered.,* 76, 146, 1985.

48. **Guillemot, F., Billault, A., Pourquie, O., Ghislaine, B., Chausse, A., Zoorob, R., Kreibich, G., and Auffray, C.**, A molecular map of the chicken major histocompatibility complex: the class II beta genes are closely linked to the class I gene and the nucleolar organizer, *EMBO J.,* 7, 2775, 1988.

49. **Guillemot, F., Billault, A., and Auffray, C.**, Physical linkage of a guanine nucleotide-binding protein-related gene to the chicken major histocompatibility complex, *Proc. Natl. Acad. Sci. U.S.A.,* 86, 4594, 1989.

50. **Bourlet, Y., Behar, G., Guillemot, F., Frechin, A., Billault, A., Chausse, A., Zoorob, R., and Auffray, C.**, Isolation of chicken major histocompatibility complex class II (B-L) beta chain sequences: comparison with mammalian beta chians and expression in lymphoid organs, *EMBO J.,* 7, 1030, 1988.

51. **Goto, R., Miyada, C. G., Young, S., Wallace, R. B., Abplanalp, H., Bloom, S. E., Briles, W. E., and Miller, M. M.**, Isolation of a cDNA clone from the B-G subregion of the chicken histocompatibility (*B*) complex, *Immunogenetics,* 27, 102, 1988.

52. **Pink, J. R. L., Kieran, M. W., Rijnbeck, A. M., and Longenecker, B. M.**, Monoclonal antibody against chicken MHC class I (*B-F*) antigens, *Immunogenetics,* 21, 293, 1985.

53. **Lillehoj, H. S., Kim, S., Lillehoj, E. P., and Bacon, L. D.**, Quantitative differences in Ia antigen expression in the spleens of $15I_5$-*B* congenic and inbred chickens as defined by a new monoclonal antibody, *Poult. Sci.,* 67, 1525, 1988.

54. **Miller, M. M., Goto, R., and Briles, W. L.**, Biochemical confirmation of recombination within the B-G subregion of the chicken major histocompatibility complex, *Immunogenetics,* 27, 127, 1988.

55. **Hala, K., Vilhelmova, M., and Hartmanova, J.**, Probable crossing-over in the *B* blood group system of chickens, *Immunogenetics,* 3, 97, 1976.

56. **Lee, R. W. H. and Nordskog, A. W.**, Role of the immune-response region of the *B*-complex in the control of the graft-vs-host reaction in chickens, *Immunogenetics,* 13, 85, 1981.

57. **Benacerraf, B. and McDevitt, H. O.**, Histocompatibility-linked immune response genes, *Science,* 175, 273, 1972.

58. **Benedict, A. A., Pollard, L. W., Morrow, P. R., Abpalnalp, H. A., Mauer, P. H., and Briles, W. E.**, Genetic control of immune responses in chickens. I. Responses to a terpolymer of poly (Glu^{60} Ala^{30} Tyr^{10}) associated with the major histocompatibility complex, *Immunogenetics,* 2, 313, 1975.

59. **Pevzner, I. Y., Trowbridge, C. L., and Nordskog, A. W.,** Recombination between genes coding for immune response and the serologically determined antigens in the chicken B system, *Immunogenetics,* 7, 25, 1978.

60. **Vainio, O., Koch, C., and Toivanen, A.,** B-L antigens (class II) of the chicken major histocompatibility complex control T-B cell interaction, *Immunogentics,* 19, 131, 1984.

61. **Maccubbin, D. A. and Schierman, L.,** MHC-restricted cytotoxic response of chicken T cells: expression, augumentation, and clonal characterization, *J. Immunol.,* 136, 12, 1986.

62. **Weinstock, D. and Schat, K.,** Virus-specific syngenic killing of reticuloendotheliosis virus transformed cell line target cells by spleen cells, in *Avian Immunology,* Vol 2, Weber, W. T. and Ewert, D. L., Eds., Alan R. Liss, New YOrk, 1987, 253.

63. **Collins, W. M., Briles, W. E., Zsigray, R. M., Dunlop, W. R., Corbett, A. C., Clark, K. K., Marks, J. L., and McGrail, T. P.,** The *B* locus (MHC) in the chicken: association with the fate of RSV-induced tumors, *Immunogenetics,* 5, 333, 1977.

64. **Schierman, L. W., Watanabe, D. H., and McBride, R. A.,** Genetic control of Rous sarcoma regression in chicken: linkage with the major histocompatibility complex, *Immunogenetics,* 5, 325, 1977.

65. **Joyner, L. P.,** Host and site specificity, in *The Biology of Coccidia,* Long, P. L., Ed., University Park Press, Baltimore, 1982, 32.

66. **Fernando, M. A., Rose, M. E., and Millard, B. J.,** *Eimeria* spp. of the domestic fowl: the migration of sporozoites intra- and extra-enterically, *J. Parasitol.,* 73, 561, 1987.

67. **Riley, D. and Fernando, M. A.,** *Eimeria maxima* (Apicomplex): a comparison of sporozoite transport in naive and immune chickens, *J. Parasitol.,* 74, 103, 1988.

68. **Lillehoj, H. S. and Ruff, M. D.,** Comparison of diseases susceptibility and subclass-specific antibody response in SC and FP chickens experimentally inoculated with *Eimeria tenella, E. acervulina,* of *E. macima, Avian Dis.,* 31, 112, 1987.

69. **Lillehoj, H. S.,** Influence of inoculation dose, inoculation schedule, host age, and host genetics on disease susceptibility and development of *Eimeria tenella* infection, *Avian Dis.,* 32, 437, 1987.

70. **Rose, M. E.,** *Eimeria, Isospora* and *Cryptosporidium* in *Immune Response in Parasitic Infections: Immunology, Immunopathology, Immunoprophylaxis,* Soulsby, E. J. L., Ed., CRC Press, Boca Raton, FL, 1987, 275.

71. **Wiesner, J.,** Biliary IgA from infected chickens as agglutinating factor for *Eimeria tenella* sporozoites, *J. Protozool.,* 26, 46A, 1979.

72. **Lillehoj, H. S.,** Secretory IgA response in SC and FP chickens experimentally inoculated with *E. tenella* and *E. acervulina,* in *Recent Developments in Mucosal Immunology,* Mestechy, J., McGhee, J. R., Ogra, P. L., and Bienenstock, J., Eds., Plenum Press, New York, 1987, 977.

73. **Davis, P. J., Parry, S. H., and Porter, P.,** The role of secretory IgA in anticoccidial immunity in the chicken, *Immunology,* 34, 879, 1978.

74. **Mockett, A. P. A. and Rose, M. E.,** Immune response to *Eimeria*: quantitation of antibody isotypes of *Eimeria tenella* chicken serum and bile by means of the ELISA, *Parasite Immunol.,* in press.

75. **Tanielian, Z., Abu Ali, N., Channoum, B. J., Sokolic, A., Borojevic, D., and Movsesijan, M.,** Circulating antibody response in chickens to homologous and heterologous antigens of *Eimeria tenella, E. necatrix,* and *E. brunetti, Acta Parasitol. Yugosl.,* 7, 79, 1976.

76. **Lillehoj, H. S.,** Immune response during coccidiosis in SC and FP chickens. I. *In vitro* assessment of T cell proliferation to stage-specific parasite antigens, *Vet. Immunol. Immunopathol.,* 13, 321, 1986.

77. **Rose, M. E., Hesketh, P., and Ogilvie, B. M.,** Peripheral blood leucocyte response to coccidial infections: a comparison of the response in rats and chickens and its correlation with resistance to reinfection, *Immunology,* 36, 71, 1979.

78. **Rose, M. E.,** Immune responses in infection with coccidia: macrophage activity, *Infect. Immun.,* 10, 862, 1974.

79. **Rose, M. E. and Hesketh, P.,** Immunity to coccidiosis: further investigations in T-lymphocyte and B-lymphocyte-deficient animals, *Infect. Immun.,* 26, 630, 1979.

80. **Giambrone, J. J., Klesius, P. H., Eckamm, M. K., and Edgar, S. A.,** Influence of hormonal and chemical bursectomy on the development of acquired immunity to coccidia in broiler chickens, *Poult. Sci.,* 60, 2612, 1981.

81. **Rose, M. E.,** Immunity to coccidiosis: effects of betamethasone treatment of fowls on *Eimeria mivati* infections, *Parasitology,* 60, 137, 1970.

82. **Lillehoj, H. S., Jenkins, M. C., Bacon, L. D., Fetterer, R. H., and Briles, W.E.,** *Eimeria acervulina*: genetic control of the immune responses to the recombinant coccidial antigens in B-congenic chickens, *Exp. Paratisol.,* 68, 148, 1988.

83. **Lillehoj, H. S., Ruff, M. D., Bacon, L. D., Lamont, S. J., and Jeffers, T. K.,** Genetic control of immunity to *Eimeria tenella.* Interaction of MHC genes and non-MHC linked genes influence levels of disease susceptibility, *Vet. Immunol. Immunopathol.,* 20, 135, 1989.

84. **Rose, M. E.,** Protective antibodies in infections with *Eimeria maxima:* the reduction of pathogenic effects *in vivo* and a comparison between oral and subcutaneous administration of antiserum, *Parasitology,* 68, 285, 1974.

85. **Davis, P. J. and Porter, P.,** A mechanism for secretory IgA mediated inhibition of the cell penetration and intracellular development of *Eimeria tenella, Immunology,* 36, 471, 1979.

86. **Augustine, P. C. and Danforth, H. D.,** Effects of hybridoma antibodies on invasion of cultured cells by sporozoites of *Eimeria, Avian Dis.,* 29, 1212, 1985.

87. **Horton-Smith, C., Long, P. L., Pierce, A. E., and Rose, M. E.,** Immunity to coccidia in domestic animals, in *Immunity to Protozoa,* Garnham, P. C. C., Pierce, A. E., and Roitt, I., Eds., Blackwell Scientific, Oxford, 1963, 273.

88. **Rose, M. E. and Hesketh, P.,** Immunity to coccidiosis: stages of the life cycle of *Eimeria maxima* which induce, and are affected by, the response of the host, *Parasitoloty,* 73, 25, 1976.

89. **Leathem, W. D. and Burns, W. C.,** Effects of the immune chicken on the endogenous stages of *Eimeria tenella, J. Parasitol.,* 53, 180, 1967.

90. **Eugui, E. M. and Allison, A. C.,** Differences in susceptibility of various mouse strains to haemoprotozoan infections: possible correlation with natural killer activity, *Parasite Immunol.,* 2, 277, 1980.

91. **Solomon, J. B.,** Natural cytotoxicity for *Plasmodium berghei in vitro* by spleen cells from susceptible and resistant mice, *Immunology,* 59, 277, 1986.

92. **Lillehoj, H. S., Kang, S. Y., Keller, L., and Sevoian, M.,** *Eimeria tenella* and *Eimeria tenella* and *Eimeria acervulina:* Lymphokines secreted by an avian T cell lymphoma or by sporozoite-stimulated immune T lymphocytes protect chickens against avian coccidiosis, *Exp. Parasitol.,* 69, 54, 1989.

93. **Ortaldo, J. R., Mason, A., and Overton, R.,** Lymphokine-activated killer cells: analysis of progenitors and effectors, *J. Exp. Med.,* 164, 1193, 1986.

94. **Herberman, R. B., Reynolds, C. W., and Ortaldo, J. R.,** Mechanisms of cytotoxicity by natural killer cells, *Annu. Rev. Immunol.,* 4, 651, 1986.

95. **Lanier, L. L. and Phillips, J. H.,** Evidence for three types of human cytotoxic lymphocytes, *Immunol. Today,* 7, 132, 1986.

96. **Welsh, R. M.,** Regulation of virus infections by natural killer cells, *Nat. Immunol. Cell Growth Regul.,* 5, 169, 1986.

97. **Mandi, Y., Seprenyi, G., Pusztai, R., and Beladi, I.,** Are granulocytes the main effector cells of natural cytotoxicity in chickens?, *Immunobiology,* 170, 284, 1985.

98. **Huff, D. and Clark, D. T.,** Cellular aspects of the resistance of chickens to *Eimeria tenella* infections, *J. Protozool.,* 17, 35, 1970.

99. **Onaga, H. and Ishii, T.,** Leukocyte migration inhibition in chickens immunized with *Eimeria tenella, Jpn. J. Vet. Sci.,* 42, 345, 1980.

100. **Onaga, H., Tajima, M., and Ishii, T.,** Activation of macrophages by cultures of antigen-stimulated spleen cells collected from chickens immunized with *Eimeria tenella, Vet. Parasitol.,* 13, 1, 1983.

101. **Rose, M. E.,** *Eimeria tenella:* skin hypersensitivity to injected antigen in the fowl, *Exp. Parasitol.,* 42, 129, 1977.

102. **Long, P. L. and Milne, B. S.,** The effect of an interferon inducer on *Eimeria maxima* in the chicken, *Parasitology,* 62, 295, 1971.

103. **Ferreiro, A., Schoefield, L., Enea, V., Schillekens, H., Van der Meide, P., Collins, W. E., Nussenzweig, R. S., and Nussenzweig, V.,** Inhibition of gamma-interferon, *Science,* 232, 881, 1986.

104. **Pfefferkorn, E. R., Eckel, M., and Rebhun, S.,** Interferon-gamma suppresses the growth of *Toxoplasma gondii* in human fibroblasts through starvation for tryptophan, *Mol. Biochem. Parastiol.,* 20, 215, 1986.

105. **Reyes, L. and Frenkel, J. R.,** Specific and non-specific mediation of protective immunity to *Toxoplasma gondii, Infect. Immun.,* 55, 856, 1987.

106. **Klesius, P. H. and Giambrone, J. J.,** Adoptive transfer of delayed hypersensitivity and protective immunity to *Eimeria tenella* with chicken-derived transfer factor, *Poult. Sci.,* 63, 1333, 1984.

107. **Prowse, S. J. and Pallister, J.,** Immunity to coccidiosis: interferon release by spleen and mucosal lymphoid cells from immune chickens, in *Coccidia and Intestinal Coccidiomorphs,* 5th Int. Coccidiosis Conf., INRA, Tours, France, 1989, 541.

108. **Morita, C., Tsutsumi, Y., and Soekawa, M.,** Migration inhibition test of splenic cells of chickens infected with *Eimeria tenella, J. Parasitol.,* 59, 199, 1973.

109. **Klesius, P. H. and Kristensen, F.,** Bovine transfer factor: effect on bovine and rabbit coccidiosis, *Clin. Immunol. Immunopathol.,* 7, 240, 1977.

110. **Wilson, G. B., Poindexter, C., Fort, J. D., and Ludden, K. D.,** *De novo* initiation of specific cell-mediated immune responsiveness in chickens by transfer factor (specific immunity inducer) obtained from bovine colostrum and milk, *Acta Virol.,* 32, 6, 1988.

111. **Kogut, M. H. and Lange, C.,** Interferon-gamma-mediated inhibition of the development of *Eimeria tenella* in cultured cells, *J. Parasitol.,* 75, 313, 1989.

112. **Munch, D. and Sevoian, M.,** Growth and characterization of and immunological response of chickens to a cell line established from JMV lymphoblastic leukemia, *Avian Dis.,* 24, 23, 1980.

113. **Keller, L. H., Beldon, K. A., and Sevoian, M.,** Immunization of chickens against Marek's disease with cell-free supernatant from JMV-1 lymphoblastoid cell line, in *Avian Immunology II,* Weber, W. T. and Ewert, D. L., Eds., Alan R. Liss, New York, 1987, 265.

114. **Speer, C. A., Reduker, D. W., Burgess, D. E., Whitmore, W. M., and Splitter, G. A.,** Lymphokine-induced inhibition of growth of *Eimeria bovis* and *Eimeria papillata* (Apicomplexa) in cultured bovine monocytes, *Infect. Immun.,* 50, 566, 1985.

115. **Hughes, H. P. A., Speer, C. A., Kyle, J. E., and Dubey, J. P.,** Activation of murine macrophages and a bovine monocyte cell line by bovine lymphokines to kill intracellular pathogens *(Eimeria, Toxoplasma), Infect. Immun.,* 55, 1987, 784.

116. **Remington, J. S., Krahenbuhl, J. L., and Mendenhall, J. W.,** Role for activated macrophages in resistance to infection with *Toxoplasma, Infect. Immun.,* 6, 829, 1972.

117. **Sethi, K. K., Pelster, B., Suzuki, N., Piekarski, G., and Brandis, H.,** Immunity to *Toxoplasma gondii* induced *in vitro* in non-immune mouse macrophages with specifically immune lymphocytes, *J. Immunol.,* 115, 1151, 1975.

118. **Anderson, S. E., Bautista, S., and Remington, J. S.,** Induction of resistance to *Toxoplasma gondii* in human macrophages by soluble lymphocyte products, *J. Immunol.,* 117, 381, 1976.

119. **Hoover, D. L., Finbloom, D. S., Crawford, R. M., Nacy, C. A., Gilbreath, M., and Meltzer, M. S.,** A lymphokine distinct from interferon-gamma that activates human monocytes to kill *Leishmania donovani in vitro, J. Immunol.,* 136, 1329, 1986.

120. **Ortaldo, J. R., Mathieson, B. J., and Wiltrout, R. H.,** Characterization and functions of natural killer cells, *Ann. Inst. Pasteur Immunol.,* 139, 44, 1988.

121. **Johnson, L. W. and Edgar, S. A.,** Ea-B and Ea-C cellular antigen genes in leghorn lines resistant and susceptible to acute cecal coccidiosis, *Poult. Sci.,* 65, 241, 1986.

122. **Clare, R. A., Strout, R. G., Taylor, R. L., Jr., Collins, W. M., and Briles, W. E.,** Major histocompatibility (B) complex effects on acquired immunity to cecal coccidiosis, *Immunogenetics,* 22, 593, 1985.

123. **Bumstead, N. and Millard, B.,** Genetics of resistance to coccidiosis: response of inbred chicken lines to infection by *Eimeria tenella* and *Eimeria maxima, Br. Poult. Sci.,* 28, 705, 1985.

124. **Bedrnik, P. and Hala, K.,** Sensitivity of different inbred lines of hens to *Eimeria tenella* infection, in *Proc. Int. Symp. Coccidia,* Prague, 1979, 221.

125. **Wassom, D. L.,** Genetic control of the host response to parasitic helminth infection, in *Genetic Control of Host Resistance to Infection and Malignancy,* Skameni, E., Ed., Alan R. Liss, New York, 1985, 449.

126. **Wassom, D. L., Brooks, B. O., and Cypress, R. H.,** A survey of susceptibility to infection with *Trichinella spiralis* of inbred mouse strains sharing common H-2 alleles but different genetic backgrounds, *J. Parasitol.,* 69, 1033, 1983.

127. **Bell, R. G., Adam, L. S., and Ogden, R. W.,** *Trichinella spiralis:* genetics of worm expulsion in inbred and F_1 mice infected with different worm doses, *Exp. Parasitol.,* 58, 345, 1984.

128. **Bacon, L. D., Ismail, N., and Motta, J. M.,** Allograft and antibody responses of $15I_5$-B congenic chickens, in *Avian Immunology,* Weber, W. T. and Ewert, D. L., Eds., Alan R. Liss, New York, 1986, 219.

129. **Ruff, M. D. and Bacon, L. D.,** *Eimeria acervulina* and *Eimeria tenella* in 15.B-congenic White Leghorns, *Poult. Sci.,* 68, 380, 1989.

130. **Jenkins, M. C., Lillehoj, H. S., and Dame, J. H.,** *Eimeria acervulina:* DNA cloning and characterization of recombinant sporozoite and merozoite antigens, *Exp. Parasitol.,* 66, 96, 1987.

131. **Parry, S. H., Barratt, M. E. J., Davis, P. J., and Jones, S.,** Theoretical and practical aspects of vaccination against coccidiosis, in *Coccidia and Intestinal Coccidiomorphs,* 5th Int. Coccidiosis Conf., INRA, Tours, France, 1989, 617.

132. **Davis, P. J., Barratt, M. E. J., Morgan, M., and Parry, S. H.,** Immune response of chickens to oral immunization by 'trickle' infections with *Eimeria,* in *Research in Avian Coccidiosis,* McDougald, L. R., Joyner, L. P., and Long, P., Eds., University of Georgia, AThens, 1985, 618.

133. **Jeffers, T. K.,** Attenuation of coccidia — a review, in *Research in Avian Coccidiosis,* McDougald, L. R., Joyner, L. P., and Long, P., Eds., University of Georgia, Atlanta, 1985, 482.

134. **Lillehoj, H. S. and Jenkins, M. C.,** Effects of MHC genes and various antigen presentations on protective host immunity following eimerian infections and immunization with a recombinant coccidial antigen: a review, in *Coccidia and Intestinal Coccidiomorphs,* 5th Int. Coccidiosis Conf., INRA, Tours, France, 1989, 634.

135. **Kim, K. S., Jenkins, M. C., and Lillehoj, H. S.,** Immunization of chickens with live *Escherichia coli* expressing *Eimeria acervulina* merozoite recombinant antigen induces partial protection against coccidiosis, *Infect. Immun.,* 57, 2434, 1989.

136. **Danforth, H. D.,** Antigenic make-up of *Eimeria,* in *Coccidia and Intestinal Coccidiomorphs,* INRA, Tours, France, 1989, 99.

137. **Jenkins, M. C. and Dame, J. B.**, Identification of immunodominant surface antigens of *Eimeria acervulina* sporozoites and merozoites, *Mol. Biochem. Parasitol.*, 25, 155, 1987.

138. **Wallach, M. C., Mencher, D., Yarus, S., Pillemer, G., Halabi, A., and Pugatsh, T.**, *Eimeria maxima:* identification of gametocytes protein antigens, *Exp. Parasitol.*, 68, 49, 1989.

139. **Danforth, H. D., Augustine, P. C., Strohlein, D. A., Jenkins, M. C., Strausberg, R. L., and Ruff, M. D.**, The use of genetically engineered antigens in eliciting protective immune response to *Eimeria acervulina* and *Eimeria tenella* in *Coccidia and Intestinal Coccidiomorphs*, INRA, Tours, France, 1989, 645.

140. **Schwartz, R. H.**, The value of synthetic peptides as vaccines for eliciting T-cell immunity, in *Curr. Top. Microbiol. Immunol.*, 130, 79, 1989.

141. **Good, M. F., Berzofsky, J. A., Maloy, W. L., Hayashi, Y., Fujii, N., Hockmeyer, W. T., and Miller, L. H.**, Genetic control of the immune response in mice to a *Plasmodium falciparum* sporozoite vaccine. Widespread nonresponsiveness to single malaria T epitope in highly repetitive vaccine, *J. Exp. Med.*, 164, 655, 1986.

142. **Turner, M. J.**, Progress towards a subunit vaccine for coccidiosis, in Proc. UCLA Symp. Parasites: Molecular Biology, Drug and Vaccine Design, Keystone, CO, April 3 to 10, 1989.

143. **Bhogal, B. S., Nollstadt, K. H., Karkhanis, Y. D., Schmatz, D. M., and Jacobson, E. B.**, Anti-idiotypic antibody with potential use as an *Eimeria tenella* sporozoite antigen surrogate for vaccination of chickens against coccidiosis, *Infect. Immun.*, 56, 1113, 1988.

144. **Current, W. L.**, *Cryptosporidium:* its biology and potential for environmental transmission, *Crit. Rev. Environ. Control*, 17, 21, 1986.

145. **Fayer, R. and Ungar, B. L. P.**, *Cryptosporidium* spp. and cryptosporidiosis, *Microbiol. Rev.*, 458, 1986.

146. **Current, W. L., Reese, N. C., Ernst, J. V., Bailey, W. S., Heyman, M. B., and Weinstin, W. M.**, Human cryptosporidiosis in immunocompetent and immunodeficient persons: studies of an outbreak and experimental transmission, *N. Engl. J. Med.*, 308, 1252, 1983.

147. **Tyzzer, E. E.**, Coccidiosis in gallinaceous birds, *Am. J. Hyg.*, 10, 269, 1929.

148. **Slavin, D.**, *Cryptosporidium meleagridis* (sp. nov.), *J. Comp. Pathol.*, 65, 262, 1955.

149. **Current, W. L., Upton, S. J., and Haynes, T. B.**, The life cycle of *Cryptosporidium baileyi* n. sp. (Apicomplexa, Cryptosporidiidae) infecting chickens, *J. Protozool.*, 33, 289, 1986.

150. **Hoerr, F. J., Current, W. L., and Haynes, T. B.**, Fatal cryptosporidiosis in quail, *Avian Dis.*, 30, 421, 1986.

151. **Fletcher, O. J., Munnell, J. F., and Page, R. K.**, Cryptosporidiosis of the bursa of Fabricius of chickens, *Avian Dis.*, 19, 630, 1985.

152. **Lindsay, D. S., Blagburn, B. L., and Ernst, J. A.**, Experimental *Cryptosporidium parvum* infections in chickens, *J. Parasitol.*, 73, 242, 1987.

153. **Goodwin, M. A. and Brown, J.**, Light-microscopic lesions associated with naturally occurring bursal cryptosporidiosis in chickens, *Avian Dis.*, 33, 74, 1989.

154. **Marcial, M. A. and Madara, J. L.**, *Cryptosporidium:* cellular localization, structural analysis of absorptive cell-parasite membrane-membrane interactions in guinea pigs, and suggestion of protozoan transport by M cells, *Gastroenterology*, 90, 583, 1986.

155. **Campbell, P. N. and Current, W. L.**, Demonstration of serum antibodies to *Cryptosporidium* sp. in normal and immunodeficient humans with confirmed infections, *J. Clin. Microbiol.*, 18, 165, 1983.

156. **Current, W. L., Reese, N. C., Ernst, J. V., Bailey, W. S., Heyman, M. B., and Weinstein, W. M.**, Human cryptosporidiosis in immunocompetent and immunodeficient persons: studies of an outbreak and experimental transmission, *N. Engl. J. Med.*, 308, 1252, 1987.

157. **Heins, J., Moon, H. W., and Woodmansee, D. B.**, Persistent cryptosporidiosis infection in congenitally athymic (nude) mice, *Infect. Immun.*, 43, 856, 1984.

158. **Current, W. L.**, *Cryptosporidium* sp. in chickens: parasite life cycle and aspects of acquired immunity, in *Research in Coccidiosis*, McDougald, L. R., Long, P. L., Joyner, L. P., Eds., University of Georgia, Athens, 1985, 124.

159. **Current, W. L. and Snyder, D. B.**, Development of and serologic evaluation of acquired immunity to *Cryptosporidium baileyi* by broiler chickens, *Poult. Sci.*, 67, 720, 1985.

160. **Lindsay, D. S., Blagburn, B.L., Sunderman, C. A., and Giambrone, J. J.**, Effect of broiler chicken age on susceptibility to experimentally induced *Cryptosporidium baileyi* infection, *Am. J. Vet. Res.*, 49, 1412, 1988.

161. **Blagburn, B. L., Lindsay, D. S., Giambrone, J. J., Sundermann, C. A., and Hoerr, F. J.**, Experimental Cryptosporidiosis in broiler chickens, *Poult. Sci.*, 66, 442, 1987.

162. **Mathis, C. and Leger, M.**, *Leucocytozoon* de la poule, *C.R. Soc. Biol.*, Paris, 67, 470, 1909.

163. **Akiba, K., Kawashima, H., Inui, S., and Ishii, S.**, Studies on Leucocytozoon of chickens in Japan. I. Natural infection of *L. caulleryi*, *Bull. Natl. Inst. Anim. Health*, 34, 163, 1958.

164. **Akiba, K.,** Current statis of studies on Leucocytozoonosis of chickens, especially on species, epidemiology, life cycle immunity, control and chemotherapy of *L. caulleryi* infection, in *Coccidia and Intestinal Coccidiomorphs,* INRA, Tours, France, 1989, 65.

165. **Morii, T. and Kitaoka, S.,** Some aspects on immunity to *Akiba caulleryi* infection in chickens, *Natl. Inst. Anim. Heatlh (Jpn.),* 10, 151, 1970.

166. **Morii, T., Matsui, T., Kobayashi, F., and Iijima, T.,** Some aspects of *Leucocytozoon caulleryi* reinfection in chickens, *Parasitol. Res.,* 75, 194, 1989.

167. **Isobe, T. and Akiba, K.,** Development of erythrocytic merozoites to gametocytes in chickens recovered from sporozoite infection with *Leucocytozoon caulleryi, J. Parasitol.,* 72, 190, 1986.

168. **Isobe, T. and Suzuki, K.,** Enzyme-linked immunosorbent assay for detection of antibody to *Leucocytozoon caulleryi, Avian Pathol.,* 15, 199, 1986.

169. **Isobe, T. and Suzuki, K.,** Detection of serum antibody to *Leucocytozoon caulleryi* in naturally infected chickens by enzyme-linked immunosorbent assay, *Jpn. J. Vet. Sci.,* 49, 165, 1987.

170. **Isobe, T., Kohno, M., Suzuki, K., and Yoshihara, S.,** *Leucocytozoon caulleryi,* infection in bursectomized chickens, in *Coccidia and Intestinal Coccidiomorphs,* INRA, Tours, France, 1989, 79.

171. **Snoeyenbos, G. H.,** Pullorum disease, in *Diseases of Poultry,* 8th ed., Hofstad, M. S., Barnes, H. John, Calnek, B. W., Reid, W. M., Yoder, H. W., Jr., Eds., Iowa State University, Ames, 1984, 66.

172. **Pomeroy, B. S.,** Fowl typhoid, in *Diseases of Poultry,* 8th ed., Hofstad, M. S., Barnes, H. J., Calnek, B. W., Reid, W. M., and Yoder, H. W., Eds., Iowa State University Press, Ames, 1984, 79.

173. **Eisenstein, T. K. and Sultzer, B. M.,** Immunity to *Salmonella* infection, *Adv. Exp. Med. Biol.,* 162, 261, 1983.

174. **Fultz, M. J., Finkelman, F. D., and Metcalf, E. S.,** Altered expression of the *Salmonella typhimurium*-specific B-cell repertoire in mice chronically treated with antibodies to immunoglobulin D, *Infect. Immun.,* 57, 432, 1989.

175. **Popiel, I. and Turnbull, P. C.,** Passage of *Salmonella enteritidis* and *Salmonella thompson* through chick illeocecal mucosa, *Infect. Immun.,* 47, 786, 1985.

176. **Lee, G. M., Jackson, G. D. F., and Cooper, G. N.,** Infection and immune responses in chickens exposed to *Salmonella typhimurium, Avian Dis.,* 27, 577, 1983.

177. **Chamdron, N. J. D., Moses, J. S., Dorairajan, N., and Balaprakasam, R. A.,** Cell mediated immune response in chicks against salmonellosis, *Cheiron* 12, 6294, 1983.

178. **O'Brien, A. D.,** Influence of host genes on resistance of inbred mice to lethal infection with *Salmonella typhimurium, Curr. Top. Microbiol. Immunol.,* 124, 37, 1986.

179. **O'Brien, A. D., Rosentreich, D. L., and Taylor, B. A.,** Control of natural resistance to *Salmonella typhimurium* and *Leishmania donovani* in mice by closely linked but distinct genetic loci, *Nature (London),* 287, 440, 1980.

180. **Skamene, E., Gros, P., Forget, P. A., Kongshavn, P. A. L., St. Charles, C., and Taylor, B. A.,** Genetic regulation of resistance to intracellular pathogens, *Nature (London),* 297, 506, 1982.

181. **Colwell, D. E., Michalek, S. M. and McGhee, J. R.,** *Lps* gene regulation of mucosal immunity and susceptibility to *Salmonella* infection in mice, *Curr. Top. Microbiol. Immunol.,* 124, 121, 1986.

182. **Crocker, P. R., Blackwell, J. M., and Bradly, D. J.,** Expression of the natural resistance gene *Lsh* in resident liver macrophages, *Infect. Immun.,* 43, 1033, 1984.

183. **Wicker, L. S. and Scher, I.,** X-linked immune deficiency (xid) of CBA/N mice, *Curr. Top. Microbiol. Immunol.,* 124, 87, 1986.

184. **Pevzner, I. Y., Stone, H. A., and Nordskog, A. W.,** Immune response and disease resistance in chickens. I. Selection for high and low titers to *Salmonella pullorum* antigen, *Poult. Sci.,* 60, 920, 1981.

185. **Silva, E. N., Snoeyenbos, G. H., Weinack, O. M., and Smyser, D. F.,** Studies on the use of 9R strain of *Salmonella gallinarum* as a vaccine in chickens, *Avian Dis.,* 25, 38, 1981.

186. **Smith, I. M., License, S. T., and Hill, R.,** Haematological, serological and pathological effects in chicks of one or more intravenous injections of *Salmonella gallinarum* endotoxin, *Res. Vet. Sci.,* 24, 154, 1978.

187. **Smith, H. W.,** The use of live vaccine in experimental *Salmonella galinarum* infective in chickens with observations on their interference effect, *J. Hyg.,* 54, 419, 1956.

188. **Bouzoubaa, K., Nagaraja, K. V., Kabbaj, F. Z., Newman, J. A. and Pomeroy, B. S.,** Feasibility of using proteins from *Salmonella gallinarum* vs. 9R live vaccine for the prevention of fowl thyphoid in chickens, *Avian Dis.,* 33, 385, 1989.

189. **Sadoof, J. C., Ballou, W. R., Bacon, L. S., Majarian, W. R., Brey, R. N., Hockmeyer, W. T., Young, J. F., Cruz, S., Ou, J., Lowell, G. H., and Chulay, J. D.,** Oral *Salmonella typhimurium* expressing circumsporozoite proteins protects against malaria, *Science,* 240, 336, 1988.

190. **Smith, G. L., Godson, G. N., Nussenzweig, V., Nussenzweig, R. S., Barnwell, J., and Moss, B.,** *Plasmodium knowlesi* sporozoite antigen: expression of infectious recombinant vaccinia virus, *Science,* 397, 1984.

Chapter 11

AUTOIMMUNE DISEASES

Mark H. Kaplan, Roy S. Sundick, and Noel R. Rose

TABLE OF CONTENTS

I. INTRODUCTION

The pathogenesis of autoimmune diseases in experimental animals has been the focus of much research both for their usefulness as models of analogous human diseases and for fundamental studies of breakdown in immune regulation. Avian autoimmune diseases are ideal for these studies because of the anatomical separation of T- and B-cell compartments. This separation facilitates examination of isolated humoral or cellular components of the immune system and their interactions with the organ or systemic target of autoimmune attack.

As with mammalian autoimmune diseases, disease can be spontaneous or artificially induced. Experimentally induced autoimmune conditions in birds include encephalomyelitis,[1] glomerulonephritis,[2] parathyroiditis, and thyroiditis.[3] In general, however, spontaneous autoimmune diseases have been better models for similar human conditions because of their value in understanding target-organ defects and disease initiation. The spontaneous autoimmune diseases discussed in this chapter parallel the human diseases vitiligo, scleroderma, and Hashimoto's thyroiditis and will likely be instrumental in understanding these and other autoimmune diseases.

II. THE SMYTH-DAM LINE CHICKEN

The Smyth-DAM (Delayed AMelanosis) chicken has a high incidence of pigmentation loss and shares symptoms with the human disease vitiligo.[4] In addition to a high incidence of delayed feather amelanosis, there is an increased occurrence of hypothyroidism and blindness caused by loss of retinal pigmentation.[4] Several lines of evidence suggest immune involvement in this disease. Bursectomy of DAM chickens resulted in a marked decrease in the percentage of the population exhibiting amelanosis and decreased the severity of symptoms in chickens that did develop disease.[5] A possible B-cell hyperactivity was suggested following immunization with *Brucella abortus* (a T-independent antigen) and sheep red blood cells (a T-dependent antigen). Antibody titers to both antigens were higher in amelanotic birds.[6] Additionally, there was a positive correlation between disease severity and level of antibody titers.[6] Treatment with corticosterone, an important neuroimmune modulator, also decreased disease incidence and severity.[7] Cyclosporin A treatment of Smyth-DAM chickens delayed both the onset of disease and the severity of pathology associated with disease incidence.[8] Following termination of cyclosporin A treatment, the incidence of amelanosis rose rapidly to levels higher than those seen in untreated birds. Pathology following termination of treatment was also more severe.[8] This suggested an initial decrease in both suppressor and effector T-cell functions by cyclosporin A and a lack of suppression following termination of cyclosporin A treatment. However, the relative roles of T-cell subsets or B cells in this disease is still uncertain. In addition, the role of genetic melanosomal defects in disease initiation and progress is still under investigation.[9]

III. UCD LINE 200 CHICKEN

The UCD line 200 chicken develops progressive systemic sclerosis or scleroderma with symptoms similar to those seen in human scleroderma.[10,11] While it is unlikely that the cause of the avian disorder is identical to human disease, it can still serve as an important model for studying the mechanisms of autoimmune attack and sclerotic progression.[11]

The line 200 chicken appears relatively normal for the first 2 weeks following hatching. In the following weeks the birds develop comb lesions (90% of the population by 3 weeks), polyarthritis (20% by 3 weeks, 35% by 4 weeks), and dermal lesions (20% by 5 weeks and 45% by 7 weeks).[10] There is enhanced mortality in birds which develop simultaneous comb, joint, and skin pathology, and death usually occurs within 10 weeks. The mortality rate for line 200 chickens is 55% at 10 months compared to a rate of less than 10% for normals at 1 year of age.[10]

Dermal pathology begins with an intense mononuclear cell infiltrate. The initial cells infiltrating the skin are primarily T cells.[12] Many of these cells are B-L positive, indicating an activated population. The ratio of CD4:CD8 T cells in the dermal infiltrate is 1.44:1, significantly different than the almost 3:1 ratio in the periphery. B cells infiltrate dermal lesions later in disease progression and primarily express surface immunoglobulin M (IgM).[12] The infiltration wanes over time. However, before this occurs, small vessels proliferate and fibroblasts migrate into dermal tissues; both processes likely facilitate extensive subcutaneous collagen deposition.[10] The deposition of collagen leads to thickening and occlusion of blood vessels. In older birds, this dermal pathology also occurs in other organs including heart, kidney, and esophagus.[10]

The genetic defect responsible for this disease is autosomal and recessive. Disease is not seen in a line (200 × normal) F_1 generation.[10] Disease occurs in 51% of the (F_1 × line 200) backcross. However, only 4% of the birds in the F_2 develop disease, arguing for incomplete penetrance of the genetic defect.[10]

Sera of line 200 chickens had higher circulating levels of immunoglobulin G (IgG) than normal chickens. In older birds, 20% of the population had IgG deposits in the kidney and glomerulonephritis.[10] Several types of autoantibodies were found in the line 200 chicken. At 4 months, 60% of the birds had rheumatoid factor, and at 6 months almost all had antibodies to type II collagen.[10] At 6 months, greater than one half of the birds had antinuclear and anticytoplasmic antibodies.[10,13] No antibodies were found to thymocytes, native DNA, histone, RNA, or polyadenine:uridine (A:U).[10,14] The cytoplasmic antigen was distributed in a spider web pattern at 1 month of age, but changed to a fine speckled pattern at 6 months.[13] This antigen was shared with other avian species, but not with mammalian extracts. Autoantibodies were found to single-stranded DNA. Antibodies to a saline-extractable antigen correlated with antinuclear antibodies, antibodies to single-stranded DNA, and the incidence of disease.[13] Further research on the specific antigens of these autoantibodies should help elucidate the mechanism of autoimmune induction.

IV. THE OBESE STRAIN CHICKEN

The best-studied model of avian autoimmune disease is the spontaneous thyroiditis of the Obese strain (OS) chicken, which closely simulates the human disease Hashimoto's thyroiditis. The disease was first recognized by R. K. Cole of Cornell University in 1956. Among the birds of the selected Cornell C strain (CS) of white leghorns, he noticed a few females that had distinctive clinical features of short stature and subcutaneous deposits of fat (i.e., "obesity syndrome").[15] After mating the CS males, some of the offspring showed similar signs. After several generations of selection, signs of obesity appeared not only in females, but in males as well. In 1962, Van Tienhoven and Cole[16] attributed the phenotypic change to congenital thyroid deficiency. The birds had large abdominal and subcutaneous fat deposits, small dry combs, brittle bones, and long downy feathers. These findings, which resembled those seen in thyroidectomized birds, could be reversed by administration of thyroxine. As a result of continued selection, the incidence of the trait in this closed flock is now over 90% in both males and females. Gross evidence of disease is first seen in OS chickens at about 6 weeks of age. The birds are small, docile, and sensitive to low environmental temperature. The skin has an oily feel, and the plumage is long and silky, like that of juvenile birds (Figure 1). They mature slowly and females do not lay eggs unless their diet is supplemented with thyroid hormones. Their serum shows hyperlipidemia and levels of circulating triiodothyronine (T_3) and thyroxine (T_4) are low. The production of

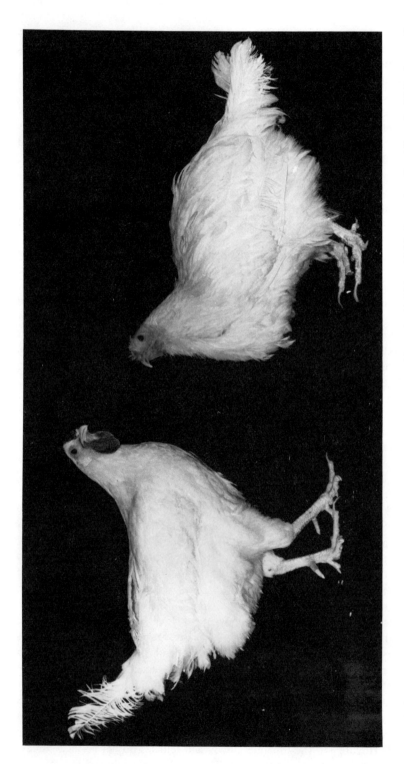

FIGURE 1.   An 18-month-old euthyroid CS hen (left) is compared to an hypothyroid 24-month-old OS hen (right). Due to hypothyroidism, the OS hen has small wattles, long silky feathers, subcutaneous accumulations of fat, and decreased height. (From Rose, N. R., Bacon, L. D., Sundick, R. S., and Kong, Y. M., in *The Menarini Series on Immunopathology: First Symposium on Organ-Specific Autoimmunity*, Vol. 1, Miescher, P. A., Ed., Schwabe & Co., Basel, Switzerland, 1978, 225. With permission.)

thyroid-stimulating hormone (TSH) is elevated. These biochemical changes are already present at 2 to 3 weeks of age.

Histological examination of the thyroid of OS chickens shows extensive infiltration by mononuclear cells and germinal center formation. The normal architecture of the thyroid gland is often obscured, giving the appearance of a lymph node. This lymphoid transformation of the gland accords with Hashimoto's original description of human thyroiditis.

Autoantibodies to chicken thyroid antigen are present in the serum of most of the chickens by 2 to 3 weeks of age. The antibodies, both IgG and IgM, are specific for chicken thyroglobulin (Tg). They do not cross-react with mammalian thyroglobulins. Thyroxine-binding antibodies are present in about 50% of the birds.[17]

Cell-mediated immunity can be demonstrated by injecting crude thyroid extract into the waddle. Swelling becomes evident 24 to 72 h later. Positive waddle reactions were observed in chickens over 12 weeks of age, but seldom in young birds. Since lesions of autoimmune thyroiditis are evident as early as 2 weeks, the waddle test seems to become positive only after thyroid pathology is well established.

A. THE IMMUNE SYSTEM OF THE OBESE STRAIN CHICKEN

A number of immune dysfunctions and abnormalities have been found in the OS chicken (Table 1). Both the T- and B-cell compartments of the chicken immune system affect disease incidence and severity. Early studies showed that a pre- or posthatch bursectomy greatly decreased thyroid infiltration,[18] while neonatal thymectomy increased infiltration and thyroglobulin antibody (Tg Ab) titer.[19,20] This increase suggested a preferential T-suppressor removal from the OS thymus, prompting early researchers to think OS spontaneous autoimmune thyroiditis was primarily a B-cell-mediated disease and to question the role of T cells in disease initiation. However, neonatally thymectomized birds treated in concert with high doses of anti-T-cell serum showed an almost complete abrogation of thyroid infiltration and Tg Ab when examined at an early age.[21] Furthermore, OS bursa cells could not transfer disease to major histocompatibility complex (MHC)-compatible CS chickens. While bursectomized OS did not have severe disease; disease was observed following histocompatible transfers of OS, CS, and (OS × CS) F_1 bursa into bursectomized OS birds.[22] Transfer of OS thymocytes to T-cell-depleted CS chicks induced disease[23] and demonstrated that control of disease is essentially T-cell mediated.

This report[23] also first described the thymocyte and T-cell hyperproliferation that was later found to be characteristic of the OS chicken.[24] This high spontaneous T-cell proliferation is already apparent during embryonic development but is present at later ages as well.[23,24] Spontaneous T-cell proliferation in OS decreases and normalizes over time, but the responses to mitogen increase and at all times are significantly higher than normal white leghorns (NWL) of the same age.[24] This hyperactivity can be demonstrated in thymus,[23] spleen, and peripheral blood cells.[24] Conditioned medium from mitogen-stimulated OS spleen or peripheral blood lymphocytes (PBLs) contain significantly higher amounts of interleukin 2 (IL-2) compared to NWL-conditioned media and less of the so-called suppressor factor (which decreases IL-2-driven chicken blast-cell proliferation when conditioned medium is used at high concentrations).[24] It was further demonstrated by IL-2 absorption studies that OS blasts display increased expression of the IL-2 receptor (IL-2R).[24] OS hyperactivity has also been seen at the effector level as thymectomized OS chicks reject skin grafts from minor histocompatibility antigen disparate donors much faster than similarly treated CS chicks.[25]

The absence, or decreased function, of suppressor T cells in OS thyroiditis has not been clearly demonstrated. Increased T-cell activity following thymectomy at hatching, demonstrable by disease severity[19-21] and allograft rejection,[25] suggests that some suppressor T-cell activity exists in untreated OS chickens. Further evidence for the presence of some suppressor

TABLE 1
Defects of the Obese Strain (OS) Chicken

Defect	Effect of Defect Expression	Genetics
T-cell hyperactivity	High spontaneous proliferation High response to Con A Increased IL-2 secretion following mitogen stimulation Increase in % of PBL that respond to Con A Increased IL-2R expression[22,23,32]	Dominant, not linked to other defects[49,73]
Increased levels of circulating corticosteroid-binding globulin	Decreased levels of hormonally active corticosterone[44]	Recessive, not linked to other defects[49,73]
Decreased corticosterone response to antigenic or GIF challenge	Reduced damping of immune response[48]	Dominant, linked to ev22 occurrence not linked to other defects[49,54]
Hypothymidinemia	Decreased nonspecific suppressor activity in serum and conditioned media[30-32]	Dominant, not linked to other defects[30,35]
Decreased T$_4$ suppressibility of thyroid function	Increased radioiodide uptake and organification of iodide under T$_4$-suppressed conditions[60]	Recessive, not linked to other defects[72,73]
Unspecified target-organ defect	Thyroid infiltration Increased level of serum Tg at hatching[39] Decreased proliferation, function of embryonic thyroid cell cultures[63]	Recessive, not linked to other defects[49,72-74]

Note: Con A = concanavalin A; IL-2 = interleukin 2; PBL = peripheral blood lymphocytes; IL-2R = interleukin-2 receptor; GIF = glucocorticoid-inducing factor; Tg = thyroglobulin; ev22 = endogenous virus, T$_4$ = thyroxine.

cell activity in OS chickens is seen following treatment with the immunosuppressive agent cyclosporin A. Surprisingly, cyclosporin A *in ovo* increased Tg Ab titers and thyroid infiltration, suggesting a selective decrease in immune suppression.[26] Treatment had no effect on disease unless it was administered *in ovo*.[26] However, because avian T-cell subsets are only beginning to be characterized both phenotypically and functionally, the cellular mechanism of disease control remains to be investigated. It was also noted that a deficiency in thymic nurse cells occurs in the OS chicken.[27] The role of these cells in thymic education has not been shown definitively. While it is intriguing to speculate that these cells are involved in tolerance induction or control of premature emigration to the periphery, these functions have not been demonstrated in any animal model.[28,29] The lack of nurse cells may play some role in the mechanism of OS T-cell hyperactivity or in the generation of thyroid antigen-specific T cells.

OS chickens also have a defect in their adherent cell populations.[30,31] As already stated, mitogen-stimulated OS splenocytes proliferate at a much increased rate compared to NWL. Proliferation of mitogen-stimulated NWL cells, when cultured in communication with stimulated OS cells, increased to an intermediate level. Conversely, OS splenocyte proliferation was reduced to this intermediate level when in communication with NWL cells.[30] The effects were attributed to a suppressive factor, termed IL-2 antagonistic activity (IAA), which had a molecular weight <10 KDa and inhibited IL-2-driven proliferation in a noncompetitive manner.[30] Production of IAA was not dependent on the presence of B or T cells and was localized to the macrophage/monocyte populations.[31] Later, it was found that PBLs were not under similar control. Similar cocultivation experiments showed that mitogen-stimulated proliferations of OS or NWL PBLs were not altered when in communication with heterologous activated splenocytes.[32] The activation state of mitogen-stimulated PBLs was assessed using a monoclonal antibody specific for an activated T-cell marker. The monoclonal recognizes an antigen exclusively expressed on activated T cells and is possibly the avian IL-2R.[33,34] More OS PBLs were activated 4 h after mitogen stimulation than OS splenocytes or any NWL cells.[32] At 36 h, OS spleen cell suspensions contained more activated cells than any other population.[32] Furthermore, while IL-2-driven proliferation of OS spleen blast cells was significantly higher than NWL spleen blasts, there was no difference in the PBL blast response of either strain to IL-2.[32] The mechanisms responsible for the differences between the activation characteristics and suppressibility of the different OS T-cell compartments are still under investigation. In view of the fact that conditioned medium made from PBLs contains little of the suppressor factor,[24] the results of the communication chamber experiments are somewhat expected. It was suggested that altered proportions of circulating concanavalin A (Con A)-activatible cells account for the difference between mitogen-induced proliferations of OS and NWL PBLs.[32] More recently, decreased circulating thymidine levels have been implicated as the nonspecific immune modulator lacking in OS chickens.[35] However, as will be discussed in later sections, this is not the sole modulator of OS immune hyperactivity. Further, the importance of any of these differences in autoimmunity has yet to be elucidated.

Analysis of thyroid-infiltrating lymphocytes (TILs) showed that 60% of the cells were T cells and 10% were activated T cells.[33,36] TILs were highly responsive to IL-2 but did not secrete IL-2 at higher levels than other resting lymphocytes.[36] Adoptive transfer experiments showed that OS TILs were more effective than spleen, thymus, or PBLs at transferring disease to irradiated MHC-compatible CS chicks.[36] The antigen specificity of thyroid-infiltrating T cells and the requirement for activated T cells in the diseased state have not been addressed. Chemically bursectomized (cyclophosphamide-treated) OS chicks still developed thyroiditis, although peak lymphoid infiltration occurred later in age and was never as severe as seen in untreated birds.[36] These treated birds showed no Tg Ab, and the percentages of cells infiltrating the thyroid that were surface immunoglobulin (Ig) positive was reduced from 19% to less than 1%. TILs from cyclophosphamide-treated birds were not as effective at transferring disease as TILs from untreated OS birds, but were still significantly better than spleen or thymus. These studies were among the first to demonstrate that lymphocytes infiltrating an autoimmune target organ can transfer organ-specific infiltration and damage to normal recipients.

The importance of B cells in OS thyroiditis should not be ignored. All studies[18-20,22,36,37] have demonstrated an important role for Tg Ab in disease severity, and there is a strong correlation between Tg Ab titer and degree of infiltration.[36-39] Furthermore, cyclophosphamide-treated birds showed a decreased level of infiltration, with peak infiltration occurring much later.[36] Other B-cell associated abnormalities have been seen in the OS chicken. These include an increase in B:T ratios compared to normal chickens[40] and an increase in Fc receptor (FcR)-bearing cells.[41] Whether some of the FcR$^+$ cells are B or T cells susceptible to FcR-mediated immunoregulation or are cells capable of antibody-dependent cellular cytotoxicity (ADCC) has not been addressed. Autoantibodies to chicken erythrocyte nuclei and other organs have also been found in the OS chicken.[42,43] It is possible that the existence of these antibodies is due to a polyclonal B-cell activation. In fact, no other autoimmune disease attributable to these antibodies has been found associated with the OS chicken. OS T-cell hyperfunction and lymphokine secretion may affect B-cell responses to external antigens. Although antibody responses following immunizations seen thus far have not demonstrated any differences in antibody titer or response times between OS and other normal chicken strains,[44] lymphokines secreted by hyperactive T cells might modulate preferential class switching, antigen-presenting capabilities, or B-cell activity and differentiation in general.

OS thyroid glands have been shown to display class II (B-L) MHC molecules on their surface.[45] While this is most likely secondary to lymphoid infiltration and lymphokine secretion, these class II molecules on thyroid epithelial cells or other cells in the thyroid could be presenting thyroglobulin or other antigenic fragments and thus serve as a source of ongoing stimulation.

B. NEUROENDOCRINE COMMUNICATION

The neuroendocrine system of the OS chicken has also been shown to be defective in some regulatory aspects. Circulating corticosterone levels have been shown to be of importance in regulation of general immune activity.[46] The OS chicken has increased levels of corticosteroid-binding globulin (CBG), while levels of total serum corticosterone (CN) are normal.[44] Therefore, OS chickens have lower levels of hormonally active CN. The binding affinity and physicochemical properties of the OS CBG are indistinguishable from CBG of normal chickens.[44,47] Additionally, the affinity of CN receptors on lymphoid tissues do not differ between OS and normal strains.[44,47] The lower level of hormonally active CN can be corrected by injection of cortisol. This treatment decreases thyroid infiltration *in vivo* by greater than 50% and reduces *in vitro* mitogen responses and IL-2 secretion to normal levels.[44] A further defect in neuroendocrine response is the lack of a transitory increase in CN following antigenic challenge, a phenomenon that is consistently observed in normal animals.[48] Injections of conditioned media from mitogen-stimulated splenocytes caused a dose-dependent increase in CN in both OS and normal chickens. The OS levels, however, were consistently lower.[48] The defect was not in the production of the glucocorticoid-inducing factor (GIF) since conditioned media produced by normal or OS splenocytes were equally effective at stimulating a CN increase.[48] Injections of synthetic adrenocorticotropic hormone (ACTH) were equally effective in both normal and OS chickens in increasing plasma corticosterone levels.[49,50] Thus, the defect in GIF hyporesponsiveness lies in the ability of the hypothalamo-hypophysial axis to stimulate the adrenal gland and not in the ability of the adrenal gland to produce corticosterone.

C. VIRAL AGENTS IN DISEASE ETIOLOGY

The role of viral pathogens in autoimmunity has been speculated upon in a number of autoimmune diseases.[51,52] Virus-like particles have been seen with the electron microscope in OS-chicken thyroid glands.[53] However, no productive infection has even been seen, and no causal relationship has ever been drawn between these particles and thyroiditis. More recently, an endogenous virus, ev22, has been identified using a Rous Sarcoma virus probe.[54] These viral sequences are found on a 5.5 kilobase (kb) SacI fragment and have only been seen in OS chickens. There is a correlation between ev22 and the OS-decreased corticosterone response, which will be discussed later. Nevertheless, there is no strict correlation between ev22[+] animals and disease incidence.

There are two autoimmune conditions in chickens known to be caused by viruses. Marek's disease virus (MDV)-infected chickens develop a peripheral neuritis.[55] MDV causes a general T-lymphocyte proliferative disorder, but some evidence exists for an antigen-specific attack. Chickens infected with MDV show a delayed-type hypersensitivity (DTH) to injected myelin.[56] Furthermore, adoptive transfer of splenocytes from infected chickens caused disease in recipients faster than infection with MDV.[57] The mechanism of autosensitization is unknown, but data suggest a nonspecific immunosuppression in MDV-infected birds.[55] The other virus-induced autoimmunity is produced by *in ovo* infection with Rous-associated virus type 7 (RAV-7) and leads to thyroiditis and pancreatitis in infected birds.[14,58] Chickens infected *in ovo* are characterized as obese with hyperlipidemia and high levels of fat deposits in the liver.[14] At 3 weeks, chickens are much smaller than uninfected hatchmates, and their thyroids show extensive infiltration.[14] However, no Tg Ab was detected in these chickens. Immunologic attack of the pancreas also occurs, another important difference between this model and OS chicken autoimmunity. RAV-7-infected chicks show low serum T_3 and T_4 and somewhat higher insulin levels. Treatment with T_4 can reduce some, but not all, of the disease symptoms.[58] Though no connection has yet been shown between viruses and OS thyroiditis, these studies suggest that viruses can be an important etiological agent in avian autoimmunity.

D. TARGET ORGAN DEFECTS

The thyroid gland of the OS chicken has a number of characteristics which distinguish it from a normal thyroid gland. The most prominent is its ability to function autonomously of pituitary stimulation. Under conditions of T_4 suppression, when synthesis of TSH is normally shut off, OS thyroid glands are still capable of radioiodide uptake.[59] This feature is shared with the CS, the parent strain of the OS.[59] The TSH autonomy is not due to the presence of thyroid-stimulating antibodies since transfer of OS serum did not increase T_4-suppressed iodide uptake in NWL chickens.[60] It is also not due to faulty TSH regulation since transplantation of OS thyroids to normal chicken chorioallantoic membranes[61] and to wing webs of normal adult chickens[62] did not alter the ability of the OS thyroids to incorporate more radioiodine than their normal transplanted counterparts. CS characteristically exhibits even greater thyroid autonomy than OS, and both are able to utilize the iodide for synthesis of T_3, T_4, and Tg.[59] Immunosuppression by cyclophosphamide treatment did not affect TSH autonomy,[59] again suggesting that autonomy was not due to the production of thyroid-stimulating antibodies.

Short-term cultures of embryonic thyroid glands also provided evidence for an organ defect. Uptake of tritiated thymidine, both for total cultures and on a per cell basis, was much lower for OS cultures than for CS and other strains.[63] The growth rate of OS thyroid cells in culture was much lower than CS cultures,[63] while there was no difference between OS and CS strains in the growth rates of other cells such as fibroblasts or myocytes. The addition of CS thyroid culture-conditioned media to OS cultures increased the growth rate and thymidine incorporation to CS culture levels.[63] Addition of OS thyroid-conditioned medium increased OS growth slightly but was far less effective than CS thyroid-conditioned medium,[63] suggesting that OS thyroid cells in culture are unable to "condition" their media.

Since thyroglobulin is the main autoantigen seen in OS chickens, Tg levels were examined in OS chickens to determine if the lack of tolerance induction was due to a decrease in circulating antigen. In fact, at hatching, OS circulating Tg levels were as much as three times the normal level.[38] These levels decreased over time up until 4 weeks, at which time cyclophosphamide-treated OS chickens had normal circulating Tg levels.[38] Binding of OS Tg Abs to OS Tg and Tg of other strains were compared to determine if any unique immunogenic epitopes exist on OS Tg. While there was a considerable degree of variation in the antibody titers and avidities of individual OS birds, there was no difference among the binding capacities for OS, CS, or normal strain Tg.[38] It is interesting to note that, in a manner similar to bursectomy, induction of tolerance to Tg greatly reduces disease severity.[39] Tolerance can be induced by a single high dose (1 to 2 mg) of Tg and is most efficacious during the first 12 h after hatch.[39]

Iodide itself is very important for disease development. CS chickens kept on a high iodide diet develop thyroiditis more rapidly than the same chicks on a normal diet.[17] CS chickens, which are susceptible to a late onset thyroiditis have naturally occurring auto-antibodies to T_3, T_4, and Tg and develop thyroiditis as adults.[64] T_4, which suppresses thyroid function, decreased OS disease severity at the early stages, but by 4 weeks had little effect.[17,38] T_4 administered simultaneously with potassium perchlorate (KClO$_4$), which inhibits active transport of iodide into the thyroid, was an effective regimen at preventing disease[65] and reducing antibody to T_4[17] and to highly iodinated Tg.[66] This evidence seems to suggest that the iodination of Tg is important in disease induction. Treatment with propylthiouracil (PTU), which prevents iodination of Tg by inhibiting thyroid peroxidase, is very effective at preventing disease.[67] Immunization of normal chicks with high iodide (HI) Tg (>60 I atoms per Tg molecule) and low iodide (LI) Tg (<13 I atoms per Tg molecule) without any adjuvant demonstrated that higly iodinated Tg was a much better immunogen.[66] Antibody from groups immunized with HI-Tg reacted with HI-Tg much better than antibody from groups immunized with LI-Tg. Neither group was particularly effective at producing antibodies reactive with LI-Tg. Additionally, HI-Tg immunized birds had significantly higher titers of antibody to T_3 and T_4.[66] In binding studies of HI-Tg antibody, 100 times the concentration of LI-Tg was needed to inhibit binding to HI-Tg and while T_4 could inhibit binding. T_3 could not.[66] In view of these results, it was enticing to speculate that the OS chicken made a highly iodinated, highly immunogenic form of the Tg molecule. However, OS serum was found to bind LI-Tg more effectively than HI-Tg, and binding to HI-Tg or LI-Tg was equally inhibited by both forms of Tg.[66] The reason for the strong OS response to LI-Tg is yet to be understood.

As already stated, alteration of various stages of thyroid function can inhibit disease. More recently, butylated hydroxyanisole (BHA) has been shown to significantly decrease OS thyroiditis.[67] BHA is an antioxidant and has no effects on either thyroid function or the immune system. The prevention of thyroiditis is only seen when BHA is administered from hatching, again demonstrating that an early event is responsible for disease induction.[67] The role of free oxygen radicals in OS thyroiditis is still speculative, but it will be interesting to see if other antioxidants have a similar effect. Additionally, other thyrostatic drugs can be used to elucidate the pathway of OS thyroid dysfunction and determine which, if any, of the thyroid functional abnormalities contribute to autosensitization or activation of the immune system.

E. GENETICS OF THE OBESE STRAIN CHICKEN

The MHC has typically been important in autoimmune conditions in determining the susceptibility of the strain to disease. Three MHC haplotypes, B^5, B^{13}, and B^{15}, have been identified in OS chickens with spontaneous autoimmune thyroiditis.[68] B^{13} has consistently been associated with severe disease,[69-71] and B^{15} has been associated with moderate to severe disease.[68-71] Birds with B^5 were first found to be low responders by Bacon et al.,[69] however, later inbreeding by Halà[68] demonstrated B^5 birds with severe disease probably due to the effect of non-MHC genes. While MHC haplotype can affect disease incidence and severity in birds within closed breeding studies,[69] there is no haplotype that has consistently conferred a low or nonresponder phenotype in the OS chicken. Breeding of OS ($B^{15}B^{15}$) and CB ($B^{12}B^{12}$), an inbred normal strain, yielded heterozygous F_1 chicks ($B^{12}B^{15}$) which did not develop thyroiditis. $F_1 \times$ OS backcrosses indicated that MHC could affect the time of disease onset, since $B^{12}B^{15}$ developed SAT later than $B^{15}B^{15}$ chicks.[72] However, this distinction is not absolute, and in the (OS $\times$ CB) F_2, homozygous B^{12} chicks developed thyroiditis and Tg Ab at the same frequency as heterozygous or B^{15} homozygous chicks.[72,73] Additionally, a lack of correlation has been shown between haplotype and other OS dysfunctions such as T-cell hyperactivity, increased levels of circulating corticosteroid-binding globulin, decreased corticosterone response, and occurrence of ev22.[49,73]

Disease occurrence is a recessive trait. F_1 from matings of OS with normal chickens do not develop disease.[72,74] Thyroiditis developed in 20 to 57% of the $F_1 \times$ OS backcrosses, while about 25% of (OS $\times$ CB) F_2 developed the disease.[72-74] This suggests that a single recessive gene might be responsible for disease induction, although the occurrence of thyroiditis in backcrosses is more variable than would be expected. Since the varying values are from studies which were performed at different times, other factors not controlled in these studies (such as iodine intake or genetic drift in the birds studied) might affect disease initiation.

The T-cell hyperactivity characteristic of OS chickens is a dominant trait. All (OS × CB) F_1 and three fourths of F_2 display this trait.[49,73] This locus seems to control all OS T-cell hyperfunctions including mitogen response, increased IL-2 secretion, and increased numbers of Con A activatible peripheral blood cells.[49] The low IL-2 antagonistic activity found in obese chickens is also a dominant trait.[30] It is not linked, nor is it the trait responsible for T-cell hyperfunction.[35] While the T-cell hyperfunction locus appears to show single gene autosomal dominant inheritance patterns, some evidence suggests a more complex case. IL-2 secretion by (OS × CB) F_1 × CB backcross shows intermediate levels in conditioned media.[49] This incomplete dominance indicates a more complicated mechanism controlling some T-cell functions. T-cell hyperactivity is not correlated with any MHC haplotype or OS neuroendocrine dysfunctions.[49,73] It can be correlated to a small degree with disease in F_2 birds which develop low-level thyroiditis.[73]

Increased uptake of radioiodine under T_4-suppressed conditions is a recessive trait.[74] This defect is not seen in (OS × CB) F_1, but is observed in about one half of F_1 × OS backcrosses.[73,74] In sharp contrast, F_1 of a CS × RLR mating show an intermediate level of radioiodide uptake under T_4 suppression.[62] This can be explained since CS are less suppressible by T_4 than OS.[59] While the OS may only have one recessive gene controlling this trait, the CS may have one or more genes showing dominance or incomplete dominance in the F_1. High radioiodide uptake was not correlated with thyroid infiltration or MHC in the F_1 × OS backcross.[73] However, it is technically difficult to assess infiltration in a bird treated with T_4, since it tends to reduce infiltration in some OS chickens.[38]

The two neuroendocrine dysfunctions segregate independently.[49] Increased circulating CBG is controlled by a single recessive gene. One quarter of F_2 have high CBG.[73] While there is no correlation in F_1 × OS backcrosses, some correlation exists between severe thyroiditis and high CBG in F_2 birds.[73] The defect in corticosterone response is a dominant trait and does not cosegregate with MHC haplotype or T-cell hyperactivity.[49] This defect does correlate with occurrence of ev22.[49] ev22 is seen in 80% of F_2 birds with severe thyroiditis.[73]

The lack of segregation of OS defects is not surprising, considering the large number of relatively small chicken chromosomes. Decreased CN response, which is correlated with ev22, is likely caused by alteration of gene expression following retroviral integration.[54] The other important observation which can be made from independent segregation of various OS dysfunctions is that these defects are primary defects in the OS chicken and do not arise as a result of autoimmunity.[73] Many of these defects contribute to spontaneous autoimmune thyroiditis in OS chicks, but the one crucial genetically determined feature for autoimmune induction remains elusive.

F. DISCUSSION: THE "THREE-GENE" CONCEPT IN RETROSPECT

Some years ago, these authors suggested that spontaneous autoimmune thyroiditis in the chicken depends upon the conjunction of at least three types of genetic lesions that have been fixed in the OS by selective breeding.[75] These genetic lesions include, as a minimum, heightened immune response to thyroglobulin, disordered thymic maturation, and abnormality of the thyroid gland. The greatest probability of disease occurs in birds with all these lesions; autoimmunity without disease or sporadic disease may be seen in chickens with one or two of these genetic traits.

This concept of multiple, unrelated genes accounting for susceptibility to spontaneous thyroiditis has been strengthened by the results described in this article. MHC-association immune response genes probably influence the severity of disease by controlling immune recognition to Tg. CS birds with "high responder" MHC genes, however, rarely develop thyroiditis emphasizing the view that MHC genes alone are insufficient to initiate disease. Abnormalities in thymus functions and resultant hyperactive T cells are characteristic of the OS flock. Although thyroiditis is the only autoimmune disease evident in OS chickens, autoantibodies to several other tissues have been identified. The thyroid gland itself shows intrinsic abnormalities. Additional genetic and nongenetic traits, such as raised levels of CBG and IL-2, also contribute to the occurrence of disease. Environmental factors further complicate the picture, and they include dietary iodine and possibly virus infection.

V. SUMMARY

The chicken offers a number of advantages for studies of autoimmune diseases. The anatomical separation of the T-cell and B-cell compartments facilitates examination of the relative contributions of the two arms of the immune response. Among the examples of genetically determined autoimmune diseases in chickens are the Smyth-DAM line, which develop amelanosis resembling human vitiligo, and the UCD line 200 chicken which develops progressive systemic sclerosis. The best-studied autoimmune disease of chickens is the hypothyroid-obesity syndrome of the OS line. These symptoms are attributable to a severe form of autoimmune thyroiditis characterized by lymphoid transformation of the thyroid and formation of autoantibodies to thyroglobulin. The disease is associated with a number of genetic traits, including MHC-related immune response genes, thymus and T-cell abnormalities, altered lymphokine production, and intrinsic defects of the thyroid gland.

As with any spontaneous autoimmune condition, an important goal of research into these avian diseases is to understand the mechanisms of autoimmune initiation and disease progression. Target-organ defects in the form of altered organ proteins, increased antigen presentation, or aberrant cellular metabolism or gene expression will likely be identified as research into these autoimmune diseases continues. Additionally, recent advances in basic avian immunology (including identification of avian T-cell markers and T-cell receptor classes, and cloning of immunoglobulin, T-cell receptor, and class II MHC genes) will undoubtedly impact on avian autoimmunity. Hopefully, they will aid in identification of T-cell subsets and other immune components involved in the development of these autoimmune diseases.

ACKNOWLEDGMENTS

Helpful discussions with Konrad Schauenstein are gratefully acknowledged. Portions of the research described in this review were supported by NIH grant DK 20028, and preparation of the review was aided by NIH grant R01AR31632-07.

REFERENCES

1. **Jankovic, B. D. and Isvaneski, M.,** Experimental allergic encaphalomyelitis in thymectomized, bursectomized and normal chickens, *Int. Arch. Allergy,* 23, 188, 1963.
2. **Bolton, W. K., Tucek, F. L., and Sturgill, B. C.,** Experimental autoimmune glomerulonephritis in chickens, *J. Clin. Lab. Immunol.,* 3, 179, 1980.
3. **Jankovic, B. D., Isvaneski, M., Popeskovic, L., and Mitrovic, K.,** Experimental allergic thyroiditis (and parathyroiditis) in neonatally thymectomized and bursectomized chickens. Participation of the thymus in the development of disease, *Int. Arch. Allergy,* 26, 18, 1965.
4. **Smyth, J. R., Jr., Boissy, R. E., and Fite, K. V.,** The DAM chicken: a spontaneous postnatal cutaneous and ocular amelanosis, *J. Hered.,* 72, 150, 1981.

5. **Lamont, S. J. and Smyth, J. R., Jr.,** Effect of bursectomy on development of a spontaneous postnatal amelanosis, *Clin. Immunol. Immunopathol.*, 21, 407, 1981.
6. **Lamont, S. J., Boissy, R. E., and Smyth, J. R., Jr.,** Humoral immune response and expression of spontaneous postnatal amelanosis in DAM line chickens, *Immunol. Commun.*, 11, 121, 1982.
7. **Boyle, M. L., III, Pardue, S. L., and Smyth, J. R., Jr.,** The effects of corticosterone on amelanosis in the DAM (Smyth) line chicken, *Poult. Sci.*, 64, (Suppl. 1), 69, 1985.
8. **Pardue, S. L., Fite, K. V., Bengston, L., Lamont, S. J., Boyle, M. L., III, and Smyth, J. R., Jr.,** Enhanced integumental and ocular amelanosis following the termination of cyclosporine administration, *J. Invest. Dermatol.*, 88, 758, 1987.
9. **Boissy, R. E., Smyth, J. R., Jr., and Fite, K. V.,** Progressive cytologic changes during the development of delayed feather amelanosis and associated choroidal defects in the DAM chicken line, *Am. J. Pathol.*, 111, 197, 1983.
10. **Gershwin, M. E., Abplanalp, H., Castles, J. J., Ikeda, R. M., Van der Water, J., Eklund, J., and Haynes, D.,** Characterization of a spontaneous disease of white leghorn chickens resembling progressing systemic sclerosis (scleroderma), *J. Exp. Med.*, 153, 1640, 1981.
11. **Van der Water, J. and Gershwin, M. E.,** Avian scleroderma: an inherited fibrotic disease of white leghorn chickens resembling progressive systemic sclerosis, *Am. J. Pathol.*, 120, 478, 1985.
12. **Van der Water, J., Haapanen, L., Boyd, R., Abplanalp, H., and Gershwin, M. E.,** Identification of T cells in early dermal infiltrates in avian scleroderma, *Arthritis Rheum.*, 32, 1031, 1989.
13. **Haynes, D. C. and Gershwin, M. E.,** Diversity of autoantibodies in avian scleroderma: an inherited fibrotic disease of white leghorn chickens, *J. Clin. Invest.*, 73, 1557, 1984.
14. **Carter, J. K., Ow, C. L., and Smith, R. E.,** Rous-associated virus type 7 induces a syndrome in chickens characterized by stunting and obesity, *Infect. Immun.*, 39, 410, 1983.
15. **Cole, R. K.,** Hereditary hypothyroidism in the domestic fowl, *Genetics*, 53, 1021, 1966.
16. **Van Tienhoven, A. and Cole, R. K.,** Endocrine disturbances in Obese chickens, *Anat. Rec.*, 142, 111, 1962.
17. **Bagchi, N., Brown, T. R., Urdanivia, E., and Sundick, R. S.,** Induction of autoimmune thyroiditis in chickens by dietary iodine, *Science*, 230, 325, 1985.
18. **Wick, G., Kite, J. H., Jr., Cole, R. K., and Witebsky, E.,** Spontaneous thyroiditis in the Obese strain of chicken. III. The effect of bursectomy on the development of disease, *J. Immunol.*, 104, 45, 1970.
19. **Welch, P., Rose, N. R., and Kite, J. H., Jr.,** Neonatal thymectomy increases spontaneous autoimmune thyroiditis, *J. Immunol.*, 110, 575, 1973.
20. **Wick, G., Kite, J. H., Jr., and Witebsky, E.,** Spontaneous thyroiditis in the Obese strain of chicken. IV. The effect of thymectomy and thymo-bursectomy on the development of disease, *J. Immunol.*, 104, 54, 1970.
21. **Pontes de Carvalho, L. C., Wick, G., and Roitt, I. M.,** Requirement of T cells for the development of spontaneous autoimmune thyroiditis in the Obese strain (OS) chickens, *J. Immunol.*, 126, 750, 1981.
22. **Polley, C. R., Bacon, L. D., and Rose, N. R.,** Spontaneous autoimmune thyroiditis in chickens. I. The effect of bursal reconstitution, *J. Immunol.*, 127, 1465, 1981.
23. **Livezey, M. D., Sundick, R. S., and Rose, N. R.,** Spontaneous autoimmune thyroiditis in chickens. II. Evidence for autoresponsive thymocytes, *J. Immunol.*, 127, 1469, 1981.
24. **Schauenstein, K., Krömer, G., Sundick, R. S., and Wick, G.,** Enhanced response to Con A and production of TCGF by lymphocytes of Obese strain (OS) chickens with spontaneous autoimmune thyroiditis, *J. Immunol.*, 134, 872, 1985.
25. **Jakobisiak, M., Sundick, R. S., Bacon, L. D., and Rose, N. R.,** Abnormal response to minor histocompatability antigens in Obese strain chickens, *Proc. Natl. Acad. Sci. U.S.A.*, 73, 2877, 1976.
26. **Wick, G., Muller, P.-U., and Schwarz, S.,** Effect of cyclosporin A on spontaneous autoimmune thyroiditis of Obese strain (OS) chickens, *Eur. J. Immunol.*, 12, 877, 1982.
27. **Boyd, R. L., Oberhüber, G., Halà, K., and Wick, G.,** Obese strain (OS) chickens with spontaneous autoimmune thyroiditis have a deficiency in thymic nurse cells, *J. Immunol.*, 132, 718, 1984.
28. **Wekerle, H. and Ketelsen, U.-P.,** Thymic nurse cells — Ia-bearing epithelium involved in T lymphocyte differentiation, *Nature (London)*, 283, 402, 1980.
29. **Wekerle, H., Ketelsen, U.-P., and Ernst, M.,** Thymic nurse cells. Lymphoepithelial cell complexes in murine thymuses: morphological and serological characterization, *J. Exp. Med.*, 151, 925, 1980.
30. **Krömer, G., Schauenstein, K., Neu, N., Stricker, K., and Wick, G.,** In vitro T cell hyperactivity in Obese strain chickens is due to a defect in nonspecific suppressor mechanisms, *J. Immunol.*, 135, 2458, 1985.
31. **Krömer, G., Schauenstein, K., Dietrich, H., Fassler, R., and Wick, G.,** Mechanisms of T cell hyperactivity in Obese strain chickens with spontaneous autoimmune thyroiditis: lack in nonspecific suppression is due to a primary adherant cell defect, *J. Immunol.*, 138, 2104, 1987.

32. **Schauenstein, K., Krömer, G., Bock, G., Rossi, K., Halà, K., and Wick, G.,** T cell hyperactivity in Obese strain (OS) chickens: different mechanisms operative in spleen and peripheral blood lymphocyte activation, *Immunobiology*, 175, 226, 1987.

33. **Halà, K., Schauenstein, K., Neu, N., Krömer, G., Wolf, H., Bock, G., and Wick, G.,** A monoclonal antibody reacting with a membrane determinant on activated chicken T lymphocytes, *Eur. J. Immunol.*, 16, 1331, 1986.

34. **Schauenstein, K., Krömer, G., Halà, K., Bock, G., and Wick, G.,** Chicken activated T lymphocyte antigen (CATLA) recognized by monoclonal antibody INN-CH16 represents the IL-2 receptor, *Dev. Comp. Immunol.*, 12, 823, 1988.

35. **Krömer, G., Klocker, H., Fässler, R., Sachsenmaier, W., and Wick, G.,** Decreased levels of thymidine in the serum of Obese strain (OS) chickens with spontaneous autoimmune thyroiditis, *Immunol. Invest.*, 17, 243, 1988.

36. **Krömer, G., Sundick, R. S., Schauenstein, K., Halà, K., and Wick, G.,** Analysis of lymphocytes infiltrating the thyroid gland of Obese strain chickens, *J. Immunol.*, 135, 2452, 1985.

37. **Jaroszewski, M., Sundick, R. S., and Rose, N. R.,** Effects of antiserum containing thyroglobulin antibody on the chicken thyroid gland, *Clin. Immunol. Immunopathol.*, 10, 95, 1978.

38. **Sanker, A. J., Sundick, R. S., and Brown, T. R.,** Analyses of the serum concentrations and antigenic determinants of thyroglobulin in chickens susceptible to autoimmune thyroiditis, *J. Immunol.*, 131, 1252, 1983.

39. **Sanker, A. J., Clark, C. R., and Sundick, R. S.,** The induction of tolerance to thyroglobulin significantly reduces the severity of thyroiditis in Obese strain chickens, *J. Immunol.*, 135, 281, 1985.

40. **Albini, B. and Wick, G.,** Proportional increase of bursa-derived cells in chickens of the Obese strain, *Nature (London)*, 249, 653, 1974.

41. **Nowak, J. S., Bacon, L. D., and Rose, N. R.,** Fc receptor bearing lymphoid cells in the chicken. II. Relative increase of Fc (IgG) receptor bearing cells in Obese strain chickens, *Immunol. Commun.*, 7, 621, 1978.

42. **Albini, B. and Wick, G.,** Erythrocyte-specific anti-nuclear factors in chickens of the Obese strain (OS), *Immunology*, 21, 957, 1971.

43. **Khoury, E. L., Bottazzo, G. F., Pontes de Carvalho, L. C., Wick, G., and Roitt, I. M.,** Predisposition to organ-specific autoimmunity in Obese strain (OS) chickens: reactivity to thyroid, gastric, adrenal and pancreatic cytoplasmic antigens, *Clin. Exp. Immunol.*, 49, 273, 1982.

44. **Fässler, R., Schauenstein, K., Krömer, G., Schwarz, S., and Wick, G.,** Elevation of corticosteroid-binding globulin in Obese strain (OS) chickens: possible implications for the disturbed immunoregulation and the development of spontaneous autoimmune thyroiditis, *J. Immunol.*, 136, 3657, 1986.

45. **Wick, G., Halà, K., Wolf, H., Boyd, R. L., and Schauenstein, K.,** Distribution and functional analysis of B-L/Ia positive cells in the chicken: expression of B-L/Ia antigens on thyroid epithelial cells in spontaneous autoimmune thyroiditis, *Mol. Immunol.*, 21, 1259, 1984.

46. **Besedovsky, H. O., Rey, A.del., and Sorkin, E.,** Integration of activated immune cell products in immune-endocrine feedback circuits, *Prog. Leukocyte Biol.*, 5, 197, 1986.

47. **Fässler, R., Dietrich, H., Krömer, G., Schwarz, S., Brezinschek, H. P., and Wick, G.,** Diminished glucocorticoid tonus in Obese strain (OS) chickens with spontaneous autoimmune thyroiditis: increased plasma levels of a physicochemically unaltered corticosteroid binding globulin but normal total corticosterone plasma concentration and normal glucocortoid receptor contents in lymphoid tissue, *J. Steroid Biochem.*, 30, 375, 1988.

48. **Schauenstein, K., Fässler, R., Dietrich, H., Schwarz, S., Krömer, G., and Wick, G.,** Disturbed immune-endocrine communication in autoimmune disease: lack of corticosterone response to immune signals in Obese strain chickens with spontaneous autoimmune thyroiditis, *J. Immunol.*, 139, 1830, 1987.

49. **Krömer, G., Fassler, R., Halà, K., Bock, G., Schauenstein, K., Brezinschek, H. P., Neu, N., Dietrich, H., Jakober, R., and Wick, G.,** Genetic analysis of extrathyroidal features of Obese strain (OS) chickens with spontaneous autoimmune thyroiditis, *Eur. J. Immunol.*, 18, 1499, 1988.

50. **Krömer, G., Brezinschek, H. P., Fässler, R., Schauenstein, K., and Wick, G.,** Physiology and pathology of an immunoendocrine feedback loop, *Immunol. Today*, 9, 163, 1988.

51. **McChesney, M. B. and Oldstone, M. B. A.,** Viruses perturb lymphocyte functions: selected principles characterizing virus-induced immunosuppression, *Annu. Rev. Immunol.*, 5, 279, 1987.

52. **Fujinami, R. S.,** Virus-induced autoimmunity through molecular mimicry, *Ann. N.Y. Acad. Sci.*, 540, 210, 1988.

53. **Wick, G. and Graf, J.,** Electron microscopic studies in chickens of the Obese strain with spontaneous hereditary autoimmune thyroiditis, *Lab. Invest.* 27, 400, 1972.

54. **Ziemiecki, A., Krömer, G., Mueller, R. G., Halà, K., and Wick, G.,** ev22, a new endogenous avian leukosis virus locus found in chickens with spontaneous autoimmune thyroiditis, *Arch. Virol.*, 100, 267, 1988.

55. **Payne, L. N., Frazier, J. A., and Powell, P. C.,** Pathogenesis of Marek's disease, *Int. Rev. Exp. Pathol.*, 16, 59, 1976.
56. **Schmahl, W., Hoffmann-Fezer, G., and Hoffmann, R.,** Zur pathogenese der Nervenlesionen bei Marekscher Krankheit des Huhnes. I. Allergische Hautreaktion gegen myelin Periphererernerven, *Z. Immunitaetsforsch. Exp. Clin. Immunol.*, 150, 175, 1975.
57. **Hoffmann-Fezer, G., Schmahl, W., and Hoffmann, R.,** Zur Pathogenese der Nervenlesionen bei Marekscher Krankheit des Huhnes. II. Ubertragbarketi von Nervenveranderungen mit milzzellen Marek-kranker Tiere, *Z. Immunitaetsforsch. Exp. Clin. Immunol.*, 150, 300, 1975.
58. **Carter, J. K. and Smith, R. E.,** Rapid induction of hypothyroidism by an avian leukosis virus, *Infect. Immun.*, 40, 795, 1983.
59. **Sundick, R. S., Bagchi, N., Livezey, M. D., Brown, T. R., and Mack, R. E.,** Abnormal thyroid regulation in chickens with autoimmune thyroiditis, *Endocrinology*, 105, 493, 1979.
60. **Sundick, R. S. and Wick, G.,** Increased 131-I uptake by the thyroid glands of Obese strain (OS) chickens derived from nonprotomone supplemented hens, *Clin. Exp. Immunol.*, 18, 127, 1974.
61. **Sundick, R. S. and Wick, G.,** Increased iodine uptake by Obese strain thyroid glands transplanted to normal chick embryos, *J. Immunol.*, 116, 1319, 1976.
62. **Livezey, M. D. and Sundick, R. S.,** Intrinsic thyroid hyperactivity in avian strains susceptible to autoimmune thyroiditis, *Dev. Comp. Endocrinol.*, 41, 243, 1980.
63. **Truden, J. L., Sundick, R. S., Levine, S., and Rose, N. R.,** The decreased growth rate of Obese strain (OS) chicken thyroid cells provides *in vitro* evidence for a primary organ abnormality in chickens susceptible to autoimmune thyroiditis, *Clin. Immunol. Immunopathol.*, 29, 294, 1983.
64. **Brown, T. R., Bagchi, N., and Sundick, R. S.,** Analysis of triiodothyronine and thyroxine binding autoantibodies in chickens susceptible to autoimmune thyroiditis, *J. Immunol.*, 134, 3845, 1985.
65. **Sundick, R. S., Herdegen, D. M., Brown, T. R., and Bagchi, N.,** Iodine depletion reduces thyroiditis in Obese strain chickens, *Endocrinology*, 121, T53, 1988.
66. **Sundick, R. S., Herdegen, D., Brown, T. R., and Bagchi, N.,** The incorporation of dietary iodine into thyroglobulin increases its immunogenicity, *Endocrinology*, 120, 2078, 1987.
67. **Bagchi, N., Brown, T. R., Herdegen, D. M., and Sundick, R. S.,** The Antioxidant Butylated Hydroxyanisole Reduces Thyroiditis in Obese Strain Chickens, Program Abstr. 71st Annu. Meet. Endocrine Soc., The Endocrine Society, Seattle, Washington, 1989, 478.
68. **Halà, K.,** Hypothesis: immunogenetic analysis of spontaneous autoimmune thyroiditis in Obese strain chickens: a two-gene family model, *Immunobiology*, 177, 354, 1988.
69. **Bacon, L. D., Polley, C. R., Cole, R. K., and Rose, N. R.,** Genetic influences on spontaneous autoimmune thyroiditis in (CS × OS) F_2 chickens, *Immunogenetics*, 12, 339, 1981.
70. **Bacon, L. D., Kite, J. H., and Rose, N. R.,** Relation between the major histocompatability (B) locus and autoimmune thyroiditis in Obese chickens, *Science*, 186, 274, 1974.
71. **Wick, G., Gundolf, R., and Halà, K.,** Genetic factors in spontaneous autoimmune thyroiditis in OS chickens, *J. Immunogenet.*, 6, 177, 1979.
72. **Neu, N., Halà, K., Dietrich, H., and Wick, G.,** Genetic background of spontaneous autoimmune thyroiditis in the Obese strain of chickens studied in hybrids with an inbred line, *Int. Arch. Allergy Appl. Immunology*, 80, 168, 1986.
73. **Krömer, G., Neu, N., Kuehr, T., Dietrich, H., Fässler, R., Halà, K., and Wick, G.,** Immunogenetic analysis of spontaneous autoimmune thyroiditis of Obese strain chickens, *Clin. Immunol. Immunopathol.*, 52, 202, 1989.
74. **Neu, N., Halà, K., Dietrich, H., and Wick, G.,** Spontaneous autoimmune thyroiditis in Obese strain chickens: a genetic analysis of target organ abnormalities, *Clin. Immunol. Immunopathol.*, 37, 397, 1985.
75. **Rose, N. R., Bacon, L. D., and Sundick, R. S.,** Genetic determinants of thyroiditis in the OS chicken, *Transplant. Rev.*, 31, 264, 1976.
76. **Rose, N. R., Bacon, L. D., Sundick, R. S., and Kong, Y. M.,** The role of genetic factors in autoimmunity, in *The Menarini Series on Immunopathology: First Symposium on Organ Specific Autoimmunity*, Vol. 1, Miescher, P. A., Ed., Schwabe & Co., Basel, Switzerland, 1978, 225.

INDEX

A

Acid phosphatase, 75
ACTH, see Adrenocorticotropic hormone
ADCC, see Antibody-dependent cell-mediated
    cytotoxicity
Adenovirus, 83, 140
Adhesion molecules, 15
Adrenocorticotropic hormone (ACTH), 190
Aflatoxin-B, 87
Agammaglobulinemia, 98, 103—109
Allergies, 120, see also specific types by name
Alloantigens, 126
Allogeneic cells, 126, 127
Allogeneic skin grafts, 124
Allogeneic transplants, 123
Allografts, 124, 127, 147
Allotype immune suppression, 103
Allotypic markers, 10
ALS, see Avian leukosis and sarcoma
Antibodies, 2, see also specific types by name
  anticytoplasmic, 185
  antinuclear, 185
  auto-, 122
  embryonic, 7
  humoral, 175
  monoclonal, 13, 15, 75
  suppression of, 7
  T-cell, 62
  T-dependent autoantiidiotypic production of, 103
  type II collagen, 185
Antibody-dependent cell-mediated cytotoxicity
    (ADCC), 52, 65, 81, 143
Antibody-forming cells, 107
Antibody-mediated immune mechanisms, 160—161
Anticytoplasmic antibodies, 185
Antigen-induced suppressor cells, 98—100
Antigen-presenting cells (APC), 26—27, 42, 128,
    160
Antigen-pulsed peripheral blood adherent cells, see
    Antigen-presenting cells (APC)
Antigens, see also specific types by name
  B-cell, 9—14
  B-cell subpopulation, 13
  B-F, 2—3
  B-L, 3—4
  Bu-1, 12
  Bu-2, 12
  bursa reticular fiber, 14
  CB1, 13
  CB2, 11
  CB3, 12
  CB4, 13
  CB5, 13
  CB7, 13
  CB8, 13
  CB9, 13
  CB10, 13
  CB11, 13
  CD1, 9
  CD2, 4—5
  CD3, 55
  CD4, 6, 43, 53, 56, 75, 158
  CD5, 5, 13, 56
  CD8, 6, 43, 53, 55, 56, 158
  CD45, 14
  cell-surface differentiation, 2
  chicken activate T-lymphocyte (CATLA), 39
  chicken fetal (CFA), 60, 113
  CT1, 5
  gut-associated mucin, 14
  HNK-1, 11
  immune associated, 141
  leukocyte common, 14—15
  lymphocyte, see Lymphocyte antigens
  MHC, see Major histocompatibility complex
    (MHC) antigens
  minor histocompatibility, 127
  myeloid, 14—15
  nonlymphoid bursal, 13—14
  parasite, 168—169
  presentation of, 160
  recombinant, 168
  T200, 14
  temperature-dependent, 100
  tumor-associated (TAAs), 74
  viral membrane, 147
Antigen-specific T cells, 27
Antimicrobial responses, 156—162
Antinuclear antibodies, 185
Anti-T antiserum, 99
Anti-thymocyte serum, 54
Antithyroglobulin, 122
APC, see Antigen-presenting cells
Arginine, 81, 86
Asbestos, 86
Assays, 54, see also specific types by name
  chromium-release (CRA), 45, 57, 64, 65, 142, 147
  graft-vs.-host (GVH), 29, 30
  in vitro, 45—46
  in vivo, 44—45
  leukocyte migration inhibition, 148
  microcytotoxicity, 144
  migration-inhibition, 141
  natural killer cells and, 52—54
  plaque-forming cell (PFC), 98
  plaque-reduction, 141
ASV, see Avian sarcoma virus
Autoantibodies, 122
Autoimmune diseases, 120, 122, 183—194, see also
    specific types by name
  in obese strain chickens, 185—194
  pathogenesis of, 184
  in Smith-DAM line chickens, 184
  in UCD line 200 chickens, 184—185
Autoimmunity, 113

Autoreactive cells, 124, 125, 128
Autoreactive clones, 121
Avian influenza, 140
Avian leukosis and sarcoma (ALS) tumors, 143—146
Avian leukosis virus (ALV), 143—144
Avian sarcoma virus (ASV), 45, 143, 145—146
Avidin, 75

B

Bacterial infections, 172—175, see also specific types by name
B-cell antigens, 9—14
B-cell lymphoma, 146
B cells, 72, see also specific types by name
  B-L antigen and, 4
  complete depletion of, 103
  developmental pathways of, 2
  development of, 24
  immune tolerance and, 121—122
  immunoglobulin positive, 25
  latent infection in, 141
  in obese strain chickens, 189
  pancreatic islet, 128
  as target of suppressor cells, 107
  T cell interactions with, 27—28
  tolerance of, 127
B-cell subpopulation antigens, 13
B-cell tumors, 73
BDM, see Bursal-derived macrophages
Benzo(a)pyrene, 86
B-F antigen, 2—3
Biochemical characterization, 7
B-L antigen, 3—4
Blood-brain barrier, 125
BMM, see Bone marrow macrophages
Bone marrow cells, 122
Bone-marrow-derived cells, 125
Bone marrow macrophages (BMM), 77
Bovine serum albumin (BSA), 102, 112
Bronchitis, 46, 140, 147
Brucella spp., 82
BSA, see Bovine serum albumin
Bu-1 antigen, 12
Bu-2 antigen, 12
Bursa cells, 53
Bursa immune agammaglobulinemia, 103—109
Bursal-derived marcophages (BDM), 77
Bursal lymphocyte antigens, 11
Bursal stem cells, 24, 126
Bursa of Fabricius, 25, 124, 144, 157
Bursa reticular fiber antigen, 14
Bursectomy, 25

C

Carrageenan, 86, 87
CATLA, see Chicken activated T-lymphocyte antigen

CB1 antigen, 13
CB2 antigen, 11
CB3 antigen, 12
CB4 antigen, 13
CB5 antigen, 13
CB7 antigen, 13
CB8 antigen, 13
CB9 antigen, 13
CB10 antigen, 13
CB11 antigen, 13
CBG, see Corticosteroid-binding globulin
CD1 antigen, 9
CD2 antigen, 4—5
CD3 antigen, 55
CD4 antigen, 6, 43, 53, 56, 75, 158
CD5 antigen, 5, 13, 56
CD8 antigen, 6, 43, 53, 55—56, 158
CD45 antigen, 14
CDR, see Complementarity determining regions
CD3/TCR proteins, 6—7
Cecal tonsils, 157
CEF, see Chicken embryo fibroblasts
Cell-mediated cytotoxicity, 36, 43, 52, 65, 81, 143
Cell-mediated immunity (CMI), 36
  in bacterial infections, 172—175
  in coccidiosis, 163—169
  in cryptosporidiosis, 169—171
  in ducks, 136
  genetic factors in, 166—167, 174
  in leucocytozoonosis, 171—172
  macrophages in, 71—88
    activation of, 80—82
    dual role of, 72—73
    environmental control of function of, 86—87
    genetic control of function of, 84—86
    identification of, 74—76
    infectious agents and, 82—84
    inflammatory responses and, 77—80
    isolation of, 76—77
    regulatory activity of, 73—74
  in neoplastic viral diseases, 140—147
  in nonneoplastic viral diseases, 147—148
  in parasitic diseases, 163—172
  in quail, 135
  RSV and, 135
  in turkeys, 134—135
Cell-surface differentiation antigens, 2
Cellular cooperation, 24—25
Cellular immune suppression, see Immune suppression
Cellular immune tolerance, see Immune tolerance
CFA, see Chicken fetal antigens
Chemoattractants, 84
Chemotaxis, 78, 84
Chicken activated T-lymphocyte antigen (CATLA), 39
Chicken embryo fibroblasts (CEF), 41
Chicken fetal antigens (CFA), 60, 113
Chicken inflammatory macrophages, 75
Chimeras, 125—126

Peripheral blood monocytes (PBM), 77
Peritoneal exudate cell (PEC), 77
Peritoneal macrophages (PM), 77
Peyer's patches, 157
PFC, see Plaque-forming cell
PHA, see Phytohemagglutinin
Phagocytosis, 79—80
Phorbol myristic acid (PMA), 78
Phytohemagglutinin (PHA), 39, 55, 74, 102
 CMI response to, 134, 136
 parasitic diseases in, 165
Plaque-forming cell (PFC) assays, 98
Plaque-reduction assays, 141
PM, see Peritoneal macrophages
PMA, see Phorbol myristic acid
PMNs, see Polymorphonuclear neutrophils
Pokeweed mitogen (PWM), 101
Polyacrylamide gel electrophoresis (PAGE), 39
Polymorphonuclear neutrophils (PMNs), 73, 79, 80
Postbursal cells, 24
Prebursal stem cells, 24
Precursor cells, 8
Professional antigen presenting cells, 26—27
Propyl gallate, 86
Prostaglandins, 73
Proteins, see also specific types by name
 CD3/TCR, 6—7
 recombinant, 168
 structural, 143
Protein tyrosin dephosphorylation, 14
PWM, see Pokeweed mitogen

R

RAV, see Rous-associated virus
RBC, see Red blood cells
Reactive oxygen intermediates (ROIs), 78, 79
Recombinant antigen, 168
Recombinant IL-2, 55
Recombinant proteins, 168
Red blood cells (RBC), 38
 aged, 73, 79
 allogeneic, 43
 B-F antigen and, 3
 sheep, see Sheep red blood cells (SRBC)
Reovirus, 83, 140
RES, see Reticuloendothelial system
Respiratory burst, 78
Reticuloendothelial system (RES), 72, 73
Reticuloendotheliosis virus (REV), 46, 98, 110, 146—147
Retroviruses, 110, 143, see also specific types by name
REV, see Reticuloendotheliosis virus
Reverse transcriptase, 143
Rheumatoid factor, 185
Ribosomal RNA, 80
RNA, 80
ROIs, see Reactive oxygen intermediates
Rotavirus, 53
Rous-associated virus type 7 (RAV-7), 190
Rous sarcoma (RS), 41, 82

Rous sarcoma virus (RSV), 41—42, 62—63, 135, 145
RS, see Rous sarcoma
RSV, see Rous sarcoma virus

S

Salmonella spp., 43, 82, 84, 173—174, 175, see also Salmonellosis
Salmonellosis, 156, 171—175, see also Salmonella spp.
SAT, see Spontaneous autoimmune thyroiditis
Scleroderma, 184
Selenium, 87
Self-antigens, 128
Self-reactive cells, 123
Self-recognition, see Immune tolerance
Self tolerance, see Immune tolerance
Semi-allogeneic grafts, 126
Sheep red blood cells (SRBC), 80, 98—99, 101, 113
 B cell response to, 112
 suppresion of response against, 102
Signal transduction pathways, 14
Silica, 87
Single oxygen, 78
Skin grafts, 29, 121, 124, 126
SM, see Splenic macrophages
Smith-DAM line chickens, 184
Specific phagocytosis, 79
Spleen cells, 127
Splenic macrophages (SM), 77
Splenic sinusoidal regions, 7
Spontaneous autoimmune thyroiditis (SAT), 113, 185, 192
Stem cells, 2, 24, 123, 126
Structural proteins, 143
Superoxide anion, 78
Suppression, see Immune suppression
Suppressive cytokines, 98
Suppressor cells, 36, 60, 74, 98, see also Immune suppression
 antigen-induced, 98—100
 B cells as target of, 107
 in bursa immune agammaglobulinemic chickens, 103—109
 characterization of, 105
 in hereditary muscular dystrophy, 110
 immune tolerance and, 122
 mitogenetic inhibition and, 146
 mitogen-induced, 101—102
 in NK inhibition, 61
 in obese strain chickens, 187
 temperature effects on, 99
 in tolerance, 112—113
 in tumor immunity, 110—112
 in virus infections, 109—110

T

TAAs, see Tumor-associated antigens
TAM, see Tumor-associated macrophages
T200 antigen, 14